基层高血压患者管理经济学评价

中英文版

Economic Evaluation of Hypertension Management in Primary Care Settings in China

国家卫生健康委卫生发展研究中心　组织编写
China National Health Development Research Center　Compilation

张艳春　主　编
Yanchun Zhang　Editor in Chief

人民卫生出版社
·北　京·

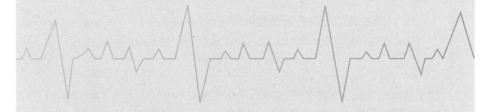

图书在版编目（CIP）数据

基层高血压患者管理经济学评价：汉英对照 / 国家卫生健康委卫生发展研究中心组织编写 .—北京：人民卫生出版社，2023.9

ISBN 978-7-117-35273-4

Ⅰ. ①基… Ⅱ. ①国… Ⅲ. ①高血压 – 病人 – 管理 – 经济评价 – 汉、英 Ⅳ. ①R544.1

中国国家版本馆 CIP 数据核字（2023）第 184142 号

基层高血压患者管理经济学评价（中英文版）

Jiceng Gaoxueya Huanzhe Guanli Jingjixue Pingjia
（Zhong Yingwen Ban）

组织编写：国家卫生健康委卫生发展研究中心
主　　编：张艳春
出版发行：人民卫生出版社（中继线 010-59780011）
地　　址：北京市朝阳区潘家园南里 19 号
邮　　编：100021
E - mail：pmph @ pmph.com
购书热线：010-59787592　010-59787584　010-65264830
印　　刷：北京印刷集团有限责任公司
经　　销：新华书店
开　　本：710 × 1000　1/16　　印张：22
字　　数：360 千字
版　　次：2023 年 9 月第 1 版
印　　次：2023 年 10 月第 1 次印刷
标准书号：ISBN 978-7-117-35273-4
定　　价：118.00 元
打击盗版举报电话：010-59787491　E-mail：WQ @ pmph.com
质量问题联系电话：010-59787234　E-mail：zhiliang @ pmph.com
数字融合服务电话：4001118166　E-mail：zengzhi @ pmph.com

基层高血压患者管理
经济学评价
中英文版

编 委 会

主　　编　张艳春

副 主 编　Peter Sheehan　　Kim Sweeny　　秦江梅

编委会成员

张艳春　Peter Sheehan　Kim Sweeny

秦江梅　张丽芳　林春梅　孟业清

王　鑫　王柯义　车文静　钱　铖

敖文华

Editorial Board of *Economic Evaluation*
of Hypertension Management
in Primary Care Settings in China

Editor in Chief　Yanchun Zhang

Deputy Editor in Chief　Peter Sheehan, Kim Sweeny, Jiangmei Qin

Member of the Editorial Committee　Yanchun Zhang, Peter Sheehan

Kim Sweeny, Jiangmei Qin

Lifang Zhang, Chunmei Lin

Yeqing Meng, Xin Wang

Keyi Wang, Wenjing Che

Cheng Qian, Wenhua Ao

前　言

为应对心血管疾病等慢性病对居民健康的挑战和威胁，2009 年我国启动了国家基本公共卫生服务项目，通过财政支持基层医疗卫生机构向居民免费提供服务，高血压患者管理是服务内容之一。2009 年以来，各级政府对基本公共卫生服务投入大量资金，但是关于该项目投入的收益分析较少。本研究利用相关国家级数据，对 2009—2015 年基本公共卫生服务项目中的高血压患者管理进行经济学评价。

基于 1991—2009 年的数据构建高血压患者血压控制率趋势模型，用于预测未实施项目下 2015 年高血压患者血压控制率。2009—2015 年，基于基本公共卫生服务项目高血压患者管理的直接效果是实际血压控制人数与预测血压控制人数的差值，测算结果显示该值为 9 532 719 人。

为开展经济学评价，研究构建了两个情境：一是假设没有实施国家基本公共卫生服务项目的情境（假设情境）；二是实施国家基本公共卫生服务项目的情境（实际情境）。通过危险因素分析构建马尔可夫（Markov）模型，预测 2016—2045 年心血管疾病发病和死亡风险，结果显示：30 年间国家基本公共卫生服务项目实施与不实施相比，高血压患者进展为冠心病、脑卒中和死亡的人数将分别减少 25 012 人、296 258 人和 744 493 人。

按照避免发病和死亡提高生产率以及劳动力增加和提高国内生产总值的逻辑框架构建标准的经济学评价模型。本研究采用净现值（net present value，NPV）法估算由于发病率和死亡率降低所节省的卫生费用以及产生的经济和社会效益。根据预测，2016—2045 年国家基本公共卫生服务项目高血压患者管理产生的经济效益是 1 698.6 亿元，如果包括社会效益，总收益达 2 673.0

亿元。按照高血压患者管理费占基本公共卫生服务项目经费总额的 14.59% 测算，基于 3.0% 和 5.0% 的贴现率，其效益成本比分别为 6.0：1.0 和 4.9：1.0；如果包括社会效益，效益成本比达 15.4：1.0 和 11.9：1.0。如果仅考虑经济效益，则内部收益率为 14.6%；如果包含社会效益，则内部收益率达 20.7%。因此，国家基本公共卫生服务项目高血压患者管理是一项成本效益极高的投入。

研究的学术贡献在于构建了适用于我国基层医疗卫生服务的健康干预项目经济学评价模型，并且在一定程度上填补了我国慢性病干预经济学评价中通过劳动力预测经济效益的空白。

本书基于主编于 2015 年 3 月—2020 年 12 月在澳大利亚维多利亚大学战略经济研究中心所做博士论文编译而成。鉴于时间紧迫、研究和编译能力有限，书中难免存在不足之处，敬请读者给予指正。

张艳春

2023 年 1 月

Foreword

To combat the challenges of cardiovascular diseases (CVDs), the Chinese government launched a program in 2009 called the National Basic Public Health Service (NBPHS). This provides disease management services in primary healthcare facilities for hypertensive patients. Although a large amount of money has been invested since 2009, little is known about the benefits of such a large investment. Based on national datasets, this study conducted an economic evaluation of hypertension management in the NBPHS from 2009 to 2015.

A trend model was built based on data from 1991 to 2009, which was used to predict hypertension control rates for 2015. The direct impact of the NBPHS on hypertensives was generated by comparing the predicted hypertension control with that of the observed levels in 2015. This generated a figure of 9, 532, 719 hypertensives who were able to get their blood pressure (BP) under control incrementally during 2009-2015.

A hypothesized scenario in which the NBPHS had not been implemented was created to compare with the NBPHS scenario. Following the pathway of risk prediction studies on CVDs, a Markov model was developed to estimate the long-term health outcomes of the NBPHS by comparing the two scenarios from 2016 to 2045. It was estimated that at the end of the 30-year projection period, there would be 25, 012, 296, 258, and 744, 493 hypertensive patients who would have avoided coronary heart disease, stroke and death, respectively, by being part of the NBPHS.

A standard model of economic evaluation was developed by estimating gross domestic product increases from labour force participation and productivity gained by averting morbidities and mortalities. Net present value (NPV) was used to estimate healthcare expenditure saved, and the economic and social benefit of morbidity and mortality averted. It was predicted that from 2016 to 2045, there would be an economic benefit of 169, 857 million CNY in NPV, or 267, 297 million CNY when including social benefit. Given that hypertension management accounts for 14.59% of the NBPHS funding: the benefit-cost ratio would be 6.0 and 4.9 at a discount rate of 3% and 5%, and if the social benefit is included, the benefit-cost ratio would be 15.4 and 14.9 at the same discount rate. The internal rate of return would be 14.6% if only the economic benefit is considered and 20.7% if the social benefit is included. This is a very high benefit investment compared to that identified in other studies.

This study contributes to academic knowledge by providing an economic framework of health interventions in primary healthcare settings in China. To some extent, it also fills a gap by addressing the economic evaluation of chronic disease interventions in China.

This book is developed totally based on the Editor-in-Chief's PhD thesis, which was done at Victoria Institute of Strategic Economic Studies, Victoria University, Melbourne, Australia from March 2015 to December 2020. Due to our limited knowledge and translation ability, and time constraints, there might be some mistakes and flaws in this book, please don't hesitate to correct me.

Yanchun Zhang

January 2023

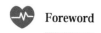

目　录

Table of Contents

1

概述

1.1 背景

20 世纪 80 年代实行社会主义市场经济之前，我国初级卫生保健体系（基层医疗卫生服务体系）在提高居民预期寿命方面一直处于世界领先地位。然而，初级卫生保健体系遇到许多问题，包括政府在卫生保健投入减少、公共卫生服务事权下放，以及基层医疗卫生服务体系的公共卫生服务职能减弱[1-2]。与此同时，随着社会的快速发展，不健康饮食习惯、缺乏运动和吸烟等高风险行为危险因素持续增加[3]。因此，我国居民的死因快速从传染病和围产期疾病转变为慢性非传染性疾病和伤害[3]。慢性非传染性疾病主要包括心血管疾病、慢性呼吸系统疾病（如慢性阻塞性肺疾病和哮喘）、糖尿病和癌症[4]。

2010 年，我国有 170 万人死于脑卒中，94.87 万人死于缺血性心脏病，93.40 万人死于慢性阻塞性肺疾病[3, 5]。《中国心血管病报告 2013》显示，我国主要心血管病是脑卒中和心肌梗死，其中，70% 的脑卒中和 50% 的心肌梗死由高血压引起[6]。2012 年，24% 的 15 岁以上人群被诊断为高血压（即全国有 2.7 亿高血压患者）[6]。心血管疾病的另一个危险因素是糖尿病，2010 年我国成人糖尿病患病率达 11.6%[5]。

基于卫生健康工作面临的主要问题，为遏制心血管疾病等慢性病的快速增长，2009 年我国出台了新的深化医药卫生体制改革的指导意见[7]，目的之一是完善基层服务体系基本医疗和基本公共卫生服务提供。促进基本公共卫生服务均等化是改革的一个重要组成部分，内容包括重大公共卫生服务项目和基本公共卫生服务项目。本论文中频繁提及的国家基本公共卫生服务项目包含由全国各地基层医疗卫生机构［基层医疗卫生机构指城市地区的社区卫生服务中心（站）及农村地区的乡镇卫生院和村卫生室］提供的一系列服务项目[8]。国家基本公共卫生服务项目的目的之一是应对慢性非传染性疾病带来的日益沉重的负担，针对慢性病的内容主要包括高血压和糖尿病健康教育、疾病管理[9]。为实施该政策，国家卫生健康委先后组织制定和修订了国家基本公共卫生服务规范[10-11]。2009 年，我国确定各级政府每年提供人均 15 元的经费用于开展国家基本公共卫生服务项目。基本公共卫生服务项目经费按照每年人均 5 元的幅度增加，从 2011 年的年人均 20 元增加到 2015 年的 40 元。据 Xiao 等[12]估计，高血压患者健康管理的费用约占国家基本公共卫生项目经费总额的 18%，是我国历年来数额最大的基层高血压患者管理投入。这些投资取得的社会和经济效益如何？这样大规模的投入是否值得长期持续下去？要回答这两个问题，我们需要进行全面的经济学评价。

我国多个研究机构曾对国家基本公共卫生服务项目进行评价。例如，2016 年，卫生部项目资金监管服务中心出版《基本公共卫生服务项目绩效评估年度报告》[13]。2014 年，中国社区卫生协会对国家基本公共卫生服务项目进行了评估[14]。Tian 等[15]开展专题研究，分析了基本公共卫生服务对成年慢性病患者的可及性及其决定因素，指出疾病管理的有效性需要提高。Yin 等[16]开发了基于工作当量的模型，计算北京市提供基本公共卫生服务的预期成本，结论是目前对国家基本公共卫生服务项目的投入尚难以满足居民需求。

尽管如此，还没有研究评估过这项大规模投资的经济和社会效益，换言之，缺乏系统的经济学评价证据。本研究针对此类干预措施构建了系统的卫生经济学评价框架，旨在评估国家基本公共卫生服务项目投资的收益和有效性，包括降低成本、提高生产率和经济效益等。具体结果采用效益成本比率和内部收益率表达。

1.2 研究目的

本研究基于 2009—2015 年三组国家数据，首次从卫生经济学的角度系统评估国家基本公共卫生服务项目在提高高血压患者管理率和血压控制率方面的效果。研究采用马尔可夫模型计算长期健康结果，并将其与血压控制的短期健康结果联系起来。因此，研究基于分析形成了经济学评价框架，评估健康结果在增加劳动参与、降低医疗卫生服务成本和为社区提供福利方面产生的经济效益和社会效益。将收益与成本进行比较，利用效益成本比或内部收益率评价项目投入产出情况。具体研究目标如下。

1. 分析 2009—2015 年国家基本公共卫生服务项目实施在提高高血压患者管理率和血压控制率方面的作用。

2. 利用马尔可夫模型，预测 2016—2045 年基于 2009—2015 年高血压控制人数增加带来的长期健康结果，包括减少心脑血管疾病发生和死亡。

3. 利用基层医疗卫生机构对高血压患者管理成本效益框架，分析国家基本公共卫生服务的投入与产出，其经济学评价指标包括效益成本比率和内部收益率。

4. 为国家通过基层医疗卫生服务体系加强慢性病干预投入提供循证依据。

选择 2009—2015 年这一时期的原因有两个：第一，在此期间，国家基本公共卫生服务项目是我国高血压患者管理的一项重要而宝贵的政策措施[17,12,8]；第二，高血压管理数据可得，进行相关趋势分析结果可靠，详见第 3 章。

1.3 国家基本公共卫生服务项目介绍

国家基本公共卫生服务项目在促进城乡居民公平获得基本公共卫生服务方面发挥着重要作用。这是 2009 年出台的新医改四个主要目标之一[18]。国家基本公共卫生服务项目由基层医疗卫生机构提供。国家卫生健康委组织研究确定国家基本公共卫生服务项目内容，其中包括高血压患者管理。

1.3.1 基层医疗卫生服务体系

如前文所述，国家基本公共卫生服务项目通过基层医疗卫生机构，即中国的初级卫生保健系统提供。医疗质量取决于基层医疗卫生机构获得的资金和资源情况。

我国基层医疗卫生服务体系建立在三级医疗卫生服务体系之上，包括社区卫生服务机构（中心或站）、乡镇卫生院、村卫生室和其他基层医疗卫生机构[18-20]。各级医疗卫生机构均授权为辖区居民，特别是老年人和慢性病患者提供基本医疗卫生服务[12]。多项研究表明，没有高质量的卫生专业人才队伍，任何卫生保健系统都无法正常运转。因此，本研究回顾了基层医疗卫生机构人才队伍建设相关政策。2006 年，我国确定了城市社区卫生服务机构设置和人员配备标准[21]，2011 年，卫生部对乡镇卫生院的配置和人员配备标准进行了修订[22]。

政策回顾显示，国家基本公共卫生服务项目是基层医疗卫生机构高血压管理中规模最大的投入和最主要的政策措施。本研究采用趋势分析和政策分析来控制由于时间变化带来的其他因素影响。

为评估国家基本公共卫生服务项目对高血压患者血压控制的影响，本研究进行了深入分析，将健康结果与基层医疗卫生机构绩效相关联，特别分析了卫生专业人员和专业知识相关内容。详见第 6 章。

1.3.2 国家基本公共卫生服务

政府为国家基本公共卫生服务项目提供资金，并通过基层医疗卫生机构向全体居民免费提供[12]，并且不论户籍是否在本地[23]。高血压患者健康管理是国家基本公共卫生服务项目之一。

2009 年《中共中央 国务院关于深化医药卫生体制改革的意见》提出，要逐步向城乡居民提供基本公共卫生服务，包括疾病预防控制、妇幼保健、健康教育等。国家基本公共卫生服务项目的人均资金投入应不低于 15 元。该项目资金投入逐年增加，2011 年为 25 元，2013 年 30 元，2014 年 35 元，2015 年 40 元。2010 年第六次全国人口普查数据显示，我国 31 个省（区、市）人口共 1 332 810 869 人。因此，该项目总投入超过 2 465.7 亿元（汇率按 6.73 元人民币兑 1 美元计算约 366.4 亿美元）。为进行经济学评价，第 5 章估算了高血压管理项目的支出。

2011 年、2013 年和 2017 年，国家卫生健康委对《国家基本公共卫生服务规范》进行了三次修订[24]，但高血压管理的内容并未发生太大变化。由于本研究使用的是 2009—2015 年数据，因此以 2013 年版《国家基本公共卫生服务规范》来解释国家基本公共卫生服务项目及其高血压控制相关内容。2013 年版《国家基本公共卫生服务规范》包括 13 类基本公共卫生服务，43

项具体服务项目。2011—2017 年三次修订均增加了服务类型和项目。基本公共卫生服务包括城乡居民健康档案管理、健康教育、老年人健康管理、高血压患者健康管理等[10]。规范提及的所有服务主要由乡镇卫生院和社区卫生服务中心负责为辖区内居民提供。

1.3.3 高血压患者管理服务规范

根据原国家卫生和计划生育委员会制订的《国家基本公共卫生服务规范》，高血压管理的目标人群是 35 岁及以上常住居民。由基层医疗卫生机构提供的服务主要包括高血压筛查和管理[10]。基层医疗卫生机构应为 35 岁及以上人群提供高血压筛查。确诊患者将接受以下管理方式。

- 对第一次到基层医疗卫生机构就诊的辖区内 35 岁及以上常住居民，测量血压。
- 对第一次发现收缩压≥140mmHg 和/或舒张压≥90mmHg 的居民在去除可能引起血压升高的因素后预约其复查，非同日 3 次测量血压均高于正常，可初步诊断为高血压。建议转诊到有条件的上级医院确诊并取得治疗方案，2 周内随访转诊结果，对已确诊的原发性高血压患者纳入高血压患者健康管理。对疑似继发性高血压患者，及时转诊。
- 向高血压高风险人群提供生活方式指导。

根据服务规范，要定期（每年至少 4 次）面对面随访高血压患者并进行血压评估。提供的服务包括测量血压并评估是否存在危急情况，确定下一次随访日期，并根据血压水平提供用药建议。该规范与《中国高血压防治指南》内容一致[25-26]。

此外，按照规范要求，对原发性高血压患者，每年进行一次较全面的健康检查，可与随访相结合。内容包括体温、脉搏、呼吸、血压、身高、体重、腰围、皮肤、浅表淋巴结、心脏、肺部、腹部等常规体格检查，并对口腔、视力、听力和运动功能等进行判断。具体内容参照《居民健康档案管理服务规范》健康体检表[10，25]。

国家卫生健康委组织制定了基本公共卫生服务项目高血压患者健康管理绩效评价指标体系，包括以下指标。

（1）高血压患者健康管理率=管理的高血压患者数/社区高血压患者数 ×100%。

（2）高血压患者规范管理率=按照规范要求管理的高血压患者人数/年内已登记的高血压患者人数 ×100%。

（3）管理人群血压控制率=年内最近一次随访血压达标人数/年内已管理的高血压患者人数 ×100%。

该评价指标体系表明，高血压管理的目标是控制血压。本研究也以此为标准评价国家基本公共卫生服务项目的效果。

1.3.4 国家基本公共卫生服务项目筹资机制和高血压控制

为了对国家基本公共卫生服务项目中高血压患者管理进行经济学评价，有必要了解其筹资机制和我国医疗卫生筹资体系。

按照国际标准，我国医疗卫生服务通过政府、社会（非政府社会保险、商业健康保险和捐赠）和个人支付三种渠道筹集资金[27]。政府资金直接转移支付给医疗卫生机构，一般用于人力、基础设施、设备采购和公共卫生服务。医疗保险基金和个人费用在个人就医时进入医疗卫生机构，医疗保险基金按以收定支原则使用[28]。

国家基本公共卫生服务项目由财政投入，政府把它作为对基层医疗卫生机构的补助[29]，居民可以免费获得基本公共卫生服务[8]。鉴于国家基本公共卫生服务项目经费由各级财政补偿给基层医疗卫生机构，按照属地化管理的原则由县区级政府对项目进行绩效评价[29]。为了更好地利用资金和提高基层医疗卫生机构工作人员的绩效，财政和卫生健康部门共同印发了关于如何将国家基本公共卫生服务资金用于基层医疗卫生机构的相关政策，明确项目经费可用于支付医务人员经费及与该服务有关的耗材，但不能用于基础设施、设备、培训和其他基础设施改善[29]。

理论上，随着国家基本公共卫生服务项目慢性病管理工作的推进，更多患者将获得服务，并因此得到更好的治疗。这将促使更多高血压患者接受更多更好的医疗服务，获得定期治疗和药物干预，从而改善高血压控制情况。因此，这种投资可能会通过健康保险和个人付费增加患者的医疗保健支出。但是，另一方面，有效落实高血压患者健康管理，可使治疗更高效、更有效，从而减少高血压的负面结果，进而可能节省医疗保健支出。国家基本公共卫生服务项目资金属于临床医疗服务以外的补充，且对接受服务者免费。图 1-1 直观展示高血压患者健康管理和高血压治疗相关服务之间的关系。

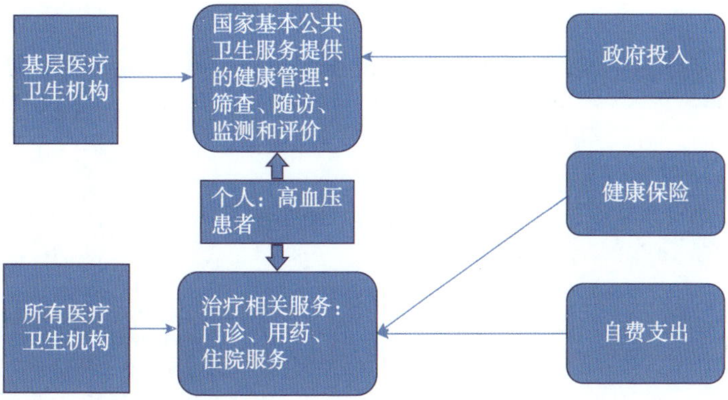

图 1-1　中国高血压患者健康管理服务提供与相关费用示意图

注：监测评价表示基本公共卫生服务监测评价

为确定国家基本公共卫生服务项目的医疗卫生服务支出是增加还是减少了，研究采用疾病成本法进行了测算与分析[30]。详见第 5 章。

1.4　概念框架、方法和数据来源

1.4.1　研究框架及概念

图 1-2 是本研究的研究框架示意图。图左侧显示研究的内容，图右侧是对应的经济学评价指标。

国家基本公共卫生服务项目于 2009 年启动，本研究采用当年的数据作为基线数据，并以 2015 年数据作为国家基本公共卫生服务项目运行 7 年的最终状态。研究以现有数据为基础，主要包括 4 个部分：一是国家基本公共卫生服务项目管理了更多患者和发挥更好的高血压控制作用；二是高血压控制带来的长期效益；三是项目的效益估计和效益成本分析；四是研究结果和政策影响分析。

1.4.2　研究内容

1.4.2.1　使用时间序列模型来确定国家基本公共卫生服务项目的贡献

本文对 1990 年至今中国高血压患病、知晓、治疗和控制情况进行系统文献综述，确定有代表性的数据用于分析我国 35 岁及以上成年人的高血压患

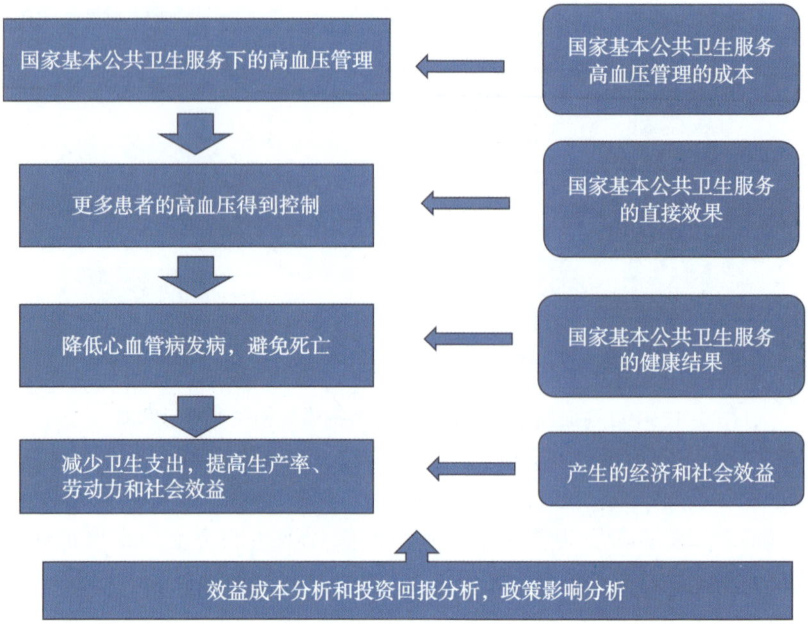

图 1-2　基层高血压患者经济学评价框架图

病率、知晓率、治疗率和控制率[31-33]。基于 R 语言操作系统采用拉格朗日插值多项式补充完善 1991—2009 年间的缺失数据[34-35]。采用专家建模进行时间序列预测分析，预测非干预状态下（未实施国家基本公共卫生服务项目）2015 年高血压患者的血压控制率。本研究认为，2015 年非干预状态的血压控制率和实际控制率之间的差异体现国家基本公共卫生服务项目的超额控制效果。研究通过文献回顾与趋势分析的估计值进行对比，验证结果的可靠性。此外，对高血压患病率、知晓率、治疗率和控制率进行年龄别分析，进而探索国家基本公共卫生服务项目在高血压管理中的增量作用。详细内容见第 3 章。

为进行比较分析，本研究设置了两种情境。一是国家基本公共卫生服务项目实施的情境，其实施效果体现为得到控制的高血压患者的增量，具体见第 3 章。二是国家基本公共卫生服务项目未实施的情境，这种情境超额增量未发生，即这些患者的血压未得到有效控制。

1.4.2.2　利用马尔可夫模型预测长期健康结果

根据 Wu 等[36]和 Zhang 等[37]的研究，高血压的致死或非致死结果主要是冠心病和脑卒中。因此，控制高血压的意义在于阻止这些相关疾病的进展。根据有关文献[38-39]，本研究采用马尔可夫模型估计国家基本公共卫生服务项目的高血压患者管理的长期结果，即由增量控制血压人数而减少不良健康事件和挽救生命的数量。

本研究将直接健康结果确定为高血压得到控制，长期健康结果确定为降低心血管疾病的发病率和减少死亡人数。相关概念解释如下。

- “高血压得到控制”：2009—2015 年血压得到控制的高血压患者总人数。这代表对患者的直接影响。
- “降低发病率”：计算了 30 年间脑卒中和冠心病发病率降低的情况，相关分析见第 4 章。
- “减少死亡”：根据避免心血管疾病死亡情况预测，反映长期健康结果。详见第 4 章。

本研究采用 2009 年中国健康与营养调查（China Health and Nutrition Survey，CHNS）数据库中高血压患者样本数据，模拟上述两种情境（其中血压得到控制的高血压患者模拟国家基本公共卫生服务项目情境下超额增加控制的高血压患者人群；血压未得到有效控制的高血压患者模拟未实施基本公共卫生服项目情境下上述人群未得到血压控制的状况）。在两个模拟组中，心血管疾病（cardiovascular and cerebravascular disease，CVD）的主要危险因素是血压水平，其中考虑了血压、血糖、血胆固醇含量、吸烟和体质量指数（body mass index，BMI）[40]。对两组性别年龄别心血管疾病特异危险因素分布的差异进行比较。统计分析使用 SPSS 22.0 软件。

基于已经开发和校准的中国心血管疾病决策模型[38, 41]相关参数，本研究构建了项目评价的马尔可夫模型。针对国家基本公共卫生服务项目实施情境，用于确定疾病转归的模型参数以最近发表的研究[38]为基础。对于未实施国家基本公共卫生服务的情境，则根据中国人群血压水平和心血管疾病风险，各项参数按照各年龄别性别分组在两种情境下的风险比进行加权获得[39]。

本研究采用马尔可夫模型并依据中国心血管疾病决策模型参数对我国 35 岁及以上高血压人群进行研究[38, 42]，马尔可夫模型的具体结构见第 4 章。无论是血压得到控制的患者还是未得到控制的患者都可能转为以下六种健康状态之一：单纯高血压、急性心脏病、急性脑卒中、慢性冠心病、慢性脑卒中和死亡。研究假设发生心脑血管事件后不会缓解到完全正常状态，即无后效性（马尔科夫性）。除了心血管疾病和死亡，研究未考虑其他健康状态或疾病。研究对冠心病和脑卒中进行分别分析，而不是以冠心病、脑卒中和两者共病的形式进行分析。根据 Gu 等[38]最近的研究，任何两种健康状态之间的转换被定义为转换率。每种状态和每个事件都有转换为其他心血管疾病状态的年转换率。高血压人群先按性别分组，再分别以 10 年为间隔划分年龄组。

中国心血管疾病决策模型描述了初始脑卒中或冠心病事件，包括心脏停搏、心肌梗死和心绞痛，以及后 28 天内发生的并发症[4, 38]。马尔可夫模型的时间间隔为一年。28 天病例死亡视作冠心病急性期或脑卒中急性期导致的直接死亡。根据 Gu 等[38]的研究，以冠心病和脑卒中的死亡率及既往患病率为基础计算一年冠心病和脑卒中病例死亡率。非心血管疾病死亡率（即除外心血管疾病的人群死亡率）等于人群全因死亡率[43]减去冠心病死亡率和脑卒中死亡率得出的差值。

本研究中，35 岁及以上高血压患者的疾病动态变化过程按照中国心血管疾病决策模型[38, 41]相关参数进行分析，详见第 4 章。

1.4.2.3 经济和社会效益估算

本研究估算高血压控制所产生健康效益的经济和社会影响，以及发病率、死亡率和其他不良健康事件减少的情况。从以下方面建模，并以货币形式计算经济和社会效益。

- 高血压控制使个人和家庭避免的疾病直接医疗费用，包括与疾病有关的医疗和其他费用、护工费、交通费和直接收入损失。
- 改善健康状况促进国内生产总值的增加，包括因避免发病和死亡而增加劳动力供给所产生的影响，以及带病工作的情况减少，从而带来劳动生产率的提高。
- 社会效益根据疾病控制对社区的影响来估算，方法是以人均 GDP 为单位估计一个统计生命年的价值，减去经济效益得到的值。根据最近的研究，每挽救一个生命相当于增加 0.5 倍人均国内生产总值的社会效益[44, 45]。

本研究采用效益成本比指标，从社会的角度评估避免发病和减少死亡带来的劳动力和国内生产总值的增长。这里的效益包括经济效益和社会效益。

估算劳动参与率增加带来的经济效益时，所采用的参加劳动的人口最大年龄为 65 岁。其社会效益按人均国内生产总值的 0.5 倍估算，参与估算人口的最大年龄为 80 岁。

经济效益：采用 2016—2045 年队列构建长期健康结果预测模型，测算死亡率和发病率。避免死亡的经济影响，按每个年龄-性别组和年份类别的劳动参与情况计算。计算经济产出贡献时，将每个年龄-性别组的人数乘以随年龄和年份变化的生产率。随后每年都利用该队列增长后的年龄人口的劳动参与率计算当年劳动力。本研究还考虑了每个年龄组人口的平均死亡率。任何一年的劳动力数据都是截至该年的所有队列人数之和。研究采用的劳动参与率按照国际劳工组织的年龄和性别类别分组[46]。每个劳动力的国内生产总值以 2017 年统计数据为基础。性别-年龄别劳动力数据以及人口和死亡率均来自联合国 2017 年中国相关数据（联合国经济和社会事务部，2017）[46]。每个年龄性别组在特定年份避免死亡的高血压患者，其平均年龄都根据 2009 年中国营养与健康调查所采用的 12 个年龄-性别类别（男/女两个性别组和 35~、45~、55~、65~、75~和 85~六个年龄组组合为 12 个年龄组）计算。人口结构也取自联合国人口报告中国数据[46]，人口数包括所有就业和失业的工作年龄人口。

社会效益：研究中，对所挽救生命年的社会价值和经济价值分别计算，因为两者在不同的投资分析中可能有不同的影响。如前文所述，在本研究中，我们认为这两部分的生命年总价值等于人均国内生产总值的 0.5 倍，是以往研究所采用范围的下限。按各国通常做法，社会价值相当于样本人均国内生产总值的一半，增加劳动参与所带来的经济效益则按本国标准计算[45]。这些假设在敏感度分析中有所不同。

避免发病的效益估算：本研究避免发病产生的效益估算仅考虑冠心病和脑卒中，因为它们是模型和前期文献研究中的主要健康结果[47]。估算避免发病的收益以避免的死亡人数为基础，根据疾病的严重程度进行加权分析[48]，详见第 5 章。

避免的疾病直接成本：根据世界卫生组织疾病经济负担计算方法[30]，对高血压、冠心病和脑卒中的直接医疗费用进行计算。直接医疗费用包括预防、诊断和治疗特定疾病的医疗费用，也称为直接成本[49]。因为数据不可得，本部分没有纳入照顾患者的相关费用。

1.4.2.4 效益成本比和内部收益率计算

为评估国家基本公共卫生服务项目的效益和成本，本研究计算了该项目的净经济效益和社会效益、效益成本比率和内部收益率。

1.4.3 数据来源

本研究采用已发表文献数据和我国政府发布的有关数据，具体如下。

- 第一组数据来自文献综述。如前所述，对 1990 年至今我国成人高血压患病率、知晓率、治疗率和控制率的文献进行系统综述，并从中选取有代表性的数据，分析国家层面 35 岁及以上成人高血压患病率、知晓率、治疗率和控制率情况[50]。
- 第二组数据来自 2009 年 CHNS。共 9 552 名人员被纳入 CHNS 分析，其中 1 025 名被调查人员由卫生专业人员诊断为高血压患者。高血压及其知晓率、治疗率和控制率的测量和定义与相关文献研究一致[51]。其中，1 017 名高血压患者年龄在 35 岁及以上。本研究利用该数据，将其分为血压控制组和血压未控制组，以血压未控制组患者的收缩压/舒张压≥140/90mmHg，作为疾病转归参数估计的基础。
- 第三个数据来源是国家卫生健康委卫生发展研究中心 2014 年在全国 17 个省（自治区、直辖市）开展的入户访谈调查。调查采用多阶段分层整群抽样方法，涵盖 20 777 个家庭，共调查 62 097 名居民。其中，确定为高血压患者的居民共 9 607 名[52]。调查数据用于分析血压控制组和未控制组患者中与高血压、冠心病和脑卒中相关的疾病成本。
- 第四个数据来源是 2012—2015 年中国高血压调查（China Hypertension Survey，CHS）。该研究采用分层多阶段随机抽样方法，在 2012 年 10 月—2015 年 12 月期间，从我国 31 个省（自治区、直辖市）收集了 451 755 名 18 岁以上人群作为样本进行分析，研究结果于 2018 年发表[33]。该数据作为高血压患病率和控制率年龄分组的依据，并根据 2010 年第六次全国人口普查数据对人群的年龄-性别结构进行标准化。

研究采用比较分析、趋势分析和建模分析等定量方法。在以上数据和概念框架的基础上，所有研究过程均做了进一步文献分析。

1.4.4 效益、效益成本比率和内部收益率计算

根据收集的成本和效益数据，计算基本公共卫生服务高血压患者管理的效益成本比和投资回报率。关于贴现率的选择，本研究主要考虑健康贴现的

最大化。根据 Claxton[53] 提供的理论框架，选择适宜的贴现率，如 0 、2% 、3% 和 5%。采用敏感度分析，通过不同预测数据的估计值来验证研究结果的合理性。

本研究采用净现值法估计血压控制获得的经济效益和社会效益。净现值是一定时期内现金流入和现金流出现值之间的差额[54]。净现值用于编制资本预算和投资规划，估计投资结果[54]，详见第 5 章。

1.5 本书结构

本书由 6 章组成。第 1 章为概述，介绍研究背景、立题依据、研究目标、概念框架以及所采用的方法。第 2 章是文献综述，重点分析高血压、高血压与心血管疾病之间的关系、高血压患者管理产生的长期健康结果以及高血压患者管理的经济学评价。文献综述为研究方法的选择提供了基础。第 3 章主要通过建立趋势分析模型来分析国家基本公共卫生服务项目在高血压控制方面的有效性。第 4 章从避免或推迟心血管疾病的发生及相关死亡的角度估算国家基本公共卫生服务项目的长期健康影响。本章还构建了基于中国心血管疾病决策模型的马尔可夫模型。第 5 章首先分析了国家基本公共卫生服务项目中高血压患者管理的成本，并在第 4 章介绍研究结果的基础上，利用创新成本效益框架开展经济学评价。第 6 章是最后一章，讨论研究结果的政策影响，包括我国政府可以采取的应对措施。此章还概述了本研究的学术贡献、研究价值和局限性，特别是所采用方法和数据的可及性与局限性。

2

高血压及其影响、健康结果及经济学评价

2.1 引言

2009年，我国启动国家基本公共卫生服务项目。2009年之前，居民患病时，包括慢性病患者，都倾向于去“大医院”看病[18]，导致慢性病医疗服务的可及性[15]、可获得性和质量均不高[55]。为了解决上述问题，强化基层卫生工作，我国启动了新一轮医药卫生体制改革[17]。国家基本公共卫生服务项目就是在这种背景下实施的，项目的另一个目标是引导慢性病患者利用基层医疗卫生服务，形成分级诊疗的就医秩序[7，15]。本研究从数量、质量、影响和经济结果等方面对国家基本公共卫生服务项目进行评估，分析通过项目开展是否实现上述政策目标。

第1章提到，国家基本公共卫生服务项目中高血压管理涉及多种干预措施，包括高血压筛查、基于循证指南的干预、团队合作管理模式、患者自我管理教育、管理过程和结果的测量和评估以及反馈[56]。国家基本公共卫生服务旨在改善患者健康，节省疾病相关并发症导致的医疗服务成本，包括门诊和住院成本、一定程度显示了其经济意义[57]。

然而，当前针对预防和公共卫生服务项目的经济学评价研究较少，传统的经济学评价方法适用性不强[58]。此外，高血压既是心血管疾病的危

险因素，又与其他危险因素有关，如年龄、性别、BMI、吸烟、糖尿病和胆固醇[37]。这使得对高血压患者管理进行经济学评价更为复杂。

为应对这一挑战，卫生经济学家们不断探索，试图为卫生保健项目的经济学评价提供一个总体框架。Tsiachristas 等[59]开发了一个通用决策分析模型，确立了疾病管理方案的五个目标：一是改善服务提供的过程；二是改善患者的生活方式和自我管理行为；三是改善生物医学、生理和临床健康结果；四是提高生活质量；五是总体健康结果。Sculpher 等[60]强调，应该利用患者数据并建立决策分析模型来开展经济学评价。

经济学评价要求在疾病管理的全程或部分过程中考虑资金配置，并将投入与产出联系起来。基于这一点，本综述旨在根据以下几个方面制订本研究的内容。

- 第一，本研究的对象是高血压，将对高血压及其影响的相关文献进行综述。
- 第二，本研究分析在开展国家基本公共卫生服务项目的背景下高血压患者管理的服务提供情况，然后将服务提供与患者生活方式或自我管理行为的改变联系起来，包括知晓、治疗和控制。这与上文讨论的 Tsiachristas 等[59]研究的第一部分和第二部分目标一致。
- 第三，本研究旨在量化 Tsiachristas 等[59]研究的第三部分。将在考虑其他流行病学因素的情况下，探索利用风险预测模型评估临床健康结果。
- 第四，本研究将在 Tsiachristas 等[59]的研究基础上，进一步量化健康结果，并将临床结果转化为长期健康结果。
- 第五，本研究的最终健康结果将转化为经济效益。本部分综述了常用的经济学评价框架，以便为本研究选择最适宜的方法。

这些内容构成本章文献综述的框架，见图 2-1。

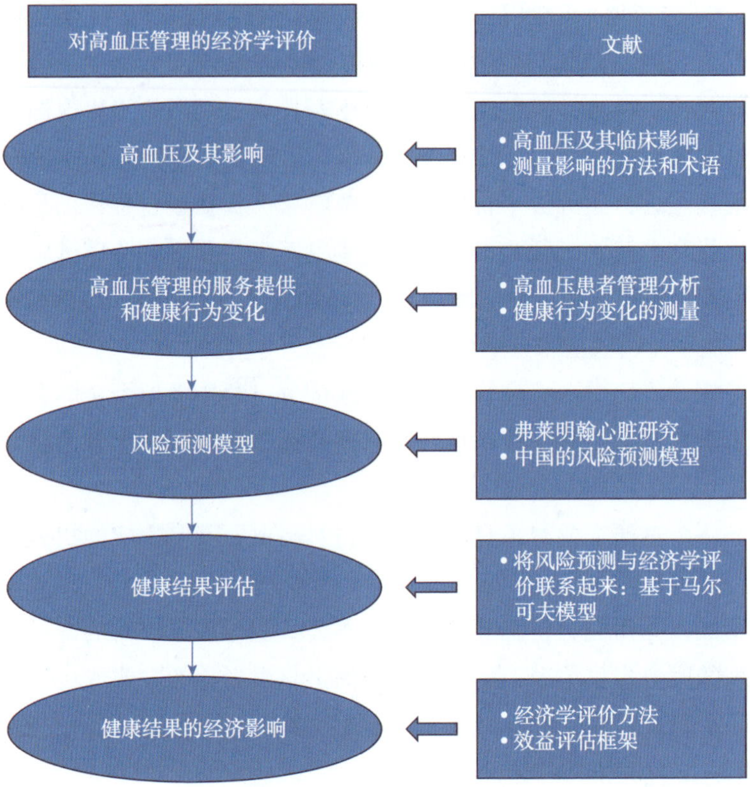

图 2-1　文献综述框架

2.2　高血压与健康影响

2.2.1　高血压和心血管疾病

血压用收缩压和舒张压表示，并以周围大气压上方的“mmHg”为单位[61]。高血压通常定义为收缩压大于等于 140mmHg，或舒张压大于等于 90mmHg。

人口调查中，通常使用血压仪直接测量高血压，或者被调查者被问及是否曾被医生诊断为高血压或目前正在接受高血压药物治疗[61-62]。该定义由世界卫生组织（2015 年）和国际高血压学会（2019 年）推荐[61-64]，并应用于国家基本公共卫生服务项目[62, 65]。

高血压治疗被定义为高血压患者目前正在服用降压药物。高血压控制是指经两次（或三次）血压测量，高血压患者的平均收缩压低于 140mmHg 且平均舒张压低于 90mmHg [33，66]。

高血压可能会导致许多健康不良事件。2016 年出版的《全球疾病负担研究》提出，高血压是全球女性疾病负担的最重要危险因素，是男性疾病负担的第二大危险因素（仅次于吸烟）[67]，根本原因是高血压是导致缺血性心脏病和脑卒中的重要危险因素。

2.2.2 高血压及其影响研究的相关指标

国家基本公共卫生服务项目的经济学评价涉及内容广，还应用了一些流行病学术语，其中一些定义如下。

- 患病率是指某特定时间内总人口中某病新旧病例所占比例，它受到新病例发生率和疾病持续时间的影响[68]。
- 发病率是指通过将某一特定时期（通常为一年）内，特定人群内新发病患者的数量除以暴露风险的人数得出的百分比数值[68]。

患病率用于描述人群疾病程度，而发病率则用来表示出现新发病例的速度。此外，患病率受带病生存时间长短的影响，而发病率通常不考虑该因素[68]。

在描述高血压的变化时，采用患病率进行总体分析，估算高血压患者数量。发病率用于描述高血压引起的并发症，主要是心血管疾病，第 3 章对此进行了具体描述。

高血压是导致心血管疾病发病和死亡的重要原因。我国心血管疾病的病死率较高[31]。相关概念定义和关系如下。

- 发病率是衡量疾病发生情况的术语。发病不代表死亡，一个人可以同时患有多种疾病。患病率用来衡量人群的患病水平。
- 死亡率是衡量死亡情况的术语。死亡率是某时期内（通常是一年）死亡人数与总人口数之比，一般用千分率表示，它与发病率和患病率均不同[69]。
- 病死率是表示一定时期内（通常为一年），患某病的全部患者中因该病死亡人数的比例。病死率通常用于预后，相对较高的病死率表明预后相对较差[70-71]。

这些定义将在本研究建模过程中应用，并将进一步解释（详见第 4 章）。

还有一些流行病学概念用来描述高血压是心脑血管病的危险因素，具体包括以下三项。

• 相对危险度（*RR*）或危险比值。为比较各组之间的风险，相对危险度是首选的统计指标。在流行病学分析中，相对危险度是暴露组发生危险的概率与未暴露组发生该危险的概率之比[72]。其计算式如下：

$$RR=[A/(A+B)]\div[C/(C+D)]=A(C+D)/C(A+B)$$

• 比值比是某事件在两组观察对象（通常是危险因素暴露组和未暴露组）中发生事件概率的比值，是比值的比较。计算公式如下：

$$OR=(A/B)\div(C/D)=AD/BC$$

其中：

A=暴露组中患某种疾病的人数；

B=暴露组中未患某种疾病的人数；

C=未暴露组中患某种疾病的人数；

D=未暴露组中未患某种疾病的人数。

因此，A/(A+B）是暴露组发病率，C/(C+D）是未暴露组发病率。比值比和相对危险度测量暴露与结果之间的关系。

比值比可用于比较不同高血压患者组别之间的心血管疾病发病风险，例如不同血压水平的患者。

• 风险比（HR）在概念上与相对危险度相似，如果风险在时间上是不恒定的，则使用风险比。风险比使用不同时间收集的数据，常用于计算随着时间推移的生存情况。例如，假设风险比为 0.5，某一组内死亡的相对危险度是另一组的一半[72]。风险比通常利用 Cox 比例风险回归模型的系数表达，因为风险与生存函数有关。

总之，关于高血压及其并发症：①患病率可用来描述两种危险因素，包括高血压和并发症，主要是心血管疾病；②发病率主要用于描述作为并发症的心血管疾病；③死亡率和病死率用来描述危险因素或并发症的终点；④风险比用于描述危险因素的强度及其与心血管疾病的定量关系。

以下 3 个概念常用于分析高血压患者的健康状况变化，围绕这些主题开展的研究较多。

• 知晓是知道自己患有高血压。在调查研究中，通常调查对象被问及“你是否曾被医生或其他卫生专业人员诊断为高血压”时回答“是的”[73]，此时即定义为该调查对象知晓高血压患病情况。

● 治疗是对高血压采取治疗或干预措施，如改变饮食、锻炼身体和服用降压药物。调查中通常定义为调查对象自我报告正在服用降压药物。

● 控制是指高血压被控制到正常水平临界以下，通常指收缩压和舒张压二者分别低于 140mmHg 和 90mmHg[61，74]。

近年来，我国高血压患病率呈上升趋势[16，52，75-76]。2012—2015 年，中国高血压调查显示，我国 18 岁及以上成年人高血压患病率是 23.2%，另有 41.3% 的人口接近患高血压的状况[33]。中国健康与营养状况调查显示，2012 年成年人高血压患病率为 25.2%[77]。但是，知晓率、治疗率和控制率都处于非常低的水平[76，78]。

上述概念可以用来对健康干预结果进行定量分析。

最近的研究更好地解释了血压与心血管疾病发病率和死亡率之间的关系[31]。与舒张压升高相比，收缩压升高与心血管疾病风险相关度更高。Gu 等[39]研究发现，将血压低于 110mmHg/75mmHg 的患者作为对照组，收缩压/舒张压为 110~119mmHg/75~79mmHg、120~129mmHg/80~84mmHg、130~139mmHg/85~89mmHg、140~159mmHg/90~99mmHg、160~179mmHg/100~109mmHg 和≥180mmHg/110mmHg 的患者心血管疾病发病的相对危险度分别为 1.09、1.25、1.49、2.15、3.01 和 4.16。因此，高血压患者管理的目标是降低血压，使血压回归正常，进而降低心血管疾病的发病率和死亡率。

对不同的高血压干预措施进行经济学评价，有助于确定每项措施对减轻疾病负担的影响。我国已开展了一些干预措施对高血压影响的研究[38，79]。2015 年，一项研究评价了降压药的影响，并进行了成本-效果分析[38]。研究结果表明，利用低成本的药物加强高血压干预治疗具有边际成本效益。2018 年的一项研究对中国高血压强化管理进行了经济学评价，结论是高血压患者强化管理比常规管理更具有成本效益[42]。但是，对高血压患者管理进行经济学评价的证据依然不足[59]。

2.3 国家基本公共卫生服务项目在高血压患者管理和血压控制中的作用

高血压患者管理指南明确指出，降低并控制血压是减少心血管疾病的关键[80-81，33]。高血压患者管理指南还对降压治疗的证据进行了文献综述，并提出了相关建议，包括改善行为生活方式因素（包括饮食和身体活动）和使用降压药物。这些指南建议的实施提高了发达国家对高血压作用的认识，并且在改善高血压控制和降低心血管疾病死亡率方面发挥了重要作用[81]。国家基本公共卫生服务项目中高血压患者健康管理也遵循这些健康干预指南。

2016 年，国家卫生和计划生育委员会发布了国家基本公共卫生服务项目指南[24]。其中，高血压患者管理规范如下。

（1）基层医疗卫生机构有义务进行高血压筛查；对所有 35 岁及以上患者在基层全科医生或其他医生就诊时，必须测量血压开展高血压筛查。将筛查结果告知患者，有助于大幅提高高血压知晓率。

（2）如果患者被诊断为高血压，基层医疗卫生机构的医生必须对这些患者进行定期（每年 4 次）随访，记录患者正在服用的药物，并在必要的情况下提供专业帮助，包括监督和提供用药建议[82]。

（3）如果病情恶化，全科医生有义务将患者转诊到上级医院接受进一步治疗。这有助于及时治疗和护理[83]。

（4）国家基本公共卫生服务项目提高了全科医疗服务的可及性[15]。在该项目实施之前，我国社区居民或患者倾向于直接去医院就诊，而大医院专科医生能够提供给每位患者的时间有限。此外，医院的临床治疗主要集中于药物治疗，非药物干预措施考虑较少[84]。

理论上，高血压患者管理可以改善知晓、治疗和控制情况。多项研究证实这些干预措施具有较好的效果[15, 66, 86]。近年来，我国多项研究基于大样本调查对高血压的知晓率、管理率和控制率进行了专门分析。2017 年的一项研究基于 170 万社区成人的调查对高血压患病率、知晓率、治疗率和控制率进行了分析[74]。其他几项研究也基于横断面调查进行了分析[25, 33, 86]。

然而，上述研究均未探讨高血压患者管理效果的动态趋势。另外两项研究对高血压患病率、知晓率、治疗率和控制率进行了动态趋势分析，且两者均使用了 2013 年和 2015 年 CHNS 数据[49, 87]。虽然这些研究为制订高血压干预措施提供了良好基础，但均不是针对国家基本公共卫生服务项目下高血压患者管理有效性开展的专门研究。如果没有评价相关项目的随机对照试验，就很难对项目提高高血压患者知晓率的影响进行量化分析。

基于通过文献综述获得的数据，本研究使用趋势分析法，以 2009 年为分界点分析国家基本公共卫生服务项目的作用。如前述研究所述，知晓率和治疗率是高血压的过程性指标，控制血压是针对高血压采取干预措施的结果性目标。因此，本研究的重点是对高血压控制状况进行分析，详见第 3 章。

2.4 如何量化高血压患者的心血管疾病发病风险

对高血压作为心血管疾病危险因素的研究开始于 20 世纪 20 年代。Paullin 等[88]根据对美国 500 名高血压患者进行的研究，认为高血压的并发症可以分为七类，分别与心脏、动脉、中枢神经系统、眼睛、肺、肾和其他器官有关。他们的研究证实，心脏肥大是高血压的首要并发症，66.4%（332/500）的患者有此并发症。1964 年，Hamilton 等[89]对高血压和脑卒中之间的关系进行了研究，结果显示控制血压可以显著减少男性多种并发症和女性脑卒中的发生。

一项 Meta 分析表明，对于 40~69 岁的成年人来说，收缩压（相当于通常的舒张压 10mmHg）每升高 20mmHg，脑卒中死亡率增加 1 倍，缺血性心脏病和其他血管病的病死率也增加 1 倍[90, 91]。随机临床试验表明，收缩压每降低 10mmHg，脑卒中和缺血性心脏病的风险降低约四分之一[92]。我国相关研究证据表明，随着血压的升高，心血管疾病发病的相对危险度明显增加[39, 93]。

2.4.1 国际风险预测方程研究

Cox 回归模型通常用于心血管疾病风险评估，最著名的研究是美国的弗莱明翰心脏研究[94]。该研究始于 1948 年，主要目的是分析导致心血管疾病的一般危险因素或特征。这项研究纳入许多尚未出现心血管疾病症状的人员。研究结果证实，心血管疾病的主要危险因素包括高血压、高胆固醇血症、糖尿病、肥胖、吸烟和缺乏运动。该研究还提供了心血管疾病风险因素的证据，包括血液甘油三酯和高密度脂蛋白（high-density lipoprotein，HDL）胆固醇水平以及年龄、性别和社会心理问题。弗莱明翰心脏研究在世界各地被广泛使用和引用，在过去的 半个世纪里，在顶级医学期刊杂志上发表了 1 200 多篇相关文章。

研究人员在估计风险因素参数时采用过各种不同的方法[95]。第一种方法是 Logistic 回归分析，用于 Benjamin 等[96]的研究中。他们采用多元 Logistic

回归模型按照特定的性别选择房颤的单个危险因素，用比值比和相对危险度描述危险因素。Singer 等[97]与 Harris 等[98]也使用相同方法开展了类似研究。第二种方法是 Cox 回归，用风险比表示所分析因素的相对危险度[99]。因为这种方法可以通过考虑时间因素更好地表达危险因素与疾病之间的风险关系。

2007 年，世界卫生组织和国际高血压学会根据性别、年龄、收缩压、吸烟状况、血液总胆固醇水平和糖尿病等因素，编制了世界卫生组织各区域（中国属于世界卫生组织西太平洋区域）致命性或非致命性心血管疾病十年风险预测图，为全球居民了解心血管疾病风险提供了一种直观、直接的方法。这也表明了弗莱明翰心脏研究风险方程在全球得到应用。

2.4.2 我国开发的风险预测模型

高血压并发心血管疾病的早期研究主要针对西方人群，研究认为冠心病是高血压的主要并发症。然而，研究显示我国心血管疾病不仅应包括冠心病，还应包括脑卒中，而且由此引发的脑卒中比冠心病造成的死亡人数更多[36-37]。许多国家开展了多项队列研究，如弗莱明翰心脏研究和世界卫生组织心血管疾病人群监测方案（名为 MONICA 项目，旨在评估心血管疾病死亡和发病的趋势以及这些趋势与危险因素水平和/或医疗保健变化之间的关系）[100]等，对导致缺血性心脏病和脑卒中的各种危险因素进行定量分析。研究人员对这些研究进行了 Meta 分析和文献研究[101-102]。近年来，用于心血管疾病风险预测的模型得到了进一步改进，纳入更多危险因素，并将时间作为影响因素进行动态分析[38, 103]。有关学者还开发了用于中国人群心血管疾病风险预测的模型，现讨论如下。

2005 年，Zhang 等[37]以中国人群队列为基础开发了心血管疾病风险预测评分模型。该模型以年龄、收缩压、总胆固醇、BMI 和吸烟为协变量，以冠心病、缺血性/出血性脑卒中为因变量。研究得出结论，针对白种人群的心血管疾病风险分层模型高估了东方人的冠心病风险，研究还提出了中国男性冠心病及缺血性和出血性脑卒中的分层评估方法。

2006 年，Wu 等[36]建立了具有特异性并经过优化的中国人群缺血性心血管疾病（包括缺血性脑卒中和冠心病）10 年风险预测模型。他们使用 Cox 比例风险回归，基于中美心血管疾病和心肺疾病流行病学合作研究数据进行了深入分析。该研究显示，男性和女性缺血性心血管疾病与年龄、收缩压、总胆固醇、BMI、当前吸烟状况和糖尿病等危险因素之间具有定量关系。

2016 年，Gu 等[38]基于 4 个中国人群队列研究，分析得出动脉粥样硬化性心血管疾病 10 年风险预测模型。该研究纳入的危险因素包括年龄、地区、城乡、当前吸烟状况、腰围、收缩压、舒张压、两周内降压治疗、总胆固醇、高密度脂蛋白、胆固醇、糖尿病、家族史等。此后，研究人员根据模型预测了动脉粥样硬化性心血管疾病 10 年风险[103]。该研究采用大样本人群数据，重点关注所有动脉粥样硬化性心血管疾病（定义为非致命性急性心肌梗死或冠心病死亡或致命性或非致命性脑卒中）。

Wu 等[36]的研究提供了一个简化的心血管疾病风险评分系统，可以很容易地将缺血性心血管疾病的风险评分转化为 10 年风险概率。Gu 等[38]的研究为中国普通人群开发了一个风险预测模型，并根据中国和世界卫生组织的统计数据校准了相关参数。2016 年的一项研究进行了类似分析，将研究结果应用于中国人口[103]。上述研究为心血管疾病长期风险预测提供了参数基础。

在 2015 年研究参数基础上，本研究探索开发一个心血管疾病长期健康结果预测模型，并且基于 CHNS 数据进行心血管疾病风险预测。详见第 4 章。

2.5 基于高血压控制评估健康结果

Moran 等[43]报告指出，适度降低收缩压可能对中国人群心血管疾病进展产生重大抑制作用。鉴于高血压是心血管疾病的主要危险因素，世界卫生组织和国际高血压学会编写了心血管疾病风险预测图，供全球各国使用[64]。收缩压每降低 10mmHg 或舒张压每降低 5mmHg，可以使 65 岁患者脑卒中的风险降低约 35%、缺血性心脏病风险降低约 25%[39, 90]。对 354 项随机试验的分析结果表明，3 种降压药物按 1/2 的标准剂量服用，可将收缩压降低 20mmHg 或舒张压降低 11mmHg，这将使得脑卒中风险降低 63% 或缺血性心脏病风险降低 46%[104]。

据估计，未得到控制的高血压每年造成 750 000 例心血管疾病患者死亡。如高血压患病率降低 25%，则可以避免 130 000 例心血管疾病患者死亡[105]。我国相关研究表明，降压干预可以使脑卒中风险降低 35%~40%、心肌梗死风险降低 20%~25%、心力衰竭风险降低 50% 以上[6]。

虽然风险方程提供了一个很好的工具，可以将高血压作为一个危险因素与致命和非致命的心血管疾病联系起来，但大多数风险预测以 10 年时间为基础，而针对高血压患者的相关分析通常以一年或更短时间为基础进行，包括患病率、发病率、病死率和死亡率等。

为开展基于生命周期的分析，研究需要长期的健康结果预测指标。因此，许多研究尝试开发相关模型，整合国内外相关的风险方程和疾病控制的长期健康结果[96]。Unal 等[105]学者开展的文献系统综述指出，到 2006 年，已开发 42 个冠心病模型并用于心血管疾病建模，其中 6 个被广泛使用[90]。在我国，心血管疾病决策模型[106]、影响分析模型[107]和马尔可夫模型[108]均得到不同程度的研究和应用。如图 2-2 所示，心血管疾病包括冠心病和脑卒中，与许多危险因素相关，包括年龄、性别、高血压和其他等风险因素。风险比描述危险因素与心血管疾病之间的关系。心血管疾病增加死亡风险，其概率将在病死率和发病率中描述。

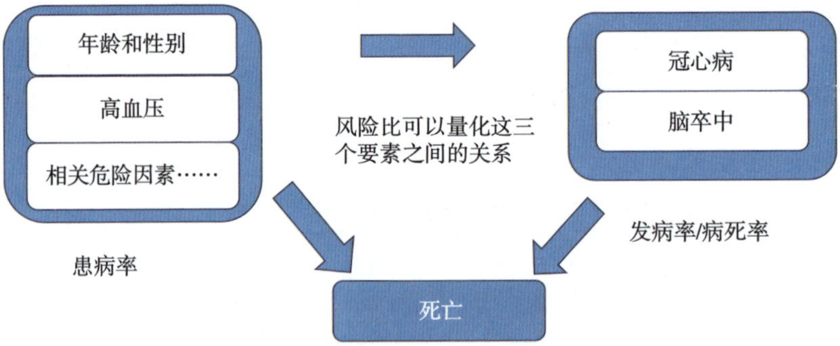

图 2-2　高血压、其他危险因素与心血管疾病之间的关系

2.5.1　冠心病决策模型及其在本研究中的应用

在对卫生健康干预项目进行经济学评价建模时，马尔可夫模型是应用最多的方法之一[109]。在我国，以马尔可夫模型为基础的冠心病决策模型在心血管疾病风险预测中得到了广泛应用和发展[38]。

冠心病决策模型是 20 世纪 80 年代开发的一种针对不同疾病之间状态转换的模型。它由 3 个子模型组成[110]：人口学/流行病学模型、桥梁模型和疾病史模型。该模型可以模拟采用不同病死率的干预措施的效果，并计算长期（可达 30 年）死亡率、发病率和费用影响。它已在美国[111]、阿根廷[112]和中国[38, 41]应用。

该模型在中国发展和应用状况较好，被称为中国心血管疾病决策模型。该方法自2008年开发出来并在我国应用，最近的应用研究于2015年开展。现将中国的研究进展回顾如下。

2008年，Moran等[113]对中国人口增长和老龄化与冠心病的关系进行了研究，建立了适合中国人群的冠心病决策模型。这项研究整合了中国特有的冠心病危险因素、发病率、病死率和患病率数据，形成了基于我国人群队列的模型，并根据特定年龄段死亡率进行校准。该研究以35~84岁的中国人口为预测对象，计算了冠心病的失能调整生命年（disability-adjusted life year，DALY）。研究结果预测，2020—2029年期间将发生780万例冠心病事件（比2000—2009年增加69%）和340万例冠心病死亡（同比增加64%），同时65岁以下成人冠心病死亡和残疾负担每年增加67%。

2010年，同一个研究团队进一步开发了冠心病决策模型[41]。这项研究预测了2010—2030年35~84岁人群的心血管疾病情况，包括冠心病和脑卒中。Moran等[42]发现，2010—2030年，老龄化和人口增长将导致心血管疾病增加一半以上，而血压、总胆固醇、糖尿病和BMI等危险因素的增长趋势可能会加速心血管疾病流行。

2012年，Chan等使用冠心病决策模型预测了2010—2030年城市化对心血管疾病的影响。他们得出结论，城市化将使冠心病发病率增加到每10万人73~81例，脑卒中发病率略有增加[114]。

2015年，Gu等主导的另一项研究，将重点置于分析我国利用低成本降压药物进行高血压控制的成本效果[38]。在这项研究中，首次将冠心病决策模型用于我国高血压干预措施的经济学评价，并对参数进行了较好的校准。作者估算了高血压筛查、实施基本药物制度及高血压患者健康管理项目的成本效用，分析了2015—2025年35~84岁未接受治疗的成人因预防心血管疾病而减少的药物支出和疾病相关支出和获得的质量调整生命年，以及因药物副作用而损失的质量调整生命年。上述冠心病决策模型基于最新流行病学参数进行了更加精准的估计，其应用为更好地构建适合我国人群的高血压健康管理提供了良好基础。更重要的是，上述研究为本研究提供了方法学指导，将心血管疾病的10年风险预测转化为年度风险预测，使得长期健康结果预测成为可能。

2.5.2 本研究的马尔可夫模型和纳入疾病

本研究基于 Gu 等[38]的研究开发了新的马尔可夫模型。马尔可夫模型是一种用于模拟随机变化系统的模型[115]。该模型假设未来的状态只取决于当前的状态，而不是过去发生的事件。该模型是模拟具有持续风险的疾病预后的便捷方法[116]。模型假设患者总是处于几种确定的健康状态之一，称为马尔可夫状态。模型将所有疾病状态纳入分析，并通过疾病状态转移概率建立一个状态和另一个状态之间的联系。在本研究中，马尔可夫模型的状态包括高血压、心血管疾病、心血管疾病死亡和非心血管疾病死亡。如第 1 章所述，从一个状态到另一个状态的转换概率可以通过风险预测模型获取。在每个疾病或者健康状态下均可分配一个效用值，一般常用失能调整生命年[117]。该效用值对整个预测周期的贡献取决于在状态中的时间长度。

高血压向心血管疾病转移的概率引自 Gu 等[38]开展的相关流行病学参数，并基于其他统计数据进行调整和校正。国家基本公共卫生服务项目服务的人群疾病风险被视为与一般人群相同。在假设未开展国家基本公共卫生服务项目的情境下，研究利用 2009 年 CHNS 数据进行模拟。然后基于 Gu 等[38]研究的流行病学参数，构建马尔可夫模型估算 30 年的长期健康结果。本研究中纳入的疾病与相关研究一致，包括以下与高血压相关的心血管疾病[106]。

- 冠心病：心肌梗死、心绞痛和其他缺血性心脏病，以及一定比例的“不明确”的已经编码的心血管疾病。
- 脑卒中：由《国际疾病分类第九次修订本》（ICD-9）编码 430~438（不包括短暂性脑缺血发作）或《国际疾病分类第十次修订本》（ICD-10）I60~I69 定义。

《国际疾病分类》是对疾病和健康状况进行分类的国际标准[118]。多数情况下，ICD-9 和 ICD-10 编码体系被用来确定特定的患者队列并评估其经过风险调整的临床结果[119]。冠心病、脑卒中发病率和患病率的数据来自中国高血压流行病学追踪调查[40]。根据世界卫生组织的研究，使用 2000—2010 年的特定年龄，冠心病决策模型对冠心病和脑卒中死亡率数据进行了预测和校验[38, 41]。

2.6 卫生健康项目的经济学评价

2.6.1 基本方法与理论

根据 Drummond 等[119-120]的研究，卫生健康项目的经济学评价主要有四种类型：成本-效果分析、成本-效用分析、成本-效益分析和最小成本分析。Drummond 等[121]对上述卫生健康项目的相关定义进一步优化，具体如下。

- 最小成本分析：在效果、效用和效益没有差别的条件下，选择成本低的方案，该分析只考虑成本，代表经济学评价的部分形式。
- 成本-效果分析，主要评价使用一定数量的卫生资源（成本）后的个人健康产出，这些产出表现为健康的结果，用非货币单位表示，包括“延长的生命年”或“正确诊断的病例数量”。
- 成本-效用分析：是成本-效益分析的一种发展，根据健康状况偏好评分或效用权重来测量项目效果，通常采用质量调整生命年或失能调整生命年来表示。成本-效用分析最常见的衡量指标是质量调整生命年。
- 成本-效益分析：在评价临床方案效果时，采用货币值分析和评估项目的实施效果。它是应用最广泛的分析形式，确定项目实施效果，进而验证成本是否合理。

2.6.2 成本-效益分析和确定效益的价值

世界卫生组织卫生经济学评价议程强调，对预防和公共卫生服务项目的经济效益关注不够[59]。

2016 年，一篇关于社区高血压患者干预经济学评价的系统综述显示[122]：从 1995—2015 年，我国只有 4 项针对上述专题的研究。在这些研究中，两项采用了成本-效果分析法[38, 75]，另外两项采用成本-效益分析法[18, 123]。2010 年，Huang[124]和 Ren[123]的研究评价了以社区为基础的脑卒中预防项目，结论是节省了疾病成本。但是，如前所述，该研究只考虑了脑卒中，而这仅仅是高血压的其中一个并发症。此外，该研究也未分析未来的成本和效益，没有明确解释该方法在经济学评价中的应用。Wang 等[17]的研究仅通过对北京市 140 名高血压患者随访一年的基础上分析高血压管理节约的成本。整体上，这两项成本效益研究并不能够为我国高血压患者管理的经济学评价提供具有代表性的证据，因为上述研究使用的方法不够全面，不完全符合经济学评价对成本-效益分析法的基本标准[120]。

为改进我国经济学评价方法，本研究采用成本-效益分析框架，其中将效益定义为卫生健康项目效果的货币价值[121]。

延长生命年对于个人是有益的，因为他们可以活更久，享受更好的生活质量。与此同时，社区也能够受益，主要体现为降低了患者的治疗费用或者挽救的生命为社会和经济做出贡献。对于生命年的价值和医疗卫生服务干预措施的效益研究很多。Drummond 等[121]在《卫生保健项目经济学评价方法（第 4 版）》中指出，人们通常采用支付意愿法来估算健康效益。该方法通过测量潜在的消费者需求和对非市场化的社会商品价值进行估算，其中社会商品包括卫生健康项目。不过，Drummond 等[121]也指出，包括支付意愿法在内的每种效益估算方法都存在优缺点。支付意愿法虽然得到普遍使用且发展得较为完备，但仍然存在两方面的主要缺陷：一是该方法基于假设，二是通过支付意愿法将质量调整生命年用于效益估算时可能不包括社会效益[121]。美国的一些研究估计，一个生命年的价值等于 15 万美元[125]，但针对该问题的观点和方法分歧较大。

为解决上述缺陷，Stenberg 等[45]开发了一个用于计算妇女和儿童健康项目的投资回报率的衡量指标，为卫生健康项目效益评估开辟了新的路径。在该模型中，卫生健康效益被认为由经济效益和社会效益组成。根据每个性别年龄组的劳动参与率和生产率，估计了劳动年龄人口劳动力参与卫生健康项目增加的经济效益。其社会效益主要来源于更长、更健康的预期寿命，其估算方法是分配一定比例的人均国内生产总值进行测算[44-45]。与支付意愿法的效益估算框架相比，这种效益估算方法解决了基于偏好的方法产生的偏倚，为效益估算提供了一个切实可行和可衡量的工具。

然而，该方法尚未应用于我国慢性非传染性疾病的干预中。因此，在 Stenberg 等[44-45]研究的基础上，本研究将该创新性模型应用于慢性非传染性疾病干预措施，即我国的基层医疗卫生机构高血压患者管理。

2.6.3　国际上对社区高血压患者干预的经济学评价研究

国际上，对基层医疗卫生机构高血压患者干预或管理措施的经济学评价研究较多。本研究回顾了几项国际研究。

在不丹，Dukpa 等[126]对世界卫生组织出台的基于初级卫生保健提供慢性非传染性疾病基本干预包[48]进行了经济学评价，应用的模型包括决策树和马尔可夫模型。研究比较了 3 种情境下终身干预成本和避免的失能调整生命年，3 种情境分别为无筛查、利用当前 WHO 提出的基本干预服务包和全人群筛查。高血压的马尔可夫模型包含 4 种健康状态：高血压未得到控制、高血压得到控制、脑卒中和死亡。队列人群的年龄范围在 40 岁或以上，每个周期为一年。使用世界卫生组织标准方法计算失能调整生命年。Dukpa 等[126]研究结果表明，初级卫生保健机构开展筛查具有较好的经济效益。

在孟加拉国，有研究从社会角度对国家高血压治疗项目进行了成本-效益分析，分别计算了到 2021 年和 2030 年为 60% 的高血压患者提供降压药物干预措施的投资回报率[127]。研究结论是，如果政府积极主动地开展高血压患者管理，到 2021 年，年投资回报率可能达到 12.7∶1；到 2030 年，年投资回报率可能达到 8.6∶1。

在希腊，Athanasakis 等[128]采用成本-效益分析的马尔可夫模型对 2014 年高血压患者控制进行了经济学评价。研究建议将促进血压控制的干预措施作为重点卫生健康政策。

在荷兰，研究者采用马尔可夫模型评估了对轻度高血压采取心血管疾病初级预防干预的经济学效果。研究发现，在 10 年期限和终身干预两种情况下，降低收缩压都具有成本效果[129]。

上述研究为本研究提供了良好的方法学和国际实践经验基础与参考。这些研究结果表明，无论是在发达国家还是发展中国家，初级卫生保健一级干预或筛查措施都具有较好的成本效益或性价比。同时，大多数经济学评价均利用马尔可夫模型开展。例如，荷兰的研究建立了马尔可夫模型，确定心血管疾病进展的 5 种状态包括健康但有高血压、急性非致命性心血管疾病、稳定的非致命性心血管疾病、心血管疾病死亡和非心血管疾病死亡[128]。这与 Gu 等[38]采用的方法类似，为高血压控制的马尔可夫建模提供了准确的参考。

2.6.4　我国的研究差距

我国对患者健康管理的经济学评价研究存在三个方面的差距。首先，几乎所有的研究均采用成本-效果分析或成本-效用分析，但缺乏成本-效益分析。例如，2000 年开展的一项对我国脑卒中干预的评价未包含成本-效益分析[130]。中国医学科学院北京协和医学院的研究对社区高血压患者管理进行了经济学评价，但未进行成本-效益分析[131-132]。其次，一些研究虽然对基层医疗卫生机构开展高血压患者管理进行了成本-效益分析，但未进行方法学讨论和深入分析。例如，一项针对糖尿病筛查项目的经济学评价研究，使用蒙特卡罗模型进行成本-效益分析，但研究只考虑获得的质量调整生命年和治疗成本，未考虑货币形式的效益，因此这种评价是不完整的[133]。另一项研究分析了社区卫生服务管理模式下高血压患者的治疗效果和成本效益，但没有进行敏感度分析[134]。最后，在经济学评价过程中，很少考虑个体对社会的经济影响[135]。

2015 年，顾东风等学者的研究部分解决了上述差距[38]。但是，依然还有两方面的研究空白需要填补。一是目前尚没有研究证据提供国家基本公共卫生服务项目的投资回报率，更不用说高血压患者健康管理的投资回报研究证据。二是多项研究表明基层医疗卫生机构一级干预措施将为经济增长和社会发展带来高回报[9, 136]，但 Gu 等[38]研究发现加强高血压治疗在我国的成本效益并不明确。从这个角度看，本研究将开展更加深入、完整的分析，提供成本-效益分析证据。

2.7 小结

本章文献综述涵盖高血压及其健康后果、高血压对心血管疾病的影响、基于风险方程的健康结果预测以及对卫生健康项目的经济学评价方法。本研究旨在评估高血压控制带来的健康收益，以及能够避免的发病和死亡。通过文献综述确定了本研究采用的方法。

研究基于不同的数据来源，采用比较分析法和趋势分析法评估国家基本公共卫生服务项目在高血压管理中的作用。这些正向的分析结果为进一步开展经济学评价和投资回报分析奠定了良好基础。详见第 3 章。

关于风险方程和长期健康结果预测，本研究在已有研究基础上开发了马尔可夫模型，详见第 4 章。

正如前述讨论分析，几项国际研究对高血压患者管理措施进行了经济学评价，如荷兰[129]、希腊[128]、不丹[126]和越南[137]等研究。借鉴这些国际研究经验，本研究将健康结果评估过程与成本和效益分析相结合，形成了本研究的马尔可夫模型框架。同时，参考相关研究形成成本-效益分析框架[44-45]。

从以下方面分析国家基本公共卫生服务项目对高血压患者管理所产生的经济和社会效益。

（1）从长期来看，健康收益增加国内生产总值，包括因死亡或患病减少而增加劳动力供应增加，因病误工减少而提高的劳动生产力，以及健康状况改善增加了更健康、更有活力的劳动力相关的投资效应。

（2）社会效益是根据疾病控制对社区的作用来估算的，其方法是以人均 GDP 为单位估计一个统计生命年的价值，减去经济效益得到的值[45]。为比较效益和成本研究计算了净社会效益、效益成本比和内部收益率。经济学评价具体过程详见第 5 章。

（3）个人和家庭节省的直接费用，包括疾病治疗、陪护人员、交通等相关成本。详见第 5 章。

3

国家基本公共卫生服务项目对高血压控制的影响

3.1 概述

高血压控制是减少心血管疾病的主要手段之一[77，137]，而以社区为基础的高血压干预是广受认可、有效且具有成本效益的措施。作为国家基本公共卫生服务项目的一部分，高血压患者管理自 2009 年开始在全国层面实施，但是没有干预控制的试点研究[15]。数据显示，截至 2017 年年底，高血压患者管理人数达到 1.01 亿[24]。尽管如此，评价高血压管理效果的基线数据并不可得。全国统计数据显示，2009—2015 年高血压患者数量逐年上升[139]。此外，由于该项目管理高血压患者基于患者自愿，因此患者有可能随时参加或退出管理。因而，测算项目的参与率非常困难。

针对构建公共卫生服务项目经济学评价模型的系统综述指出，开展经济学评价时，明确公共卫生服务干预措施的影响至关重要[57]。然而，分析患者随访、药物和非药物治疗对高血压患者管理的影响研究很少[138-140]。因此，开展基层高血压干预措施有效性评估的难点在于建立项目参与情况与长期健康结局之间的联系。

另外，由于社会经济发展等其他混杂因素的影响，量化国家基本公共卫生服务项目中实施高血压控制的增量效果更为困难。原因主要有两个：一是随着社会经济的不断发展，基层医疗卫生服务质量和居民高血压知晓情况持续改善；二是除了国家基本公共卫生服务项目，还有许多国家和地方的项目同步实施，很难区分各个项目各自的影响。为了克服这些障碍，本研究利用2009年之前的数据，通过时间序列趋势分析预测2015年高血压患者的控制情况。

为了估算高血压患者管理的效果，本研究分析了高血压患病率、知晓率、治疗率和控制率（以下简称“四率”）之间的关系。根据国家基本公共卫生服务项目规范，基层医疗卫生机构负责开展高血压患者筛查、提供治疗和转诊服务、建立健康档案、评估危险因素以及定期随访管理（至少每三个月一次）[10，25]。因此，理论上，高血压管理应提升其知晓率、治疗率和控制率，这一结论已经在研究中得到证实[15，66，85]。

为了达到研究目的，本研究需要找到能够反映2009年前后高血压患病率、知晓率、治疗率和控制率的时间序列数据，并在此基础上进一步开展测算。本章分为5个部分。“3.2”对1990年以来有关高血压患病率、知晓率、治疗率和控制率相关数据进行了文献综述。“3.3”对文献提取的数据进行年龄别特征及趋势分析。“3.4”利用拉格朗日插值法补齐了1990—2009年的缺失数据。同时，利用2009年之前的数据构建时间序列预测模型，通过该模型预测2015年高血压控制率，研究认为该预测值与2015年高血压控制率的实际值之间的差值体现国家基本公共卫生服务项目的效果。“3.5”比较了“3.4”的计算结果与相关文献研究结果，并围绕相关内容进行讨论。最后两个部分，“3.6”和“3.7”对本章进行了整体讨论并得出结论。

3.2 高血压患病率、知晓率、治疗率和控制率的文献研究（1990年至今）

3.2.1 文献检索策略

2018年11月22日，本研究通过PubMed检索了高血压患病率、知晓率、治疗率和控制率的相关文献。关键词包括（hypertension OR high blood pressure）AND（prevalence OR epidemiology OR awareness OR treatment OR control）AND（China OR Chinese），检索要求文献有全文，发表日期为2000年1月1日至2018年12月31日，共检索到5 553篇文献。此外，作者通过其他途径（与该领域内学者个人交流）获取文献3篇，共计5 556篇文献，通过题目与摘要进行了综述。

3.2.2 纳入排除标准

文献纳入标准：①采用多阶段分层整群随机抽样方法的国家代表性调查；②目标人群年龄为18岁及以上成人；③调查人群根据国家或者国际人口结构进行标准化；④血压值通过现场调查测量获取，测量人员经过专业培训，并且取2~3次的平均值；⑤文章以英语或者中文作为发表语言；⑥高血压定义为收缩压≥140mmHg或舒张压≥90mmHg，和/或正在使用降压药物。

高血压知晓定义为调查者自报其为经医生明确诊断的高血压人群。高血压治疗定义为患者自报调查前两周内一直在使用降压药物。高血压控制定义为收缩压<140mmHg和舒张压<90mmHg。香港特别行政区、澳门特别行政区和台湾省的相关研究没有纳入分析。

排除标准：针对特定民族、职业或者一定年龄范围的人群调查；研究对象不能代表18岁及以上成人的调查；如果两篇或多篇文章针对同一主题和年龄范围，则纳入影响因子较高的文章；作为增刊发表的文章也被排除研究。

3.2.3 文献分析

经过初步筛选，得到117篇相关文献，对摘要和全文深入分析，最终有30篇文献符合纳入标准，其中15篇用于数据提取，15篇用于与高血压管理效果进行对比分析（见3.5讨论）。文献筛选过程见图3-1，纳入分析的文献见表3-1。

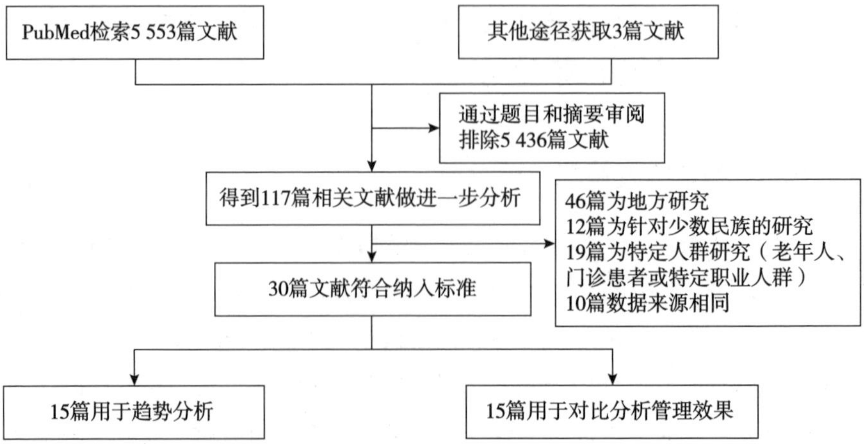

图3-1 文献筛选过程

表 3-1　1991—2018 年我国高血压患病率、知晓率、治疗率和控制率文献汇总

序号	发表文章的题目	调查年份	调查设计	年龄范围	分析方法	样本量
1	Trends in prevalence，awareness，treatment and control of hypertension in the middle-aged population of China，1992-1998[141]	1992—1994，1998	中国心血管疾病流行状况多中心调查：随机整群抽样	35~59	1992 年和 1998 年高血压患者四率比较分析	18 746 人（1992—1994 年）13 504 人（1998 年）
2	Hypertension burden and control in China[33]	2003—2012	综述	18+	系统综述	不适用
3	Prevalence，awareness，treatment，and control of hypertension in China[142]	2002	中国国家营养与健康调查（China National Nutrition and Health Survey）	18+	对比分析	141 892 人
4	Prevalence，awareness，treatment，and control of hypertension in China[143]	2000—2001	InterASIA；四阶段分层抽样	35~74	描述性分析（均数，标准差）	19 012 人
5	Trends in prevalence，awareness，treatment，and control of hypertension among Chinese adults 1991-2009[87]	1991—2009	中国健康与营养调查（CHNS）	18+	趋势分析	8 426~8 503 人
6	Hypertension prevalence，awareness，treatment，and control in 115 rural and urban communities involving 47 000 people from China[144]	2005—2009	前瞻性城乡流行病学调查（prospective，standardized collaborative study，PURE）	35~70	广义线性模型	153 996 人
7	Prevalence of hypertension in China：A cross-sectional study[86]	2007—2008	横断面调查	20+	我国高血压患病率分析	46 239 人

续表

序号	发表文章的题目	调查年份	调查设计	年龄范围	分析方法	样本量
8	Hypertension among older adults in low-and middle-income countries: Prevalence, awareness, and contro [145]	2007—2010	SAGE	50+	描述性分析	13 348 人
9	Prevalence, awareness, treatment, and control of hypertension in China: Results from a national survey [65]	2009—2010	多阶段分层抽样	18+	我国高血压患者四率分析	50 171 人
10	Hypertension and related CVD burden in China [146]	2010	2010 年中国非传染性疾病监测	18+	文献综述（2010 年中国非传染性疾病监测）	不适用
11	The dynamics of hypertension prevalence, awareness, treatment, control and associated factors in Chinese adults: Results from CHNS 1991-2011 [51]	2011	中国健康与营养调查（CHNS）	18+	中国健康与营养调查队列数据	8 658~12 474 人
12	China cardiovascular diseases report 2015: a summary [77]	2011	中国健康与营养调查（CHNS）	18+	文献综述	不适用
13	Report on Chinese Residents' Chronic Diseases and Nutrition [147]	2012	多阶段分层抽样	18+	描述性分析	不适用
14	Status of hypertension in China: Results From the China Hypertension Survey, 2012-2015 [33]	2012—2015	中国高血压调查	18+	*t* 检验和多元 Logistic 回归分析	451 755 人
15	Burden of hypertension in China: A nationally representative survey of 174 621 adults [148]	2013—2014	2013—2014 年中国慢性病与危险因素监测（CCDRFS）	18+	多元线性回归分析和 Logistic 回归分析	174 621 人

本部分分析了1991—2013年我国18岁及以上或者20岁及以上成人高血压的患病率、知晓率、治疗率、控制率。由于其研究对象年龄不符合要求，表3.1中第1、4、6、8篇文章未纳入分析。

CHNS数据是连续性最好的数据，该调查是全国范围的大型连续性横断面调查。该调查旨在分析我国居民健康和营养状况及其社会和经济影响因素[149]。根据国家基本公共卫生服务项目指南，高血压筛查与管理的主要目标人群是35岁及以上成年人。CHNS数据库不仅为进一步分析提供了长期数据，而且可以提供35岁以上高血压患者分析所需数据。此外，2016年的一项研究[144]和2012—2015年的中国高血压调查[33]也提供了可供分析的国家级数据。

因此，本研究利用1991—2011年CHNS发表数据和相关文献的数据进一步分析。所有数据均以2010年全国人口普查数据为基础进行年龄标准化。

本研究应用了1991—2015年CHNS全部调查数据。调查对象小于18岁，或年龄、性别、收缩压和舒张压数据存在缺失值的个案不纳入分析。

研究最终纳入24 410名调查对象的75 526条数据。2015年CHNS数据中，35岁及以上调查对象11 525名。本文综述了7篇不同来源的文献，涉及1991—2015年高血压患者患病率、知晓率、治疗率和控制率的情况（表3-2），每一年份数据均标注了调查年份、样本量和调查对象的年龄范围。为了分析高血压知晓率、治疗率和控制率之间的关系，研究分析了知晓治疗率（治疗率/知晓率）和治疗控制率（控制率/治疗率）。

如表3-2所示，1991年以来高血压患病率、知晓率、治疗率和控制率均呈上升趋势。1991—2015年，高血压患病率从14.13%上升至23.20%；知晓率从23.19%上升至46.90%；治疗率从10.88%上升至40.70%；控制率的水平一直较低，但也从2.75%上升至15.30%。

本研究进一步分析了知晓率、治疗率和控制率之间的关系。研究表明：①知晓治疗率高于治疗控制率。1991—2015年，治疗控制率最高值不超过0.45，知晓治疗率最低值大于0.5；②1997年以后，知晓治疗率高于0.70（70%），即如果患者知晓高血压患病情况则大概率会选择治疗；③治疗控制率持续上升，表明患者依从性提升，卫生服务体系和其他因素可能起到了积极作用。

表3-2显示，2015年CHNS数据并不可靠。首先，2009和2011年

表 3-2　高血压知晓率、治疗率和控制率之间的关系

调查年份	调查名称	样本量/人	年龄范围	患病率/%	知晓率/%*	治疗率/%*	控制率/%*	知晓治疗率 **	治疗控制率 **	参考文献或数据来源
1991	CHNS	8 436	18+	14.13	23.19	10.88	2.75	0.536	0.250	CHNS ***（1991—2011）
1993	CHNS	7 906	18+	15.23	18.46	9.45	2.71	0.543	0.257	
1997	CHNS	8 496	18+	17.51	13.87	8.13	1.70	0.738	0.177	
2000	CHNS	9 500	18+	17.42	21.28	12.58	3.09	0.697	0.243	
2004	CHNS	8 843	18+	19.90	23.47	16.18	4.72	0.772	0.277	
2006	CHNS	8 974	18+	18.58	28.39	19.00	5.10	0.742	0.237	
2009	CHNS	8 411	18+	21.92	26.46	20.53	6.12	0.874	0.268	
2011	CHNS	12 490	18+	19.85	36.11	26.52	9.31	0.734	0.351	
2002	CNNHS	141 892	18+	18.00	25.00	20.00	5.00	0.800	0.250	（Wu et al，2008）
2003—2012	文献系统综述	N/A	20+	26.70	44.60	35.20	11.20	0.789	0.318	（Li et al.，2015）
2009—2010	中国慢性肾病调查	50 171	18+	29.60	42.60	34.10	9.30	0.800	0.273	（Wang et al.，2014）
2010	中国慢性病调查	98 658	18+	33.70	33.30	23.90	3.90	0.718	0.163	（Xu Y，2013）
2013—2014	中国慢性病与危险因素监测	173 621	18+	27.80	31.90	26.40	9.15	0.828	0.347	（Li et al.，2017）
2012—2015	中国高血压调查	451 755	18+	23.20	46.90	40.70	15.30	0.868	0.376	（Wang et al.，2018）
2015	CHNS****	13 980	18+	45.37	19.65	16.12	6.71	0.82	0.416	CHNS 数据库，2019 年 5 月 26 日进行数据处理

备注：* 知晓率、治疗率和控制率均以高血压患病人数作为分母进行分析；** 知晓治疗率是知晓人群中治疗患者人数占比，治疗控制率指治疗人群中的血压控制患者人数占比，均以百分比表示；*** CHNS 数据以 2000 年（2000 年之前数据）和 2010 年（2000 年之后数据）全国人口普查数据进行年龄标化；****CHNS 数据中 18~35 岁年龄组高血压患病率极高，与其他研究相比数据较反常。由于 2015 年数据为新发布数据，需要进一步确认。因此，后续分析中只分析 35 岁及以上年龄人群数据，与其他研究保持一致。

CHNS 数据显示，成人高血压患病率大约为 20%，2015 年 CHNS 数据显示为 45.37%。同时，2015 年高血压知晓率和治疗率均远低于 2009 和 2011 年 CHNS 数据。其次，在另外一个同期调查（2012—2015 年中国高血压调查）中，高血压患病率、知晓率、治疗率和控制率和 1991—2011 年 CHNS 数据结果比较接近，且样本量远大于 2015 年 CHNS 数据结果。因此，在本研究后续分析中，采取中国高血压调查 2012—2015 年数据作为实际值进行分析。

3.3　年龄别高血压四率分析

年龄是心血管疾病的重要影响因素[150]。因此，本部分分析了 1991—2009 年共 19 年间，不同年龄组高血压患病率、知晓率、治疗率和控制率的发展趋势。

附表 A1 列出了高血压知晓率、治疗率和控制率。1991—2015 年，35 岁及以上高血压患者中，知晓率从 27.10% 上升至 44.91%，治疗率从 14.44% 上升至 38.42%，控制率从 2.87% 上升至 14.72%。2015 年，在知晓患病的患者中 85.5% 接受了降压治疗，1991—2015 年该值上升了 32.2 个百分点。在接受治疗的患者中，控制率从 1991 年的 19.9% 上升至 2015 年的 38.3%。见表 3-3。

表 3-3　1991—2015 年 35 岁及以上高血压患者四率趋势分析数据

年份	患病率/%	知晓率/%[a]	治疗率/%[a]	控制率/%[a]	知晓治疗率	治疗控制率
1991	22.18	27.10	14.44	2.87	0.533	0.199
1993	22.59	26.29	14.00	2.73	0.533	0.195
1997	26.10	18.78	12.12	2.95	0.645	0.243
2000	26.33	30.82	19.81	4.55	0.643	0.230
2004	27.46	33.33	23.95	6.95	0.719	0.290
2006	25.96	37.42	27.91	7.41	0.746	0.265
2007[b]	41.90	41.60	34.40	8.20	0.827	0.238
2009	30.47	37.85	29.54	8.61	0.780	0.291
2011	28.19	50.93	40.05	14.31	0.786	0.357
2015[c]	32.62	44.91	38.42	14.72	0.855	0.383

备注：a. 知晓率、治疗率和控制率的分母均为高血压患病人数，知晓治疗率和治疗控制率同表 3.1；b. 2007 年对 115 个城市和农村社区 47 000 人的高血压四率的一项调查[144]；c. 数据来源于中国高血压调查 CHS 2012—2015（Z. Wang et al.，2018）。

本研究描述了1991—2015年不同年龄组高血压的四率。结果显示，1991—2015年所有年龄组人群的高血压患病率、知晓率、治疗率和控制率均呈上升趋势。75岁及以上年龄组人群高血压患病率最高，而65~74岁年龄组人群的知晓率、治疗率和控制率最高，见图3-2至图3-5。

数据显示：①1991—2009年35岁及以上成人不同年龄组高血压四率均呈上升趋势；②高血压患病率随着年龄增加而增加，35岁及以上人群患病率

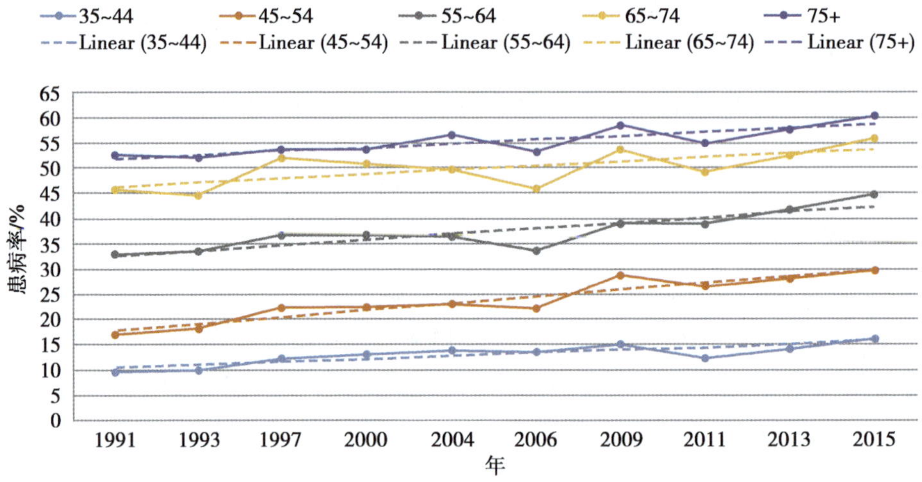

图3-2 1991—2015年间多年份不同年龄组高血压患病率

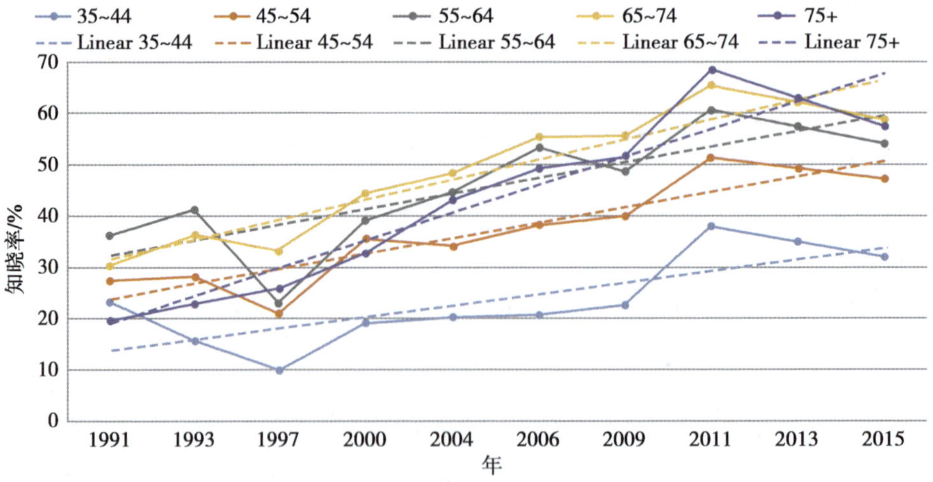

图3-3 1991—2015年间多年份不同年龄组高血压患者知晓率

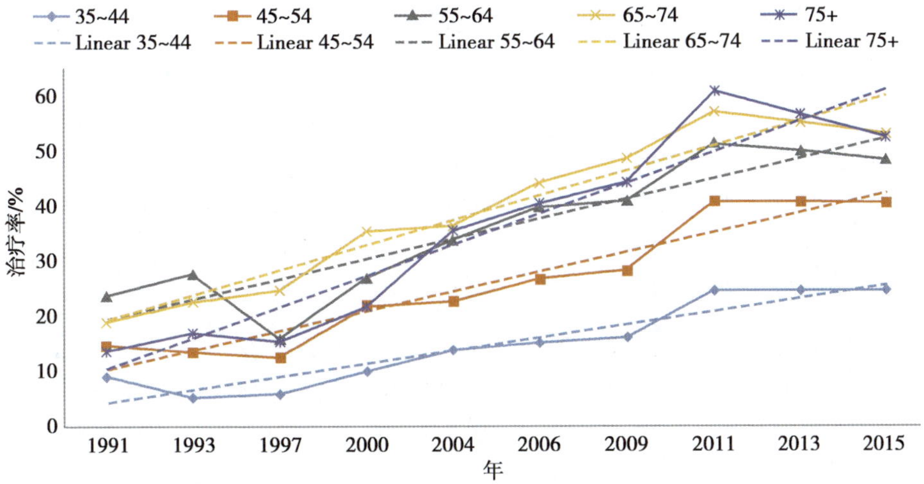

图 3-4　1991—2015 年间多年份不同年龄组高血压患者治疗率

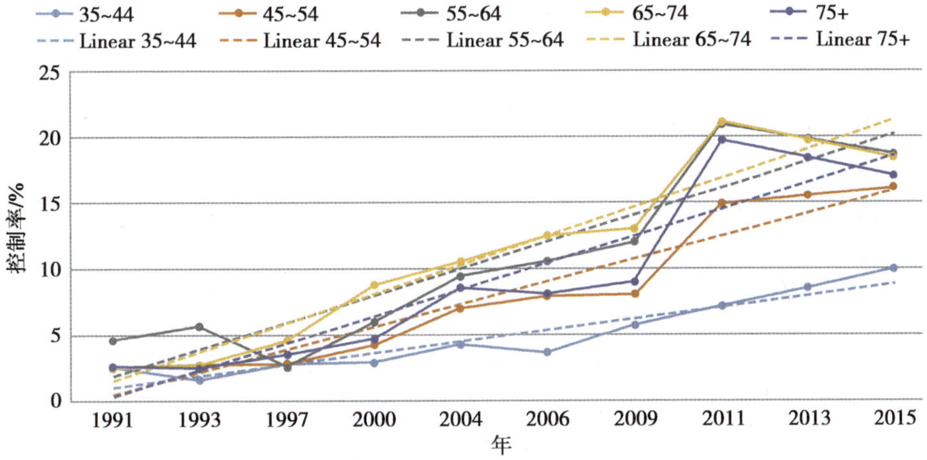

图 3-5　1991—2015 年间多年份不同年龄组高血压患者血压控制率

高于 10% 且快速上升，75 岁及以上年龄组高血压患病率最高；③尽管 75 岁及以上年龄组高血压患病率最高，但其知晓率、治疗率和控制率却不是最高。知晓率和治疗率最高的年龄组为 65~74 岁，控制率最高的年龄组为 55~64 岁。与 65~74 岁年龄组人群相比，75 岁及以上年龄组人群知晓率、治疗率和控制率明显偏低。尽管高血压患病率随着年龄增加而增加，知晓率、治疗率和控制率随着年龄增加而增加，但是低年龄组的治疗控制率高于高年龄组，35~44 岁、45~54 岁、55~64 岁、65~74 岁和 75 岁及以上年龄组分别为 40.4%、40.0%、38.7%、34.8% 和 32.6%，见图 3-6。

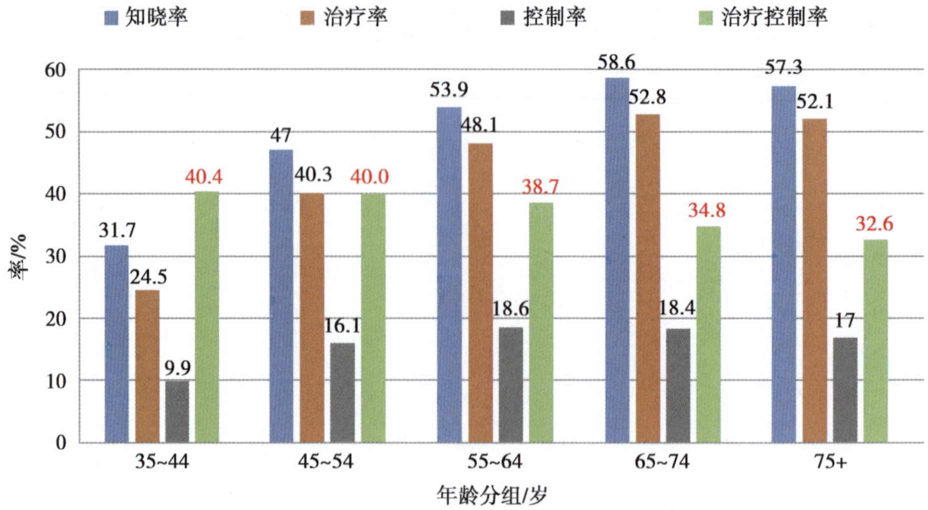

图 3-6　2012—2015 年调查 35 岁及以上年龄组高血压知晓率、治疗率、控制率和治疗控制率

数据来源：WANG Z，CHEN Z，ZHANG L，et al. Status of Hypertension in China：Results From the China Hypertension Survey，2012-2015［J］. Circulation，2018，137（22）：2344-2356.

如表 3-3 所示，从 1991—2015 年，知晓治疗率持续上升。2015 年，该比率为 0.855，远高于治疗控制率。该结果表明，如果患者知晓自己患高血压，则他们更愿意接受治疗，而接受治疗是控制高血压的关键[31，33]。根据国家基本公共卫生服务项目规范要求，高血压管理的第一步就是在基层医疗卫生机构实行“首诊测血压”。如表 3.3 所示，1991—2015 年治疗控制率远低于知晓治疗率。因此，尽管国家基本公共卫生服务项目的定量效果难以精确测算，但是根据图 3.2~图 3.5 的趋势变化可以看出，2015 年与 2009 年相比，在患病率没有明显变化的情况下，知晓率、治疗率和控制率增加比较明显。

知晓治疗率用来反映高血压患者的治疗意愿，而治疗控制率反映高血压患者的治疗效果[33]。2009 年之前和 2009 年之后的数据比较显示，高血压患者的知晓治疗率变化不大，均在 80% 左右。该结果进一步表明，患者知晓患有高血压后大概率会接受医疗服务。2009 年之后的治疗控制率高于 2009 年之前，可能是由于国家基本公共卫生服务项目实施后医疗服务的可得性和可及性提高。

由于高血压患者管理的目标是有效控制血压，而对知晓率和治疗率的影响都可以转化为血压控制，因此接下来的分析围绕血压控制展开。

3.4 高血压控制率的时间序列分析

3.4.1 数据来源

利用1991—2009年CHNS数据进行了时间序列分析[51, 87]。由于CHNS数据并不是规律连续数据，因此研究还使用了一些其他具有全国代表性的研究数据，产生了一组时间序列数据集。1991—2015年35岁及以上成人高血压四率数据如表3.3和图3.2~图3.5所示。

按照2010年中国人口统计调查数据对2010年之前的高血压四率进行年龄标准化。研究还对高血压控制进行了年龄别分析，详见附表D。

3.4.2 统计分析

研究考虑年龄和时间两大因素，针对高血压四率进行了描述性分析。

尽管研究对1991—2011年CHNS数据进行了系统提取并且全面收集了文献数据，但是1991—2009年并不是每年都有数据，其中只有10年数据可以获得用于时间序列分析。因此，本研究借鉴两项采用小样本时间序列分析方法的研究[34-35]，基于R语言操作系统利用拉格朗日插值法，基于1991、1993、1997和2000年的数据生成1995年数据，基于1997、2000、2004和2006年数据生成2002年的数据。见表3-4。

基于R语言操作系统利用拉格朗日插值法补齐1991—2009年高血压控制率数据（R语言操作过程见附表B）。

对1991—2009年数据进行趋势分析，并根据趋势分析产生的公式预测2015年的数据。根据2012—2015年高血压调查数据估计2015年高血压实际（观测）控制率[33]。比较实际（观测）值和预测值得出高血压患者控制人数差值，研究认为该差值代表国家基本公共卫生服务项目实施的增量效果。

3.4.3 结果

3.4.3.1 高血压四率初步趋势分析

2014年的一项研究[149]指出，2000—2001年间，我国高血压患者血压控制率为8.1%（n=15 540），而另一项研究显示2005—2009年的血压控制率为 8.2%（n=18 915）。综上所述，我国 2000—2009 年之间高血压患者的血压控制率保持在较低的水平。图 3-7 展示了 1991—2013 年我国 35 岁及以上成人高血压知晓率、治疗率和控制率的发展趋势。2009—2011 年，高血压控制率明显上升，为进一步分析国家基本公共卫生服务项目干预效果提供了重要基础。

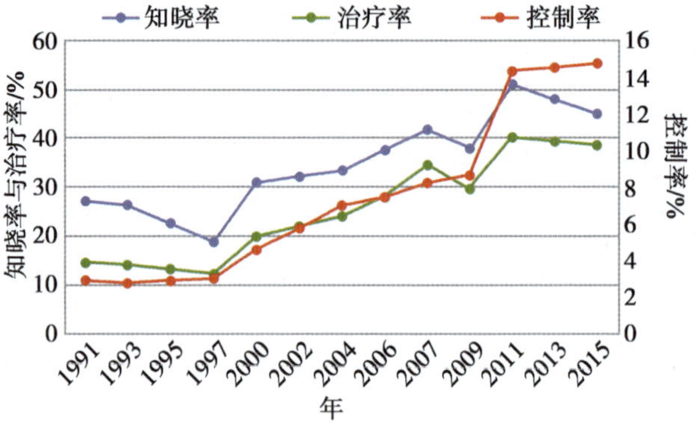

图 3-7　1991—2015 年间多年份 35 岁及以上成人高血压知晓率、治疗率和控制率

3.4.3.2　高血压控制率趋势分析和 2015 年控制状况预测

利用拉格朗日插值法补齐 1991—2009 年高血压控制率数据，见表 3-4。

表 3-4　1991—2009 年高血压控制率

年份	控制率/%	年份	控制率/%
1991	2.94	2001	5.26
1992	2.92	2002	5.90
1993	2.85	2003	6.48
1994	2.78	2004	6.95
1995	2.74	2005	7.10
1996	2.78	2006	7.41
1997	2.94	2007	8.20
1998	3.37	2008	8.26
1999	3.95	2009	8.61
2000	4.60		

注：利用拉格朗日插值法插入 1995 年和 2002 年的数据。

由于趋势分析的数据少于 20 个，研究进行了小样本时间序列分析，并且事前用拉格朗日插值法进行了小样本数据处理。采用 SPSS 22.0 统计软件，基于专家建模法（expert-modeler method）进行时间序列预测分析，得出 2015 年我国高血压患者的预测控制率。如表 3-5 和图 3-8，利用布朗指数平滑模型进行线性趋势预测。

自相关函数残差表明各数据呈现随机分布且没有异常值，表明模型曲线拟合度较好（详见附录 B）。

表 3-5　高血压控制率时间序列预测模型建模情况

模型	预测数（Number of predictors）	模型拟合统计		Ljung-Box Q（18）			异常值数据量
		静态 R^2	R^2	统计值	自由度	P 值（Sig.）	
控制率-model_1	0	0.162	0.990	3.852	17	1.000	0

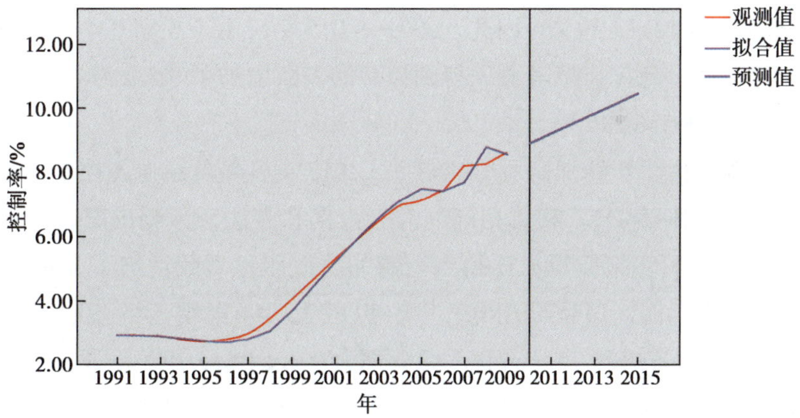

图 3-8　1991—2009 年高血压控制率时间序列趋势和 2010—2015 年预测分析

表 3.6 列出了基于 1991—2009 年数据趋势分析模型估计的 2010—2015 年高血压预测控制率，并列出了预测值上限和下限。按照 1991—2009 年数据，预测 2015 年高血压控制率将为 10.46%［95%*CI*（7.33%，13.59%）］。

表 3-6 模型预测 2010—2015 年高血压控制率 单位：%

模型	2010 年	2011 年	2012 年	2013 年	2014 年	2015 年
预测值	8.92	9.22	9.53	9.84	10.15	10.46
UCL*	9.40	10.13	10.93	11.80	12.73	13.71
LCL**	8.43	8.32	8.13	7.88	7.57	7.20

注：*UCL 为上限值，**LCL 为下限值。

3.4.3.3 国家基本公共卫生服务项目效果估计

本研究利用 2009—2015 年高血压控制率的实际值和预测值之间的差值反映国家基本公共卫生服务项目的效果。按照 2010 年第六次全国人口普查数据，31 个省（自治区、直辖市）35 岁及以上成年人口数为 685 998 627 人。

根据 2012—2015 年中国高血压调查，2015 年 35 岁及以上高血压患病率为 32.6%[33]，高血压患病人数为 223 772 752 人。根据 2015 年高血压控制率预测值 10.46%［95%*CI*（7.20%，13.71%）］和实际值 14.72% 之间差值，国家基本公共卫生服务项目的实施使得高血压控制率提升了 4.26 个百分点［95%*CI*（1.13，7.39）］。因此，2009—2015 年，由于国家基本公共卫生服务项目的实施，高血压患者血压得到控制的人数增加了 9 532 719 人［95%*CI*（2 528 632，16 536 806）］。

研究还分析了年龄别高血压控制率，2015 年各年龄组血压控制率的实际值和预测值见附表 D3。利用相同的人口数据和方法，预测出国家基本公共卫生服务项目的实施使得血压得到控制的高血压患者数增加了 8 009 449 人（95%*CI*：1 581 856，13 065 018），其中男性 35~44 岁组、45~54 岁组、55~64 岁组、65~74 岁组和 75 岁及以上组分别为 0 人、1 635 397 人、1 564 164 人、170 388 人和 617 939 人；女性各年龄组分别为 0 人、1 568 221 人、1 523 002 人、169 167 人和 761 170 人。尽管分年龄组的预测数据加和与全年龄组分析存在明显差别，但是按照两个数据分析产生的效益成本差别不大，均能显示项目的效果（具体在第 5 章讨论）。

此外，由于 2012—2015 年中国高血压调查原始数据库未能获得，研究无法获取性别年龄别高血压患病率和控制率，因此男性和女性的患病率和控制率视为相同；同时，未能获得 75~84 岁和 85 岁及以上年龄组分组数据，所以将两个年龄组合并为一组（75 岁及以上组），这可能进一步降低数据的精确性。因此，本研究用了全部年龄组数据进行分析（详见附录 D）。

为了检验利用 2012—2015 年中国高血压调查原始数据库进行趋势分析预测结果的可靠性，本文作者还检索了其他相关文献，提供了多个国家基本公共卫生服务项目的高血压控制效果数据。详见 3.5 部分的内容。

3.4.3.4 灵敏度分析

为了评价趋势分析预测模型的灵敏度，本研究进行了两项分析：一是计算模型的预测数据的 95%*CI* 和上、下限值，见表 3.6（上限值和下限值）；二是基于 1991—2009 年数据进行直接线性模拟，并将研究结果与曲线趋势分析模型进行对比（图 3-9）。直接线性模拟分析结果显示，2015 年我国 35 岁及以上高血压控制率预测值为 10.66%，比指数回归分析模型预测值 10.46%［95%*CI*（7.20%，13.71%）］高 0.2 个百分点，两者差异小于 5%，且直接线性回归模型的预测值在指数回归分析的 95%*CI* 内。基于此，按照直接线性回归模型预测得出 2009—2015 年通过国家基本公共卫生服务项目的实施，9 085 173 人血压得到控制，而指数预测模型的预测值为 9 532 719 人，这个结果依然在指数预测模型的 95%*CI*（2 528 632，16 536 806）内。

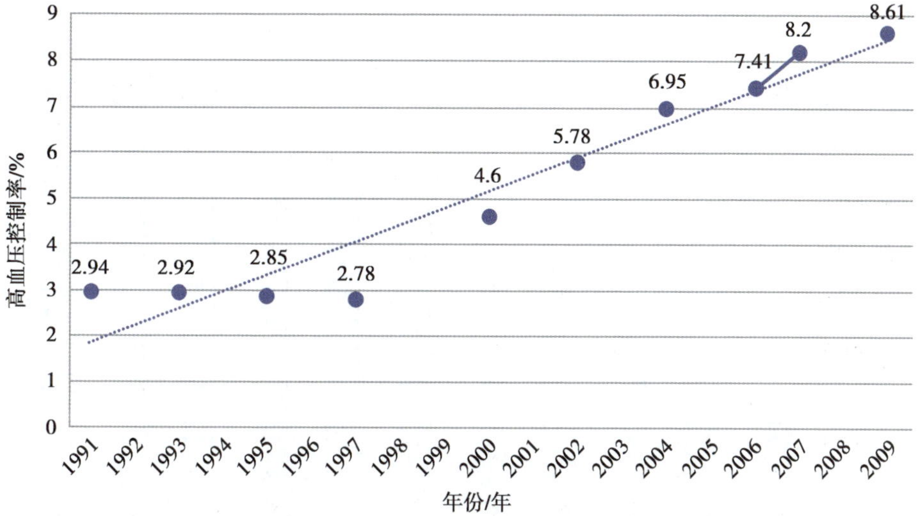

图 3-9　1991—2009 年 35 岁及以上成人高血压控制率直接线性趋势分析

注：线性趋势模型分析公式：y=0.367 2x+1.483 6，R^2=0.924 8

3.5 国家基本公共卫生服务项目高血压控制效果的相关研究结果

3.5.1 高血压管理的统计分析

量化高血压患者控制的效果，首先需要了解国家基本公共卫生服务项目管理的高血压患者人数，根据国务院医改办的数据，我国基层医疗卫生机构管理的高血压患者人数从2010年的1 480万人增加至2013年的8 503万人，如图3-10所示。2017年底，国家基本公共卫生服务项目管理的高血压患者人数达10 104万人，项目财政投入经费达人均55元。截至2018年，国家基本公共卫生服务项目投入合计约4 528亿元，其中2 483亿元来自中央财政投入。

本研究基于1991年以后基层高血压患者管理的研究结果和国家官方公布的纳入国家基本公共卫生服务项目管理的高血压患者人数，估算国家基本公共卫生服务项目管理效果。利用统计数据中的高血压管理人数乘以高血压控

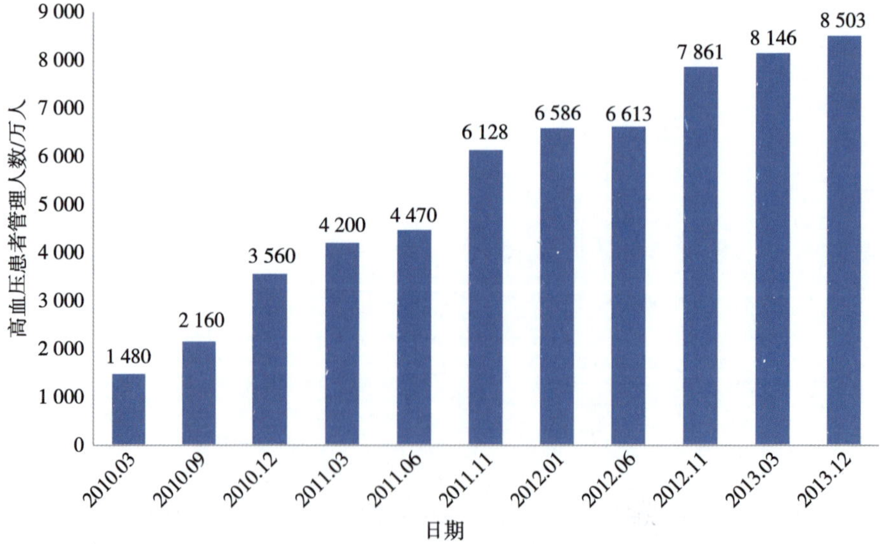

图3-10 2009—2013年国家基本公共卫生服务项目高血压患者管理人数

数据来源：国务院医改办，2015年医疗卫生改革监测，2016年4月15日引用。

制率，那么就可以得出血压得到控制的患者人数，该数据可以与趋势分析所得数据进行对比分析。

如前所述，2015 年 35 岁及以上成人高血压患病率和知晓率分别为 32.62% 和 44.91%[33]，据此估计 2015 年我国 35 岁及以上高血压患者数为 223 772 752 人，其中 100 496 343 人知晓其患有高血压状况。而按照国家基本公共卫生服务项目统计数据，截至 2015 年底，我国有 8 835 万人接受国家基本公共卫生服务项目管理，照此推算我国 88% 的高血压知晓患者已经纳入国家基本公共卫生服务项目管理。因此，利用中国高血压调查[33]估算的知晓国家基本公共卫生服务项目管理的高血压患者人数具有一定的代表性。

3.5.2 其他研究分析国家基本公共卫生服务项目的高血压控制情况

国内外多项研究尝试分析高血压管理项目的效果，主要结果指标为血压降低程度和高血压控制状况。为了验证趋势分析结果的可信赖程度，本文对高血压患者管理的血压控制效果的文献进行了综述。

与一般人群高血压四率趋势分析结果对比而言，本部分文献是针对 2009 年启动的新一轮医改背景下国家基本公共卫生服务项目效果进行的分析。

如表 3-7 所示，四项不同的研究估算了国家基本公共卫生服务项目高血压管理的影响与效果。

按照 3.5.1 的分析，国家基本公共卫生服务项目管理的高血压患者数为 8 835 万，四项研究估算结果，高血压控制人数应在 6 979 650~16 212 225 人（表 3-7）。

3.5.2.1 国家基本公共卫生服务项目的效果估算（以 2009 年前的数据进行估算）

有两项研究评价了 2009 年国家基本公共卫生服务项目开始前基层医疗卫生机构慢性病管理效果。一项研究是在北京以高血压管理规范为基础的追踪评价，研究对象是基层医疗卫生机构管理的 50 岁及以上的脑卒中高危人群，结果显示高血压知晓率、治疗率和控制率分别为 70.0%、62.1% 和 29.6%[151]，该研究表明通过基层医疗卫生机构开展高血压患者管理可以有效提高患者知晓率，进而提高血压控制率；另一项研究样本代表性较好，以我国 1 000 个城市社区卫生服务中心管理的 249 830 名高血压患者作为研究对象，评价了

表 3-7　不同研究估计的基层医疗卫生机构高血压患者控制情况

参数	年份	研究对象	样本量	人群年龄范围/岁	研究设计	控制率	国家基本公共卫生服务项目贡献率 **	国家基本公共卫生服务项目增加控制的高血压患者人数/人 ***
我国基层高血压控制情况	2007—2010	基层医疗卫生机构	249 830	18~79	目的抽样	27.0%（*SE*=0.7%）	提高了 11.7 个百分点	10 336 950
国家基本公共卫生服务项目的影响分析	2011、2013	基层医疗卫生机构	4 958	≥45	中国健康与养老追踪调查（CHARLS）	控制率改善了 7.9%（*SE*=2.9%）	控制率提高了 7.9%	6 979 650
我国新医改之下高血压四率分析	2008、2012	医疗机构	1 961 和 1 836	≥45	CHARLS	21.7%~36.4%	提高了 15.3 个百分点	13 517 550
国家基本公共卫生服务项目可及性和对成人慢性病的影响分析	2013	基层医疗卫生机构	1 367	25~95	多阶段分层随机抽样	33.65%*（*SE*=1.28%）	提高了 18.35 个百分点	16 212 225

注：* 慢性病控制率表示的是高血压和 2 型糖尿病两者的情况，两类疾病没有分别表达；**2012—2015 年中国高血压调查显示 18 岁及以上成人高血压的控制率为 15.3%[33]。而根据该标准，国家基本公共卫生服务项目的贡献为估算值减去一般人群的血压控制率（即基层医疗卫生机构血压控制率减去一般人群血压控制率，该估算可能存在低估的情况）；*** 利用国家基本公共卫生服务项目改进的血压控制率乘以 8 835 万人，即得出高血压控制人数增加值。

高血压患者社区药物干预和血压控制之间的关系（表 3-7）。研究显示，社区卫生服务机构管理的高血压患者治疗率为 37%，其中，36.5% 的患者接受单一药物治疗，63.5% 的接受联合用药，两者的血压控制率分别为 27.7% 和 24.1%[139]。基于同一作者的另一项分析发现，35 岁及以上人群血压控制率为 14.72%[33]。基层医疗卫生机构管理的高血压患者血压控制率减去全人群的血压控制率，差值为 12.28%，以 2013 年管理的高血压患者人数乘以该差值则得出增加控制的高血压患者数为 1 044 万人（8 503 万人 ×12.28%）。

3.5.2.2 基于前后对比分析的研究

按照本研究文献纳入标准，只搜索到两篇在国家层面评价国家基本公共卫生服务项目的文献，两篇文章均利用了中国健康与养老追踪调查（China Health and Retirement Longitudinal Study，CHARLS）数据，均基于浙江省和甘肃省的数据进行了前后对比分析。Zhang 等研究发现，由于国家基本公共卫生服务项目的实施，2011—2013 年两省高血压控制率提升了 7.9%（*SE*=2.9%）[152]。Hou 等研究显示，2008—2012 年两省基层医疗卫生机构管理的高血压患者血压控制率从 21.7% 提高至 36.4%，提高了 14.7 个百分点[66]。这两项研究提供了基于国家基本公共卫生服务项目管理规范评价高血压管理效果的方法，将重点置于高血压知晓率、治疗率和控制率。尽管如此，CHARLS 的调查人群年龄范围为 45 岁及以上，与国家基本公共卫生服务项目管理的高血压患者与高危人群（35 岁及以上）并不完全一致。因此，本研究无法用 CHARLS 的数据来全面评估项目的实施情况。因此，上述两个项目虽然一定程度上提供了项目评价证据，但是并不能全面反映项目实施情况。在第一项研究中[152]，作者将接受免费健康体检的高血压患者作为纳入项目管理的标准；而第二项研究将高血压知晓、治疗和控制作为纳入项目管理的标准进行分析[66]。

上述两项分析提供了 2011—2013 年和 2008—2012 年两个时间段高血压控制率变化的情况，估算值分别为 7.9% 和 14.7%。如果按照上述结果进行粗算，以 2013 年国家基本公共卫生服务项目的高血压人数 8 503 万人为基础，得出项目增加血压控制的高血压患者数在 672 万~1 250 万人。

3.5.2.3 一项针对国家基本公共卫生服务项目的评价

2015 年开展的一项研究针对国家基本公共卫生服务项目高血压和糖尿病管理开展了针对性评价，利用横断面调查数据分析了国家基本公共卫生服务项目的可及性和效果[15]。研究将高血压规范管理定义为定期随访和检查，分析发现国家基本公共卫生服务项目管理人群以中老年人为主，平均年龄为65.26岁。调查患者中，33.65%的患者血压和血糖得到有效控制（过去3个月内）。尽管该研究[15]并没有用病例对照或者队列研究，但是它提供了高血压控制状况的全面信息，也是专门针对国家基本公共卫生服务项目的评价。

该研究显示，管理人群血压控制率为33.65%，而前述研究显示一般人群血压控制率为14.72%，二者差值为18.93个百分点。按照管理人群8 503万人计算，理论上，项目实施增加血压控制的高血压患者人数为1 610万人。

其他相关研究显示，基层医疗卫生机构管理的高血压患者具有较高的血压控制率，但主要是针对我国发达地区的研究，不能够代表我国整体情况。例如，北京一项研究分析了基于高血压管理规范的基层患者管理项目效果，从4个社区卫生服务中心选择了140名高血压患者进行了12个月的追踪，研究结果显示城市患者血压控制率从40.0%上升至70.7%，农村患者血压控制率从27.9%上升至72.9%[153]。针对上海市徐汇区和深圳市较发达地区的研究显示，国家基本公共卫生服务项目的实施使得高血压基层管理率从36.1%提升至83.2%[82]。在成都市玉林社区卫生服务中心开展的一项追踪研究[（33±25）个月]显示，高血压患者的血压控制率从32%提高到85%[154]。

该部分通过文献分析讨论了高血压控制效果的数值范围。这些研究均基于基层医疗卫生机构相关研究，并且用了卫生健康行政部门上报的数据进行分析。结果显示，截至2015年，通过国家基本公共卫生服务项目实施增加的血压控制患者人数分别为1 044万、672万~1 250万和1 610万人，其他文献显示数据范围是672万~1 610万人。

上文“3.4”分析的高血压控制人数预测值为9 532 719人[95%*CI*（2 528 632，16 536 806）]，该结果在文献分析的数值区间。

3.6 讨论

本章分析了通过国家基本公共卫生服务项目实施所增加的血压得到控制的患者人数。时间序列分析显示，2009—2015年血压控制人数增加953万人，并通过其他相关文献分析进行验证，结论是国家基本公共卫生服务项目实施所增加的血压得到控制的患者数应在672万~1610万人之间，进一步验证了本研究的可信性。

深入分析发现，知晓率是提升高血压控制率的关键影响因素，患者知晓后才会寻求医疗服务，国家基本公共卫生服务项目的实施在提高知晓率方面发挥了重要作用，进而改善了血压控制率。

分析还发现知晓率、治疗率和控制率随着年龄增加而提高。尽管如此，年轻患者的治疗控制率更高，35~44 岁组、45~54 岁组、55~64 岁组、65~74 岁组和 75 岁及以上组治疗控制率分别为 40.4%、40.0%、38.7%、34.8% 和 32.6%。这表明国家基本公共卫生服务项目中，较低年龄组患者尚未得到很好管理，但是其知晓率、治疗率和控制率的小幅改善就可能带来血压控制的较大幅度提升。然而，国家基本公共卫生服务项目在 35~44 岁年龄组患者未发挥有效作用（附录 D）。

研究发现，尽管高血压控制率有所改善，但是改善幅度并不理想[32,38]。我国的治疗控制率在 0.163~0.376 之间，但治疗控制率远低于同期国际水平[32, 38]。尽管中国高血压基层管理指南（2014 年修订版）与国际指南相契合[155]，但是纳入国家基本公共卫生服务项目的高血压患者血压没有控制到理想水平，可能存在管理不到位的情况，可能由于基层服务提供不足[19, 15]，尤其是基层卫生人力不足[19, 66]。与国际比较分析显示，我国高血压知晓率依然有待大幅度提升[63]。

有研究认为，我国抗高血压药物在可得性、成本和处方开具方面存在缺陷[79]。收入水平较低和医疗保险成本较高可能影响国家基本公共卫生服务项目在高血压控制方面的效果[79]。

此外，我国地域广阔、人口众多，城乡和区域间发展不均衡是我国社会经济发展的主要问题且将长期存在[157]。证据表明，文化水平、地理、健康状况、职业和其他因素是卫生服务体系公平性和影响受益的重要因素[158]。对基层医疗卫生服务和高血压患者管理而言，这些影响因素同样发挥着重要作用[32, 159-160]。据报道，我国仅有少数高血压患者得到确诊，得到有效控制的患者更是少之又少[31]。从这个意义上说，国家基本公共卫生服务项目的实施依然任重道远。卫生改革有待进一步深化，特别是在完善投入补偿机制、人才队伍建设、改进基本药物的可得性和可及性以及缩小地区差距等方面。

通过趋势分析开展高血压四率分析的研究较多，对比而言，多项研究进行了比较相似的分析，例如基于 CHNS 数据的两项研究[51, 87]。然而，以 2009 年我国新医改为节点进行的前后对比分析的研究较少，因此本研究在一定程度上填补了该领域的空白。

此外，中国地域广阔，各地经济水平、人口学特征、气候、习俗等差异较大。因此，开展基于全国人口的分析可能会被认为是没有意义的。但是，国家基本公共卫生服务项目自 2009 年开始在全国实施，针对该项投入具有明确的管理规范和指南标准，同时该项目还是国家公共卫生服务均等化的重要内容。尽管项目的人均投入数额看起来并不大，但这是迄今为止我国针对基本公共卫生服务的最大投入。因此，编者认为有必要在国家层面开展基本公共卫生服务项目的评价，特别是分析提高高血压患者的知晓率、治疗率和控制率方面的效果。

3.7 局限性分析

第一，时间序列模型所使用的数据来源不同，以年为单位的数据并不连续，可能导致预测的精确度。但是，本研究进行了文献综述，并且使用拉格朗日插值法改进了可信度，并且每项预测值都提供了 95% 的置信区间范围，具体结果见第 5 章。第二，如前所述，我国区域间差别较大，增加了从国家层面评价国家基本公共卫生服务项目效果的难度。该缺陷只能通过具有连续、完整的数据来完善。尽管 CHNS 数据库提供了最全面和连续的高血压患者四率数据，但是这项调查并不是最具有代表性的数据。因此，该研究采用了 2012—2015 年中国高血压调查的数据进行分析，但是这导致了数据来源不一致、不连续。

尽管如此，分析显示 2009 年之前的 CHNS 数据与相关调查数据具有高度的一致性。例如，1991 年 CHNS 数据显示，18 岁及以上成人年龄标化高血压患病率、知晓率、治疗率和控制率分别为 14.13%、23.19%、10.88% 和 2.75%；而同期中国高血压调查的结果显示 15 岁及以上人口上述四率分别为 13.6%、26.3%、12.1% 和 2.8%[33]。另一项研究采用 2006 年和 2009 年 CHNS 数据与 2005—2009 年中国 115 个城市和农村社区对 47 000 名调查人口的高血压四率数据进行对比分析，结果显示二者的结果也是相似的[144]。

但是，2009 年之后 CHNS 和其他国家级具有代表性的数据之间出现较大的差异。例如，2009 年之后的中国高血压调查数据显示 2012 年和 2015 年我国成人高血压控制率分别为 13.8% 和 16.8%[33]。而 2015 年 CHNS 数据显示

35 岁及以上成人高血压控制率为 12.7%，而 2011 年 CHNS 数据显示控制率为 14.72%，2012—2015 年中国高血压调查显示控制率为 14.72%，即 2009 年之后的 CHNS 数据可信度较差。因此，针对 2009 年之后的分析，本研究采用中国高血压调查数据进行。

3.8 小结

国家基本公共卫生服务项目的实施有效地改善了高血压患者的知晓率、治疗率和控制率。据估算，2009—2015 年间，由于项目的实施增加血压控制的患者人数为 9 532 719 人［95%*CI*（2 528 632，16 536 806）］。项目还有效改善了高血压患者的知晓率，该效果在 55 岁及以上人口中最显著。尽管如此，我国基层高血压患者管理在提升知晓率、治疗率和治疗控制率方面依然面临艰巨的任务，特别是对年轻患者的管理。下一步政策重点应该关注低年龄组人群的早期发现、干预和治疗，主要措施是加强基层医疗卫生服务能力建设，特别应加强基层卫生人力、提高医疗保险的效率和改善药物可及性。

4

基于马尔可夫模型估计国家基本公共卫生服务项目的健康产出

4.1 项目介绍

第 3 章基于血压控制状况分析了国家基本公共卫生服务项目对高血压患者管理的效果，并对基本公共卫生服务项目工作机制进行了探讨。上述分析估计了 2009—2015 年间国家基本公共卫生服务项目实施效果，即高血压控制人数增加了 9 532 719 人。本章将分析高血压控制的长期健康产出。研究假设如果国家基本公共卫生服务项目未实施，则 9 532 719 名高血压患者的血压将得不到控制，这种情境被称为未实施国家基本公共卫生服务项目的情境。而实际（观测）情况则是实施国家基本公共卫生服务项目情境。在两种情境（实施国家基本公共卫生服务项目和未实施国家基本公共卫生服务项目）下，分析高血压控制和未控制的长期健康产出。二者之间的差值反映国家基本公共卫生服务项目实施的健康产出。

正如第 2 章所讨论的，心血管疾病常作为高血压干预评估结果指标。然而，如果将心血管疾病作为主要评估结果指标，那么除了高血压之外，其他危险因素也很重要。本研究使用 2009 年 CHNS 调查数据，从高血压患者样本数据中获得这两种情境下的其他因素（即年龄、性别、血压、血胆固醇、糖尿病、BMI 以及吸烟情况）相关信息。基于多因素分析，确定两种情境下心血管疾病发病的风险水平。为了比较实施国家基本公共卫生服务项目情境和未实施国家基本公共卫生服务项目情境下的风险水平，利用已发表的高血压流行病学分析和相关模型研究来确定模型中疾病状态转移的参数[40, 107, 114]。对于未实施国家基本公共卫生服务项目的情境，将实施国家基本公共卫生服务项目情境的参数利用计算的相对比率进行加权。

2015年，Gu等[38]对低成本药物控制高血压的干预进行了成本-效果分析，建立了高血压控制风险预测和长期健康结果模型。该模型已在中国近期一项针对强化高血压控制的经济学评价中得到应用和验证[42]。基于上述研究，本研究建立马尔可夫模型来模拟高血压的长期进展，并估计相关的发病率和死亡率。这是本章讨论的重点。

本章还有其他3个部分的内容：第4.2节基于文献综述和CHNS 2009的数据，进行了两种情境下心血管疾病风险的多因素分析；第4.3节介绍了两组的马尔可夫模型和参数估计；第4.4节概述了未来30年内冠心病、脑卒中和死亡的长期预测与估计。

4.2 高血压患者心血管疾病风险分析

4.2.1 危险因素分析

如第2章所述，年龄、性别、血压、BMI、总胆固醇、吸烟和糖尿病已被确定为缺血性心血管疾病（ischemic cardioovascular disease，ICVD）的独立危险因素，缺血性心血管疾病主要是指冠心病和脑卒中[36, 40, 103]。然而，不同研究分析的危险因素不尽相同。例如，Wu等[36]通过年龄、收缩压（systolic blood pressure，SBP）、BMI、总胆固醇、吸烟和糖尿病等因素建立了用于评估缺血性心脑血管病的Cox模型。Yang等使用年龄、收缩压、总胆固醇、低密度脂蛋白（LDL-C）、腰围、吸烟状况、糖尿病、城乡差异和动脉粥样硬化性心血管疾病（atherosclerotic cardiovascular disease，ASCVD）家族史作为危险因素，开发了预测中国人群ASCVD的工具[161]。2007年，WHO/ISH以年龄、性别、收缩压、总胆固醇、吸烟状况和糖尿病作为独立因素，制订了适用于全球不同区域的心血管疾病风险预测图[47]。

为了模拟两种情境的相对比率，必须使用包含危险因素信息的数据库。唯一可访问且符合要求的数据库为2009年“中国营养与健康调查”（CHNS）数据库。CHNS旨在获得关键公共卫生危险因素、人口、社会和经济因素以及健康结果的信息，这是一项以家庭为基础的调查，从 1989—2015 年开展了十轮调查。CHNS 采用多阶段、随机整群抽样法进行抽样[149]，尽管最新的数据已于 2015 年发布，但本研究针对心血管疾病风险分析所必需的生物标志物信息仍未公开发布，我们目前无法获得这些生物标志物信息。

2009 年 CHNS 数据共有 9 552 名 18 岁及以上被调查人员，其中 1 025 名由卫生专业人员诊断为高血压患者。高血压患病率、知晓率、治疗率和控制率的测量和定义已在前述章节进行了解释[51]。本研究在确诊的 1 025 名高血压患者中，1 017 名 35 岁及以上患者的数据用作进一步分析，这些患者被分为血压控制组和未控制组（血压未控制指 SBP/DBP≥140/90mmHg，否则为已控制）。

为了进行心血管疾病风险预测，我们从 2009 年 CHNS 数据库中获得 1 017 名 35 岁及以上高血压患者的年龄、性别、收缩压、舒张压、BMI 和总胆固醇的平均值。对于每个年龄性别组，使用风险评估公式计算吸烟率和糖尿病患病率。根据 WHO 标准（2011），本研究糖尿病的确认标准是糖化血红蛋白值大于 6.5%，或接受降糖治疗，或对“医生是否曾告知您，您患有糖尿病（U24a）”的问题回答为“是”的调查对象。关于吸烟状况，我们根据对问题“你还抽烟吗？（U27）”的回答来确定。

首先进行描述性分析。G1 和 G2 分别代表实施国家基本公共卫生服务项目情境中血压得到控制的高血压患者和未实施国家基本公共卫生服务项目情境下血压未得到控制的高血压患者。将两者在特定年龄性别层面上的每个危险因素进行分析，比较年龄、收缩压、舒张压、总胆固醇、高密度脂蛋白和低密度脂蛋白胆固醇的平均值。采用 t 检验来确定差异是否具有统计学意义（$P<0.05$）。Pearson 卡方检验用于检验两组之间吸烟率和糖尿病患病率的差异是否具有统计学意义（$P<0.05$）。本研究计算了每十岁一组的年龄组别间中国成年人心血管疾病危险因素的平均值和比例，并对两组特定年龄性别情况下的危险因素分布的差异进行比较。使用 SPSS 22.0 统计软件进行统计学分析。图 4-1 显示了本研究为进行比较而建立两种情境的决策树。从左边的第一个单元格开始，上面分支代表实施国家基本公共卫生服务项目情境，下面分支代表未实施国家基本公共卫生服务项目情境。

4.2.2 危险因素分析结果

在 35 岁及以上被诊断为高血压的 1 017 名患者中，男性占 44.05%，女性

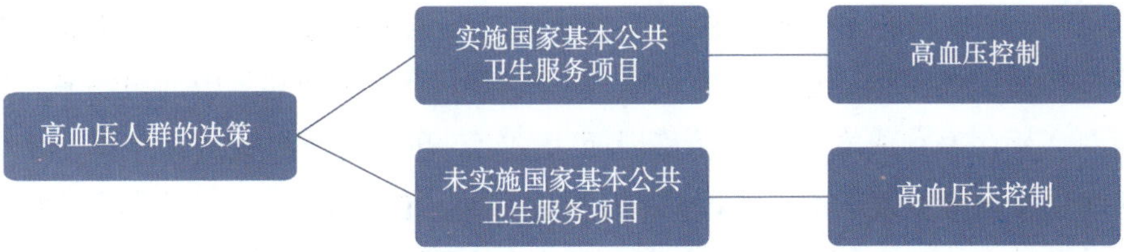

图 4-1 实施国家基本公共卫生服务项目和未实施国家基本公共卫生服务项目的高血压人群决策树

占 55.05%；血压得到控制的占 68.53%，血压未得到控制的占 31.47%。各年龄性别组高血压患者血压控制组与未控制组收缩压和舒张压比较，差异均有统计学意义（$P<0.05$）。在血压控制组中，男性和女性患者的平均收缩压约为 127mmHg；而在高血压未控制组中，男性和女性患者的收缩压平均值范围为 147~169mmHg。两组在年龄、总胆固醇、高密度脂蛋白、BMI、糖尿病发病率、吸烟率等方面比较，差异均无统计学意义（$P>0.05$）。

综合以上分析，在被认为是心血管疾病独立危险因素的 8 个变量中，仅血压值存在差异，为进一步分析两组间的心血管疾病患病风险提供了基础。

作者针对上述分析撰写了一篇文章，并在 2018 年发表于《中国全科医学》杂志[162]，详细信息见参考文献。

4.3 方法：马尔可夫模型研究

在近期研究中，中国心血管疾病决策模型（Cardiovascular Disease Policy Model-China model）是发展最完善且应用最广泛的心血管疾病风险预测模型[38, 41, 113]。因此，本研究基于中国心血管疾病决策模型建立了预测长期心血管疾病风险的马尔可夫模型。

为了评估国家基本公共卫生服务项目实施对高血压患者管理结果的影响，在预测的 30 年期间，在两种情境下分别建立了马尔可夫模型。本研究结果分析了在国家基本公共卫生服务项目管理下，封闭队列中模拟的整个高血压人群以及不同年龄和性别组的健康结果。

4.3.1 马尔可夫模型的建立

马尔可夫模型是一种状态转移模型，通常用于评估抗高血压治疗的结果[56，163]。中国心血管疾病决策模型是基于马尔可夫模型建立的，它是一个状态转移数学模型，用于研究中国成年人群中冠心病和脑卒中的患病率、发病率、死亡率和成本，状态转移周期为一年。研究者已经证实，中国心血管疾病决策模型可以应用于模拟封闭队列[38，40]。在这项研究中，依据上述模型相关参数，构建中国35岁以上高血压患者人群马尔可夫模型[38，41]。马尔可夫模型的结构如图4-2所示。在本研究中，心血管疾病包括脑卒中和冠心病两类疾病，因此图4-2中将其作为一种状态进行表述。

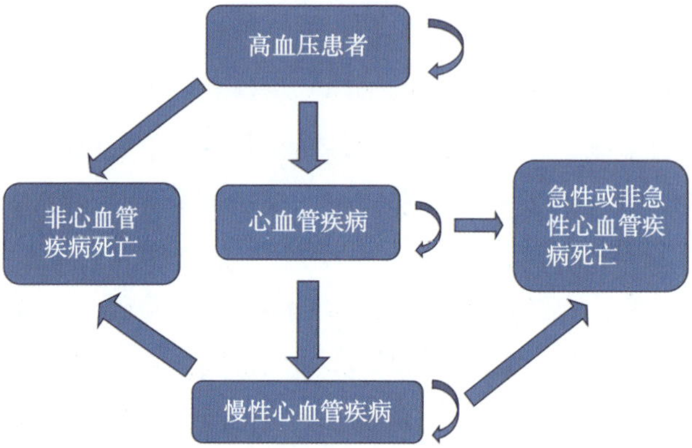

图4-2 高血压患者的心血管疾病进展的马尔可夫模型

高血压控制组和未控制组患者均在这六种健康状态中进行转移，即单纯高血压、急性心脏病、急性脑卒中、慢性冠心病、慢性脑卒中或死亡。

在中国心血管疾病决策模型中，描述了脑卒中或冠心病事件首次发病及其28天内的后遗症[38，41]。

马尔可夫模型的状态转移周期为一年。28天病死定义为冠心病或脑卒中导致的急性死亡。与顾东风等学者[38]的研究方法一致，本研究一年期冠心病和脑卒中病死率也是根据冠心病和脑卒中死亡率及其既往患病率进行计算。

非心血管疾病死亡率等于人群全因死亡率减去冠心病死亡率和脑卒中死亡率[163]。

同样，中国心血管疾病决策模型下冠心病和脑卒中的定义与已有研究一致[38]。研究假设：①心血管疾病事件发生后，无法缓解至未患心血管疾病的状态；②未考虑其他健康状况或疾病；③冠心病和脑卒中进行独立分析，而不是分为冠心病、脑卒中及其组合三种形式进行分析。根据顾东风等[38]的研究结果确定任意两种健康状态之间的转移概率。处于每种心血管疾病状态的患者每年都有转移到其他不同状态的可能性。高血压患者人群按每 10 岁一个年龄组和性别进行分层。

本研究中，35 岁以上高血压患者的动态变化过程按照中国心血管疾病决策模型相关参数进行模拟[38，41]。患者处于基线状态，直至发生致命或非致命性心血管疾病事件，或其他非心血管疾病相关原因导致的死亡。以 1 年为基本模拟周期，从稳定性心血管疾病状态开始，患者随后可能会发生致命或非致命心血管疾病事件，或非心血管疾病原因的死亡。如图 4.3 所示，共有 6 种健康状态：高血压、冠心病、冠心病死亡、脑卒中、脑卒中死亡和非心血管疾病死亡。死亡状态来自 3 个原因，即冠心病、脑卒中和非心血管疾病原因。上一个周期的高血压、冠心病和脑卒中分别进入下一个周期。

采用 TreeAge Pro 2019 R1.1 软件（TreeAge Software，Inc.，Williamstown，MA，USA）进行马尔可夫模型运算，模型结构如图 4-3 所示。

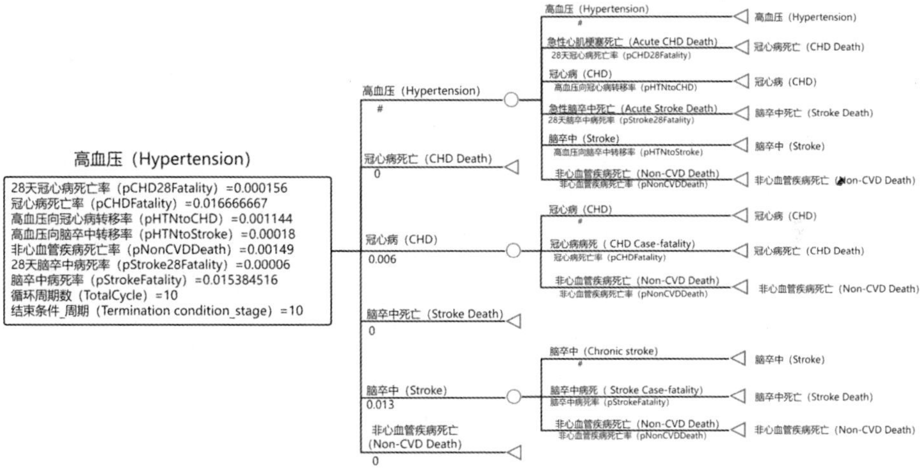

图 4-3　以男性、高血压控制组、年龄 35~45 岁为例的马尔可夫模型结构

注：# 表示为同一级别下第一个分支在本级别中的比例，同一级别所有分支比例之和为 1；“○”代表循环；“△”代表结束（死亡）。

4.3.2　目标人群

如第三章所述，据估计因国家基本公共卫生服务项目实施，全人群中增加的高血压控制的患者人数为 9 532 719 名。由于没有针对该人群开展全国范围内的代表性调查，本研究采用2012—2015年中国高血压调查（CHS 2012—2015）数据来代表目标人群的年龄性别结构、高血压患病率和控制情况。2012年10月—2015年12月，中国高血压调查采用分层多阶段随机抽样方法，抽取全国31个省份的451 755名18岁及以上居民的全国代表性样本，调查结果于2018年发布[33]。依据2010年第六次全国人口普查数据对年龄性别结构进行标化。国家基本公共卫生服务项目的效果通过高血压控制人数来表示。CHS 2012—2015中，本研究假设高血压得到控制的患者年龄性别结构与研究人群相同。采取该假设的另一个依据是基于第三章的讨论分析，据该分析估计，35岁以上具有一定知晓水平的高血压患者中，约有88%的在国家基本公共卫生服务项目中接受了一定形式的健康管理（表4-1）。

表4-1 用于对目标人群进行年龄标准化的数据 单位：%

分组	人群占比[a]	实际患病率[b]	实际控制率[b**]
男性/岁			
35~44	10.2	17.8	9.9
45~54	13.1	30.0	16.1
55~64	14.0	43.5	18.6
65~74	8.9	53.8	18.4
75~84	4.5	56.8	17.0
85+*	0.7	56.8	17.0
女性/岁			
35~44	5.9	10.8	9.9
45~54	11.6	27.8	16.1
55~64	14.2	45.0	18.6
65~74	9.8	58.0	18.4
75~84	5.7	62.7	17.0
85+*	1.3	62.7	17.0

注：*《中国高血压调查》中没有列出85岁以上人群的高血压患病率和控制率，本研究假设85岁以上人群的高血压患病率和控制率与75岁以上年龄组一样，分别为62.7%和17.0%。

**《中国高血压调查》中未给出特定年龄-性别的实际控制率，本研究假设相同年龄组男性和女性的控制率相同。

资料来源：a. 2010年第六次全国人口普查数据，中国国家统计局。b.《中国高血压调查》[33]。

根据2012—2015年中国高血压调查和2010年中国第六次人口普查数据，进一步假设：①因国家基本公共卫生服务项目而使血压得到控制的9 532 719名高血压患者的性别年龄别结构与CHS 2012—2015调查[35]中高血压患者的性别年龄结构相同；②在未实施国家基本公共卫生服务项目的情境中，高血压未得到控制的9 532 719名高血压患者也具有与2012—2015年中国高血压调查患者相同的性别年龄结构；③由于85岁以上年龄组的高血压患病率无法通过2012—2015年中国高血压调查获得，因此假设85岁组的高血压患病率和控制率与75~84岁组相同。

计算各年龄性别组的高血压人数：首先，根据2010年第六次全国人口普查各年龄性别组的人口结构，对各年龄-性别组的高血压患病率和控制率（取自CHS 2012—2015）进行加权；然后，将各年龄-性别组的构成乘以9 532 719。结果如表4-2所示。

表4-2　35岁以上目标高血压患者的加权结构和数量

分组	构成/%*	高血压患者人数/人
男性/岁		
35~44	6.11	582 276
45~54	12.71	1 211 554
55~64	16.04	1 529 342
65~74	10.29	981 285
75~84	4.64	442 566
85+	0.79	75 476
女性/岁		
35~44	3.55	338 476
45~54	11.29	1 076 590
55~64	16.16	1 540 445
65~74	11.02	1 050 308
75~84	5.96	568 066
85+	1.43	136 336
总计	100	9 532 719

资料来源：* 来自2010年中国第六次人口普查分年龄性别人口构成和2012—2015中国高血压调查各年龄组患病率[33]。

4.3.3 估计长期健康结果的参数

假设将 9 532 719 名高血压患者放置于高血压控制组和未控制组这两种情境下的封闭队列，中期和长期健康结果由可避免的心血管疾病和可避免的死亡表示。

假设在实施国家基本公共卫生服务项目情境（G1）中，9 532 719 名高血压患者的血压得到控制，决定疾病状态转移模型的参数与从前期研究中提取的一般人群模型的参数相同[38]。在未实施国家基本公共卫生服务项目情境（G2）中，9 532 719 名高血压患者的血压未得到控制，决定疾病状态转移的模型参数通过两组各性别年龄别的年度风险比标化（加权）获得。

如前所述，在血压控制组和未控制组两组在年龄、总胆固醇、高密度脂蛋白、BMI、糖尿病发病率、吸烟率等方面差异均无统计学意义，有统计学意义的是两组的血压水平。基于中国人群的血压和心血管疾病风险[39]，根据 G2 到 G1 的相对风险，按照收缩压水平对 G2 的参数进行加权。如 2009 年 CHNS 数据显示，两组的收缩压水平已在本章第 1 节进行了描述，该章节还描述了心血管疾病的危险因素。根据收缩压水平估算冠心病和脑卒中的相对风险[39]。还对 G1 与 G2 的风险比进行估算，通过比较 G2 和 G1 的相对比率，得出每个年龄-性别组的风险比，具体见表 4-3。

表 4-3 G1 和 G2 收缩压水平和发生冠心病和脑卒中的相对风险

分组	收缩压/mmHg*		多变量调整 *RR* 表示为 Gu et al.（2008）					
			冠心病			脑卒中		
	G1	G2	G1	G2	G2 与 G1 的比值	G1	G2	G2 与 G1 的比值
男性/岁								
35~44	127	147	1.23	2.03	**1.65**	1.76	3.62	**2.06**
45~54	127	149	1.23	2.03	**1.65**	1.76	3.62	**2.06**
55~64	129	152	1.23	2.03	**1.65**	1.76	3.62	**2.06**
65~74	127	157	1.23	2.03	**1.65**	1.76	3.62	**2.06**
75~84	126	160	1.23	2.84	**2.31**	1.76	5.83	**3.31**
85+	127	157	1.23	2.03	**1.65**	1.76	3.62	**2.06**

续表

分组	收缩压/mmHg*		多变量调整 *RR* 表示为 Gu et al.（2008）					
			冠心病			脑卒中		
	G1	G2	G1	G2	G2 与 G1 的比值	G1	G2	G2 与 G1 的比值
女性/岁								
35~44	131	155	1.17	1.63	**1.39**	1.98	3.32	**1.68**
45~54	125	152	1.16	1.63	**1.41**	1.59	3.32	**2.09**
55~64	127	156	1.16	1.63	**1.41**	1.59	3.32	**2.09**
65~74	131	156	1.17	1.63	**1.39**	1.98	3.32	**1.68**
75~84	126	164	1.16	2.00	**1.72**	1.59	4.96	**3.12**
85+	138	164	1.17	2.00	**1.71**	1.98	4.96	**2.51**

注：* 各年龄-性别组的收缩压水平取自 2009 CHNS。

马尔可夫模型的参数如下。

- 正文 4.3.2 部分描述了高血压人群的性别年龄结构。
- 既往的心肌梗死（myocardial infarction，MI）、冠心病和脑卒中的发病率，28 天急性冠心病和脑卒中的病死率和死亡率指标均来源于近期相关流行病学和模型研究[38，105]，这些研究均对数据进行了校准。假设研究人群中既往心肌梗死或脑卒中与一般人群相同。
- 根据 2013 年城乡性别年龄别疾病死亡率统计数据[43]对非心血管疾病死亡率进行计算，人口结构采用 2010 年全国第六次人口普查数据。由于无法获得城市和农村人口的年龄性别结构相关参数数据，本研究假设城市和农村人口结构差异没有统计学意义。本研究调整了 2013 年的城乡别死亡率，并得出了性别年龄别的全因死亡率[43]。按性别年龄别调整的非心血管疾病死亡率见附录表 B3。
- 冠心病和脑卒中的死亡率来自 Chan 等[106]的研究，适用于 85 岁以下的高血压患者。死亡率是在规定的时间段内（通常是 1 年）用死亡人数除以处于风险中的人口数[98]。85 岁以上成人冠心病和脑卒中死亡率根据《2014 中国卫生和计划生育统计年鉴》[43]中的城乡性别年龄别疾病死亡率计算，其中性别年龄结构根据 2010 年中国人口普查数据进行调整。

• 28 天病死率用于反映急性心血管疾病引发的死亡，是根据 Chan 等[106]的研究每个周期为 1 年。病死率是指特定时间段内被诊断出患特定疾病的所有个体中因该疾病死亡的比例，病死率用特定时间（1 年）内因所分析疾病导致的死亡人数除以该期间患有该疾病的人数得出。

• 冠心病或脑卒中的病死率由冠心病或脑卒中死亡率以及既往心肌梗死或既往脑卒中的患病率（用作冠心病或脑卒中的一般患病率）得出。这是通过将冠心病或脑卒中死亡率减去既往冠心病或脑卒中 28 天病死率获得。

详见表 4-4 和附表 B4。

表 4-4　参数和数据来源

参数	来源
不同年龄-性别组的高血压患者比例	2010 年第六次全国人口普查；Wang et al., 2018[33]
冠心病	
既往冠心病	（Gu et al.，2015）[38]
G1 情境下冠心病发病率	（Gu et al.，2015）[38]
G2 情境下冠心病发病率	计算得出
28 天病死率	（Gu et al.，2015）[38]
冠心病死亡率	（Gu et al.，2015）[38]
冠心病病死率（每年）	计算得出
脑卒中	
既往脑卒中	（Gu et al.，2015）[38]
G1 情境下脑卒中发病率	（Gu et al.，2015a）[38]
G2 情境下脑卒中发病率	计算得出
28 天病死率	（Gu et al.，2015a）[38]
脑卒中死亡率	（Gu et al.，2015a）[38]
脑卒中病死率（每年）	计算得出
非心血管疾病死亡率	《2014 中国卫生和计划生育统计年鉴》[43]

马尔可夫过程以 1 年为周期运行，模型里的所有流行病学参数都是按照每 10 岁一个年龄组赋予。运行 10 个周期后，将其更改为下一个 10 岁年龄组的参数。将前 10 个周期的高血压、冠心病、脑卒中的健康结果，冠心病或脑卒中导致的死亡和非心血管疾病死亡输入下一个 10 岁年龄性别组。具体信息详见附录表 B4。

该模型以 4 种状态开始：单纯高血压、既往心肌梗死、既往脑卒中和死亡（初始时点为 0）。在两种情境下（实施国家基本公共卫生服务项目和未实施国家基本公共卫生服务项目）估计目标人群中每个年龄-性别组冠心病、脑卒中的累计发病率，每个年龄-性别组即刻（28 天）病死、慢性心血管疾病导致的死亡和非心血管疾病原因导致死亡的累积死亡率。

在马尔可夫模型中，心血管疾病、不良事件和死亡之间的转移在 30 年间的变化是显而易见的。对于 75~84 岁年龄组，仅报告了 10 年和 20 年的变化；而对于 85 岁以上年龄组，由于缺乏预期寿命数据，仅报告了 10 年的变化。在每个周期中，随着时间的推移，冠心病、脑卒中和死亡的数量与前一个周期中数据相加。

4.3.4 灵敏度分析

2009 年中国营养与健康调查（CHNS 2009）数据显示 G1（血压控制组）和 G2（血压未控制组）之间的差异主要由高血压导致的。虽然 2015 年中国营养与健康调查（CHNS 2015）没有其他血液学因素的数据，但是有血压值数据。而在 2015 年中国营养与健康调查（CHNS 2015）中血压的测量和高血压的定义与 2009 年中国营养与健康调查（CHNS 2009）完全相同。因此，采用 2015 年中国营养与健康调查（CHNS 2015）数据分析 G1（血压控制组）和 G2（血压未控制组）的收缩压水平，对 2009 年数据进行敏感度分析，结果见表 4-5-1 和表 4-5-2。除了 G1 组 35~45 岁的女性（5.47%）和 G2 组 85+岁的女性（5.62%）之外，2009 年和 2015 年 CHNS 在所有年龄组的高血压控制组和非控制组之间的差异均较小。2009 年和 2015 年，各年龄组收缩压的差异占 2009 年高血压控制组的百分比为 0.63%，高血压未控制组的百分比为 0.60%，详见表 4-5-1 和表 4-5-2。

表 4-5-1　2009 年和 2015 年 CHNS 高血压控制组收缩压情况（G1）

分组	2009 年			2015 年			2009 年和 2015 年对比，收缩压的差异占 2009 年数据比例/%
	例数	平均血压/mmHg	标准差	例数	平均血压/mmHg	标准差	
男性/岁							
35~44	10	127.13	5.675	13	129.18	10.140	1.61
45~54	28	127.33	11.195	48	124.62	7.487	−2.13
55~64	35	128.65	10.841	97	127.67	9.020	−0.76
65~74	42	127.44	9.605	117	127.30	8.405	−0.11
75~84	16	126.50	9.022	40	128.25	6.650	1.38
85~	2	127.00	5.185	2	130.67	6.600	2.89
女性/岁							
35~44	7	131.10	9.863	10	123.93	9.815	−5.47
45~54	43	125.04	9.543	57	126.66	9.751	1.30
55~64	51	126.69	11.169	123	125.52	9.539	−0.92
65~74	63	130.68	8.343	103	126.52	8.472	−3.18
75~84	22	125.52	13.155	41	129.59	7.676	3.24
85~	1	136.67	N/A	4	133.83	4.290	−2.08
总计	320	127.68	10.101	655	126.88	8.743	−0.63

注：各年龄-性别组的收缩压水平取自 CHNS 2009 和 CHNS 2015。N/A 为数据不可得。

表 4-5-2　2009 年和 2015 年 CHNS 高血压控制组收缩压情况（G2）

分组	2009 年			2015 年			2009 年和 2015 年对比，收缩压的差异占 2009 年数据比例/%
	例数	平均血压/mmHg	标准差	例数	平均血压/mmHg	标准差	
男性/岁							
35~44	14	147.24	14.556	26	148.53	14.882	0.88
45~54	55	148.63	13.642	106	148.94	15.154	0.21
55~64	74	152.15	18.032	199	152.27	14.904	0.08
65~74	78	156.64	14.886	193	154.94	16.721	−1.09
75~84	38	159.94	19.435	64	154.22	14.540	−3.58
85~	3	156.67	6.110	13	157.79	11.375	0.71

续表

分组	2009 年			2015 年			2009 年和 2015 年对比，收缩压的差异占 2009 年数据比例/%
	例数	平均血压/mmHg	标准差	例数	平均血压/mmHg	标准差	
女性/岁							
35~44	11	155.45	28.772	26	150.54	15.361	−3.16
45~54	48	151.88	14.520	111	155.88	16.421	2.63
55~64	97	156.08	14.913	208	153.96	14.788	−1.36
65~74	99	155.80	15.144	234	158.13	17.357	1.50
75~84	56	164.35	23.929	109	157.25	17.100	−4.32
85~	4	163.08	5.865	13	153.92	14.859	−5.62
总计	577	155.43	17.273	1 302	154.50	16.104	−0.60

注：各年龄-性别组的收缩压水平取自 CHNS 2009 和 CHNS 2015。N/A 为数据不可得。

4.4 长期健康结果估计

4.4.1 两组心血管疾病进展和死亡的长期趋势

在每个预测的年份，进入马尔可夫队列进展为冠心病、脑卒中数量及因心血管疾病死亡患者人数和非心血管疾病死亡人数总和恒定，死亡人数逐年增加。

图 4-4 显示为 G1 和 G2 情境下，以 35~44 岁年龄组男性和女性高血压患者为例，预测其 30 年间总死亡人数占比趋势图。这表明在预测期结束时，G2 情境中因心血管疾病导致的死亡人数高于 G1 情境。

附录 B 列出了所有其他年龄性别组在预测 30 年期间内的死亡趋势作为补充材料。

4.4.2 避免心脑血管患者数和死亡数的估计

与 G2（未实施国家基本公共卫生服务项目）相比，G1（实施国家基本公共卫生服务项目）情境下的第 10 个预测周期年末，实施基本公共卫生项目全国多增加血压控制的患者中分别避免了发生冠心病 43 386 名、脑卒中 314 004

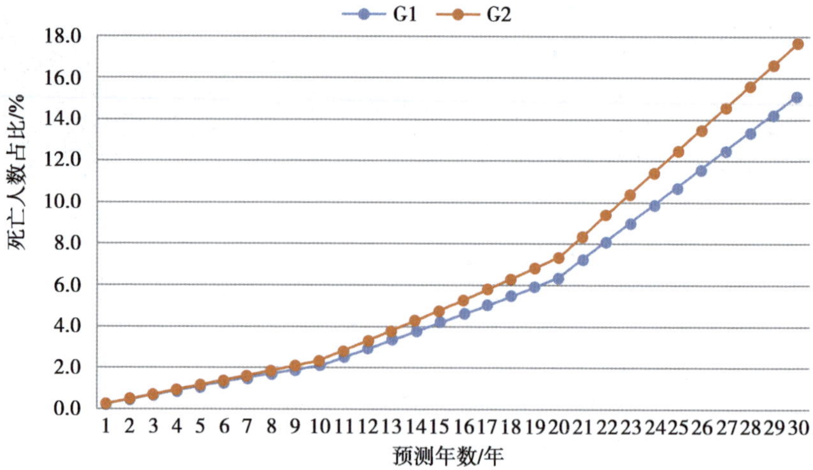

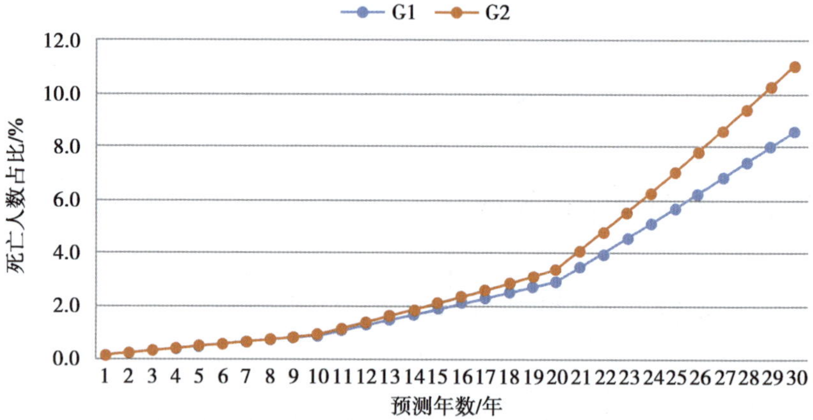

图 4-4　G1 和 G2 情境下 35~44 岁男性（上侧）和女性（下侧）的死亡百分比

名和死亡 289 644 名。在第 20 个预测周期年末，分别避免发生冠心病 45 035 名、脑卒中 400 313 名和死亡 558 625 名。在第 30 个预测周期年末，分别多避免发生冠心病 25 012 名、脑卒中 296 258 名和死亡 744 493 名。表 4-6、表 4-7 和表 4-8 中列出这些结果的详细信息。如表 4-8 所示，在为期 30 年的分析中，避免心血管疾病患者数和死亡数出现负值，主要是男女年龄较大的群体（65~74 岁和 75~84 岁年龄组）。这是因为未实施国家基本公共卫生服务项目情境中，各年龄组死于心血管疾病的患者比实施国家基本公共卫生服务项目情境的患者多，因此高年龄组心血管疾病带病生存人数相对更少，尤其是脑卒中。

表 4-6　预测至第 10 年的运行结果

单位：名

分组	G1			G2			G2-G1（避免发生心血管疾病和死亡的患者人数）		
	冠心病	脑卒中	死亡	冠心病	脑卒中	死亡	冠心病	脑卒中	死亡
男性/岁									
35~44	8 850	7 325	11 961	12 685	8 295	13 241	3 835	970	1 279
45~54	20 764	43 028	55 518	27 332	55 544	62 625	6 568	12 516	7 107
55~64	52 845	171 455	160 667	62 566	235 985	181 610	9 720	64 529	20 943
65~74	39 085	134 254	250 126	47 710	182 196	281 718	8 625	47 943	31 591
75~84	10 657	27 684	262 932	13 782	44 502	330 665	3 124	16 818	67 733
85~	196	708	63 276	214	1 017	67 247	18	310	3 971
女性/岁									
35~44	1 822	3 301	2 901	2 010	3 713	3 061	187	413	160
45~54	15 382	37 287	24 892	16 788	53 124	29 098	1 406	15 838	4 205
55~64	52 731	151 827	104 128	57 084	231 981	130 512	4 353	80 154	26 384
65~74	36 524	142 037	188 712	40 111	187 380	215 570	3 587	45 343	26 858
75~84	16 363	39 042	288 907	18 303	67 216	376 364	1 941	28 174	87 457
85~	529	1 628	105 549	550	2 626	117 503	21	998	11 954
总计							43 386	314 004	289 644

表 4-7　预测至第 20 年的运行结果

单位：名

分组	G1			G2			G2-G1（避免发生心血管疾病和死亡的患者人数）		
	冠心病	脑卒中	死亡	冠心病	脑卒中	死亡	冠心病	脑卒中	死亡
男性/岁									
35~44	11 288	11 640	36 786	17 081	18 271	42 491	5 794	6 632	5 705
45~54	27 984	87 416	165 285	39 953	147 164	191 465	11 969	59 748	26 180
55~64	49 619	176 237	501 353	63 760	270 605	575 794	14 141	94 368	74 441
65~74	16 748	49 410	689 698	19 449	76 986	812 824	2 701	27 576	123 127
75~84	464	1 683	413 651	193	1 152	434 930	–271	–531	21 278
85~	196	708	63 276	214	1 017	67 247	18	310	3 971
女性/岁									
35~44	2 675	7 595	9 779	3 278	12 979	11 345	603	5 384	1 566
45~54	21 910	86 113	89 760	25 939	153 118	115 012	4 028	67 005	25 252
55~64	47 061	199 008	362 939	52 755	295 357	438 796	5 694	96 349	75 857
65~74	22 513	66 566	633 132	23 385	109 438	779 062	873	42 872	145 930
75~84	1 058	3 309	506 396	523	2 912	549 760	–535	–397	43 364
85~	529	1 628	105 549	550	2 626	117 503	21	998	11 954
总计							45 035	400 313	558 625

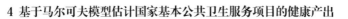

表 4-8　预测至第 30 年的运行结果

单位：名

分组	G1			G2			G2-G1（避免发生心血管疾病和死亡的患者人数）		
	冠心病	脑卒中	死亡	冠心病	脑卒中	死亡	冠心病	脑卒中	死亡
男性/岁									
35~44	14 331	34 814	87 775	21 795	63 359	102 978	7 464	28 545	15 203
45~54	33 031	113 086	412 957	45 871	191 467	482 630	12 840	78 381	69 673
55~64	23 572	67 940	1 113 669	25 708	107 119	1 301 559	2 136	39 179	187 891
65~74	740	2 721	935 116	259	1 666	970 908	−481	−1 055	35 792
75~84	464	1 683	413 651	193	1 152	434 930	−271	−531	21 278
85~	196	708	63 276	214	1 017	67 247	18	310	3 971
女性/岁									
35~44	5 111	24 123	29 135	6 516	45 658	37 457	1 405	21 535	8 323
45~54	24 115	128 254	259 680	28 452	200 737	321 327	4 337	72 483	61 647
55~64	30 398	91 952	970 678	29 347	149 716	1 189 612	−1 051	57 764	218 934
65~74	1 552	4 928	959 805	682	3 973	1 026 267	−870	−955	66 463
75~84	1 058	3 309	506 396	523	2 912	549 760	−535	−397	43 364
85~	529	1 628	105 549	550	2 626	117 503	21	998	11 954
总计							25 012	296 258	744 493

4.5 小结

基于上述分析，由于国家基本公共卫生服务项目的实施，预测未来 10 年、20 年和 30 年心血管疾病患病和心血管疾病导致的死亡均有明显下降。与 G1 情境相比，G2 情境（未实施国家基本公共卫生服务项目）下心血管疾病的发病率和死亡率要高得多，表明国家基本公共卫生服务项目在预防心血管疾病发生和避免死亡方面效果明显。

本分析假设在实施国家基本公共卫生服务项目情境下血压得到控制的患者与一般人群中血压得到控制的患者之间差异无统计学意义；在未实施国家基本公共卫生服务项目情境下的血压未控制患者和一般普通人群中血压未控制的患者二者之间差异无统计学意义。对 2009 年 CHNS 数据进行分析结果显示，血压水平随着年龄的增长而升高，这与其他研究结果相同[35, 147]，同时数据显示两个模拟组心血管疾病风险的决定因素是血压水平。

本研究是首个从该角度分析高血压患者健康管理结果的研究。如第 3 章所述，一些研究试图从提高血压控制率和降低血压水平的角度评估国家基本公共卫生服务项目高血压患者管理健康效果[15, 65, 154]。然而，关于高血压管理的中长期影响的研究较少，本研究在一定程度上填补了这一空白。

本研究先进性主要体现在以下 3 个方面：一是利用调查数据反映高血压人群危险因素的真实状况。通过使用 2009 年 CHNS 数据，比较血压控制和未控制两组高血压患者的危险因素，包括年龄、性别、血压、总胆固醇、BMI、吸烟状况和糖尿病。为使分析更具代表性，本研究采用 2012—2015 年中国高血压调查（CHS 2012—2015）数据对高血压人群进行性别年龄别结构分析。如第 3 章所述，根据 CHS 2012—2015[33]，估算 2015 年 35 岁以上的高血压患者人数为 223 772 752 人，仅有 100 496 343 名高血压患者意识到自己的病情。根据医改报告统计数据[164]，截至 2015 年底，全国约有 8 835 万高血压患者被纳入国家基本公共卫生服务项目管理。据此推算，可能有 88% 以上高血压知晓患者在一定程度上接受了国家基本公共卫生服务项目的患者管理服务。基于此，研究认为《中国高血压调查》[33] 中知晓高血压的患者可用于代表中国国家基本公共卫生服务项目在管的高血压患者。二是采用马尔可夫模型[38, 113]，结合心血管疾病风险预测参数[39, 165]，进行长期预测。这填补了我国高血压患者管理经济学评价研究领域的空白。由于高血压是一种“慢性病”，同时也是心血管疾病的危险因素，死亡多是因其导致心血管疾病引起，评价其健康管理效果不仅应关注短期控制情况，还应该从中长期角度评价，这有助于政策制定者长期决策。三是本研究提供了 30 年间所有模拟状态的清晰结构，为各种经济学评价提供了基础，包括成本-效果分析、成本-效用分析和成本-效益分析等，因为研究提供的树形透明结构可以将各年度成本、效果、效用和效益数据分配给各个状态[117, 166]。

人们可能会质疑这种假设，即在未实施国家基本公共卫生服务项目情况下，9 532 719 名患者中没有一个患者的血压得到控制。然而，这是一种可能存在的情境。如第 3 章所述，中国患者高血压的知晓率、治疗率和控制率仍然较低；而认知、治疗和控制的改善情况也远未令人满意。1991—2015 年，我国成人高血压控制率一直低于 20%，这意味着在这 25 年间内，超过 1.5 亿高血压患者的高血压未能得到有效控制。

还有人提出，在中国为所有高血压患者提供治疗服务，每年可防止约 800 000 起心血管疾病事件的发生[38]。本研究通过长期预测，并综合考虑避免心血管疾病和避免死亡，对此进行进一步估计。虽然本研究取得了一些进展，但依然有待进一步深入。最新数据显示，在 35 岁以上的高血压患者中，仅有不到 15% 的患者血压得到有效控制[33]。如果所有高血压患者的血压都得到控制，那么可避免的死亡人数将是当前估计的若干倍。

本章有效衔接了第 3 章和第 5 章的研究内容，将直接健康结果与经济结果联系起来。使用的方法有两个：一是使用 Gu 等[38, 39]研究的心血管疾病风险估计模型；二是用于长期健康影响估计的马尔可夫模型，该模型是卫生健康干预项目经济学评价的常用方法[42, 127]。国际上，对基层医疗卫生机构高血压患者管理的经济学评价开展得较多，例如在阿根廷[112]、荷兰[129]、越南[137]和英国[167]等的相关研究。但是，我国这方面的相关研究还较少，因此本研究在一定程度上填补了国内研究的空白。

本研究的局限性主要在于用于分析致死性和非致死性心血管疾病危险因素的数据比较陈旧（CHNS 2009），如果可以获得更新的数据，则可以更新所有结果。

总而言之，在 30 年的预测时间里，国家基本公共卫生服务项目的实施将冠心病、脑卒中和死亡的发生人数分别减少了 25 012、296 258 和 744 493 人。马尔可夫模型的结果提供了每个模拟年份中高血压、冠心病、脑卒中和死亡的人数，这些指标可应用于经济学评价。相关内容将在下一章继续讨论。

5 国家基本公共卫生服务项目高血压管理的成本、效益和投资回报——基于创新性方法的研究

5.1 介绍

基于第 3 章和第 4 章的讨论结果，本章对国家基本公共卫生服务项目的投入进行了经济学评价，基于成本-效益分析框架测算投资回报情况。

澳大利亚维多利亚大学经济战略研究中心（Victoria Institute of Strategic Economic Studies，VISES）开发了健康干预的投资回报研究模型，该模型通过专家同行评议，并在多个不同研究中得到应用。该模型最早开发用于母婴健康[45]和青少年健康[168]干预相关经济学评价。值得一提的是，该模型已应用于慢性病管理经济学评价，即心血管疾病评价[44]和精神疾病干预评价[169]。这些研究覆盖了包括中国在内的很多国家。近年来，该方法逐渐应用于更多的国家，如印度和布隆迪[170]。

上述研究均包括健康产出模型和经济学评价模型。这些结果均利用“统一健康工具”（One Health Tool，OHT）模拟健康产出。该方法基于马尔可夫模型研发，利用整合的方法来评估成本和健康效益[45-46，165]。本研究利用第 4 章介绍的马尔可夫模型，根据中国公布的数据，以及联合国和国际劳工组织发布的中国人口和劳动力数据，对 VISES 开发的经济模型进行了调整[44-45，169]。

经济学评价中需要确定分析角度，即个人、社会、企业或者保险[171-173]。国家基本公共卫生服务项目在全国范围内实施，目的是为全国居民提供同质化、均等化的服务，受益对象是全社会的个人、家庭以及各类组织。因此，本研究采用与国际同类研究一致的社会视角[137]。我们将国家基本公共卫生服务项目视为针对高血压患者人群的一项增量干预，其效益包括通过降低冠心病和脑卒中而节省的成本，健康状况增加的劳动力以及由此而提升的劳动生产效率，还有社会效益，这些效益都可以转化为相应的货币形式[173]。

5.2 概念框架

如第 2 章所述，卫生健康服务项目的经济学评价主要有 4 种类型（最小成本分析、成本-效用分析、成本-效果分析和成本-效益分析）。其中，成本-效益分析被认为是涵盖内容最广的分析，因为它可以确定一个项目的收益与成本的比值[120]。卫生项目的效益以货币单位进行度量[120]。

本研究概念框架如图 5-1 所示，主要包括两个部分。第一部分（粉色背景）包括直接和间接健康产出，以及其中的时间框架，第 4 章进行了具体讨论分析。第二部分（蓝色背景）代表由于健康结果改善带来的经济和社会效益测算框架。

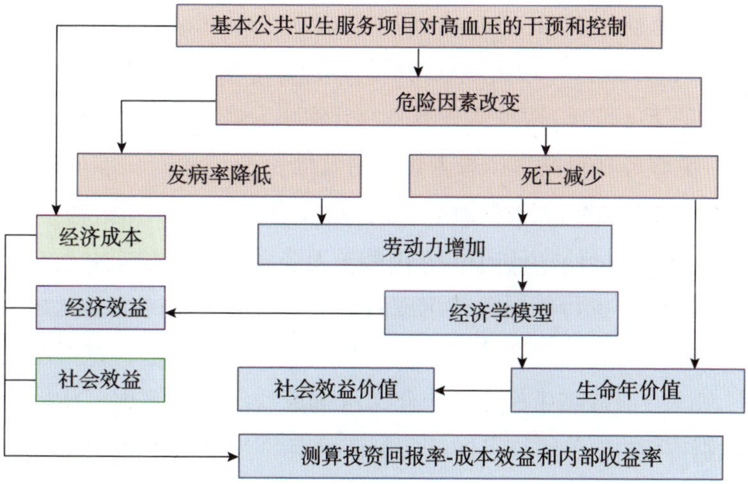

图 5-1　VISES 健康干预项目投入产出分析框架

在该框架下，经济成本是国家基本公共卫生服务项目下高血压患者健康管理的投入。然而，如第 1 章分析，由于国家基本公共卫生服务项目的实施，更多患者知晓患病状况，并获得更多、更好的治疗。对患者而言，卫生服务的利用可能增加了，因此治疗成本有可能增加。但是，另一方面，如第 4 章分析，高血压控制可能会降低冠心病和脑卒中的发病率，这又可能节省卫生服务成本。为了估算长期收益，本研究将医疗支出进行了单独分析，计算高血压控制和未控制两种情况下的医疗支出。研究采用了 WHO 的疾病成本法（cost of illness，CoI）[30]，利用国家卫生健康委卫生发展研究中心 2014 年开展的 17 个省居民健康询问调查数据进行计算[52]。

5.2.1 干预、成本和效益

5.2.1.1 干预措施与成本

本研究界定了干预的内容和范围，即 2009—2015 年国家基本公共卫生服务项目高血压患者管理。高血压患者管理内容包括 35 岁及以上成人首次到基层医疗卫生机构就诊时进行血压测量，基层医疗卫生机构对高血压患者进行定期随访、监测评估、提供血压控制治疗咨询，并在出现恶化情况时转诊至上级医院。高血压患者管理的直接健康结果是血压控制，定义为 SBP/DBP≤140/90mmHg[26]。第 3 章分析显示，2009—2015 年由于国家基本公共卫生服务项目实施超额控制的高血压患者数是 9 532 719 人。

根据 Gu 等研究的中国心血管决策模型（Cardiovascular Disease Policy Model-China model）[38] 相关参数，本研究构建了马尔可夫模型预测长期健康结果（具体见第 4 章）。两种情境下心血管疾病发病率和死亡率差异就是国家基本公共卫生服务项目高血压患者管理的效果。

5.2.1.2 构建模型估计健康结果改善的效益

劳动力人口过早死亡将会对 GDP 增长产生负面影响。如果人们带病生存可能会引起残疾，也可能导致休工或者以低劳动生产率的状态继续工作。因此，如果高血压得到控制会降低心血管疾病的发病率，那么就可以提高劳动生产参与率，进而提高生产力。老年人群健康状况的改善也可能提高劳动参与率，很多国家的相关研究已经证实了该论点[44]。因此，估算这些影响转化为劳动力和生产力、再转化为 GDP 的因素，就是经济模型构建的主要任务。为此，本研究利用 VISES 经济效益估计模型[44]，基于中国人口经济学评价指南相关数据进行深入分析[171]。

本研究将预测期限界定为2016—2045年，经济效益是这段时间干预后所降低的心血管疾病发病率和死亡率。降低死亡率产生的经济效益基于每个年龄、性别和年度的劳动力参与情况。每个年龄组增加的血压有效控制所减少死亡的人数乘以所在年龄组的劳动参与率（不同年龄和年度参数不同）就得到国家基本公共卫生服务项目高血压管理的经济效益。每个年龄组的劳动参与率都用来计算这个年龄组下一年度的劳动力。同时，该模型计算每个年龄组的平均死亡率。每个预测年度的劳动力是各年龄组预测队列中所有劳动力之和。劳动参与率是所在年龄组当年度数据，即劳动力和劳动参与率均随年龄、预测年度变化而变化。

按性别和年龄划分的劳动参与率、人口数据和死亡率均来源于国际劳工组织统计数据库[174]。GDP数据来源于世界银行发展指标数据库[175]，死亡率数据来源于联合国《世界人口展望》的预测数据[46]。

基于2009年CHNS数据库，分别计算12个年龄性别组（男性/女性、35岁、45岁、55岁、65岁、75岁和85岁以上）的高血压患者的平均年龄。本研究中的人群包括全部工作年龄人群，既包括在业人群也包括非在业（失业或者无工作）人群。根据2017年国际劳工组织数据，2016年65岁以上男性和女性的劳动参与率分别为27.6%和15.3%。因此，本研究劳动力估算的最大年龄是70岁。劳动力人口人均GDP是通过全国GDP除以劳动力人口总数计算的。

考虑到社会效益，本研究假设所节省的生命年价值的社会和经济效益可以分别计算。这种方法在以前的研究中经常使用[44-45, 169]。同样，根据这些研究中使用的参数，社会效益估算的最大年龄为80岁。

5.2.1.3 发病率降低的效益估计

本研究的疾病发病率只包括冠心病和脑卒中两种情况，对患病状态下的效益估计是基于疾病严重程度和分布计算等同于冠心病和脑卒中死亡减少而带来的经济效益。冠心病和脑卒中的慢性患病状态视为发病，而急性状态按照死亡率合并入死亡状态。最新的全球疾病负担发病率数据显示[176]，心绞痛有4种严重程度：无症状、轻度、中度和重度。轻度心绞痛为剧烈体力活动时胸痛；中度心绞痛为中等体力活动时胸痛；重度心绞痛是在轻度体力活动时就发生胸痛。重度心绞痛患者将失去劳动能力，为了便于分析，研究将其视为与死亡相同的严重程度。轻度和中度心绞痛患者被认为等同于完全健康，不包含在死亡率的效益估计中。脑卒中的死亡率分析也采用了类似的方法。慢性脑卒中的严重程度分为5级：轻度、中度、中度合并认知障碍、重度以及重度合并认知障碍[176]。后3种严重程度都将导致活动障碍（例如，吃饭穿衣困难、上床受限或者使用轮椅），或者认知能力有问题（例如，说话、思考或者记忆障碍），以及需要辅助（例如，需要在别人的帮助下吃饭、如厕或者穿衣）。本研究将轻度和中度人群视为健康人群，即完全健康。

基于严重程度的分布[48]，在项目实施和未实施两种情况下计算各年龄组每年的冠心病和脑卒中患者人数，进而估计两种状况下的经济效益，如表5-1所示。

表5-1　冠心病和脑卒中患者严重程度和分布

冠心病			脑卒中		
严重等级	分布/%	失能（残疾）权重	严重等级	分布/%	失能（残疾）权重
无症状心绞痛	30.40	0	轻度	18.60	0
轻度心绞痛	24.00	0.033	中度	42.80	0.02
中度心绞痛	12.60	0.080	中度+认知障碍	22.70	0.07
重度心绞痛	33.00	0.167	重度	11.70	0.32
			重度+认知障碍	1.60	0.55

5.2.1.4　净现值

本研究采用净现值（NPV）法估计高血压控制的经济效益和社会效益。净现值是一段时间内现金流入现值和现金流出现值之间的差额。净现值主要应用于资本预算和测算投资收益的规划项目[54]。其计算公式如下。

$$\text{NPV}=\sum_{ti=1}^{n}\frac{R_t}{(1+i)^t}$$

其中：

R_t=一个时间周期内净现金流入和流出之差；

ti=替代投资可能获得的贴现率或者回报；

t=时间周期数量，本研究采用通常做法，即以一年为一个时间周期。

研究采用了投资回报方法比较国家基本公共卫生服务项目高血压患者管

理产生的效益和成本，采用一定的贴现率计算未来预测结果。相关参数如表 5-2 所示。

表 5-2　健康产出和成本收益分析参数表

项目	单位	数值	资料来源和发表年份
增量成本	10 亿元		
估计低值		24.66	**专家咨询**
估计中等值		35.97	Jq et al.，2015；Zhao，et al.，2015
估计高值		44.38	Xiao et al.，2014
高血压控制的增量效果	患者人数	9 532 719	**第 3 章趋势分析**
2017 年人均 GDP	元	58 681	世界银行（2017）
贴现率	%	0、2、3、5	Liu et al.，2011
2013—2017 年生产率增长	N/A	N/A	世界银行（2017）
人口和死亡率	N/A	N/A	联合国经济与社会事务部，人口分部（2017）

注："N/A"表示不适用。

5.2.2　目标人群结构和估计假设

本研究围绕 9 532 719 名高血压患者展开分析，起始时间是 2016 年，分为两种情境：一种情况是这些高血压患者血压得到控制（国家基本公共卫生服务项目实施）；另一种情况是这些患者血压没有得到控制（国家基本公共卫生服务项目未实施）。假设两种情境下这些患者的年龄性别结构和分布与我国高血压患者人群一致[33]。根据联合国统计数据中的中国人口数据，对 2015—2045 年 30 年间的中国人口进行了年龄和性别预测。劳动力人口是全社会所有参与劳动和生产活动的人群，既包括在业人口，也包括失业或者非在业人口。本研究采用国际劳工组织相关预测数据，并综合考虑国家数据之间的差异，数据涵盖范围、收集和整理方法以及我国人口的其他特点。1990—2015 年的数据是估算数，而 2016—2030 年的数据是预测数。人口数据更新时间为 2017 年 7 月。2015—2050 年，按 5 岁年龄组、地区、区域和国家划分的男性和女性人口每年的死亡人数也来自联合国人口统计数据库。

有学者提出随着慢性病发病率的提高，国家的人口或者相关生产状况会受到动态影响[135]。但是，这种影响很难估计，因此动态影响在本研究中忽略不计。

5.2.3 灵敏度分析

为了解决增量成本和效益估计的不确定性问题，本研究进行了单变量敏感度分析，即，每次在控制其他变量均值或者基线水平的情况下改变一个变量。同时，为了提高数据准确性，本研究采用已有估计的最高值和最低值进行分析，包括成本和健康产出。除此以外，研究利用不同的贴现率估计成本和社会经济效益，采用的贴现率分别为0、2%、3%和5%。

5.2.4 疾病经济成本分析（CoI）

如前所述，在实施国家基本公共卫生服务项目过程中，由于增加了用于高血压控制的药物成本，医疗支出也可能增加。为了分析这可能导致的成本增加问题，本研究进行了疾病经济成本分析。

基于可获得的数据，本研究采用WHO推荐的疾病经济成本方法计算由于冠心病和脑卒中减少而降低的直接经济成本[177]。疾病直接经济成本是每一类疾病平均直接成本乘以患者人年数获得的，主要考虑疾病的就诊情况（包括自我用药、门诊和住院）。分析所使用的数据来自2014年国家卫生健康委卫生发展研究中心在全国17个省份34个基层卫生综合改革重点联系点（每个省一个城市区和一个农村县）开展的家庭健康服务询问调查。

冠心病包括心绞痛、心肌梗死和其他缺血性心脏病，脑卒中包括调查所指的脑血管疾病。直接疾病负担以年为单位计算，包括直接医疗成本和直接非医疗成本，并且细分为门诊和住院两类费用。这是根据每种疾病计算的，并考虑了每个疾病分析人群的就医概率，即本研究中的高血压、冠心病和中风[85]。非住院患者医疗支出是两周医疗费用乘以26（因为一年有52周），住院患者的费用以年为单位计算。研究假设是基于不管高血压是否控制，冠心病和脑卒中的疾病经济成本相同（即费用不同主要由于就医频率不同引起）。年度疾病经济成本是上述两类疾病的加和，具体公式如下。

直接医疗费用=（高血压患者人口 × 两周就诊率 × 人次均就诊费用 × 26+高血压患者人口 × 两周自我医疗的比例 × 平均每人两周自我医疗费用 × 26+高血压患者人口 × 住院率 × 次均住院费用）

直接非医疗费用=（高血压患者人口 × 两周就诊率 × 次均就诊非医疗费用 ×26+高血压患者人口 × 住院率 × 次均患者非医疗费用）

上述公式中每个指标的含义解释见表 5-3。

表 5-3 疾病经济负担计算指标定义

指标	定义和计算方法
两周就诊率	调查时，过去两周接受门诊服务的患者占所有高血压患者人数的比例
人次均就诊费用	高血压患者门诊就诊费用除以高血压患者人数
两周自我医疗的比例	调查时，过去两周自我医疗的患者占所有高血压患者人数的比例，主要反映患者去药店购药，自我营养治疗等措施
平均每人两周自我医疗费用	自我医疗总花费除以患者总人数
人次均就诊费用	门诊相关费用总额除以两周门诊就诊人数，主要反映交通、营养、患者照顾等费用
住院率	调查前一年内住院患者数除以调查患者总数
次均住院费用	住院费用除以住院患者总数
次均患者非医疗费用	住院患者住院相关费用总额除以住院患者总数，反映住院相关交通、营养、照护等相关费用

上述方法由 WHO 研发，并得到了广泛应用和验证。2014 年，本研究负责人与所在研究团队成员联合撰写了相关文章并发表了研究结果[52]，包括对高血压、冠心病和脑卒中疾病经济负担的分析，为本研究提供了良好基础。上述文章分析了中国 8 个典型地区慢性病患病情况和疾病经济负担。本研究采用的居民家庭健康询问调查中，共有 9 677 名高血压患者（患者自报经医疗专业人员诊断为高血压），过去一年中采取了治疗措施的患者，共计 9 166 名高血压患者、1 047 名冠心病患者和 736 名脑卒中患者[52]。

5.3 干预成本、效益和投资回报

5.3.1 国家基本公共卫生服务项目高血压管理投入

如第 2 章所述，国家基本公共卫生服务项目由政府出资在全国范围内为居民免费提供，包括高血压管理[15]。在项目实施初期，2009—2010 年项目资金仅为年人均15元。2011年增长至25元，2013年30元，2014年35元，2015年40元[178]。根据2010年第六次全国人口普查数据，中国31个省（自治区、直辖市）人口数为1 332 810 869人。据此测算，2009—2015年间，项目投资超过2 465.7亿元（约合366.4亿美元，按照人民币兑美元6.73的当时汇率）。

2009—2015年国家基本公共卫生服务项目资金用于高血压患者管理的部分就是本研究所描述的"成本"。尽管国家基本公共卫生服务项目经费总额比较容易计算，但是不同项目占用的资金差别较大。针对高血压患者管理的项目投入，不同的研究结果差异也较大。例如，2014年，世界银行的一项研究估算，约18%的项目经费被用于高血压患者管理，大约443.8亿元（或者65.9亿美元）[12]。另一项研究基于社区基本公共卫生服务工作量进行测算[179]，提出大约20.4%的资金用于慢性病患者管理，包括高血压和糖尿病患者健康管理，但是研究没有明确针对高血压患者管理的资金占比。另一项在深圳开展的研究利用相似的方法进行了估算[180]，为高血压和糖尿病患者健康管理成本估计提供了证据，研究认为高血压患者管理的费用是糖尿病的2.51倍。而世界银行[12]的研究认为高血压患者管理费用占资金总额的18%，糖尿病患者管理占7%，照此推算，高血压患者管理的费用是糖尿病的2.57倍。尽管上述两项研究得出慢性病患者管理费用占比不相同，但是两者在高血压患者管理和糖尿病患者管理费用比例方面的研究结论相似。按照2015年的研究，高血压和糖尿病患者管理费用占基本公共卫生服务经费的20.4%，而高血压费用是糖尿病费用的2.51倍，那么可以推算出高血压患者健康管理费用占基本公共卫生服务经费总额的14.59%。如果用基本公共卫生服务经费总额乘以14.59%，那么可以得出2009—2015年间用于高血压患者管理的费用为359.7亿元（约合53.4亿美元）。

尽管如此，2019年2月，本研究负责人邀请国内基本公共卫生服务相关专家进行了专题小组讨论，大家一致认为仅有10%~12%的项目经费用于高血压患者管理。因此，本研究采用10%作为最小成本估计值，即246.6亿元。综上所述，基于文献研究和专家咨询，本研究得出2009—2015年高血压患者管理费用即干预成本的3个估计值：246.6亿元、359.7亿元和443.8亿元。

5.3.2 发病和死亡人数减少的估算

为了进行效益估计，研究需将发病和死亡减少情况进行货币化转化。实施国家基本公共卫生服务项目和未实施项目两种情况下死亡人数差值作为项目干预效果之一。在基本公共卫生服务项目实施的情况下，10 年、20 年和 30 年三种情况下的高血压患者死亡人数分别为 1 519 570 人、3 577 605 人和 5 857 687 人；而如果没有实施基本公共卫生服务项目，则上述数据将分别为 1 809 214 人、4 136 230 人和 6 602 179 人（表 5-4）；减少死亡人数分别为 289 644 人、558 625 人和 744 493 人。每个预测年度的死亡人数通过马尔可夫模型计算，同时展示了预测各年度的年份、患者年龄等情况。具体见附表 C3-1 和 C3-2。

表 5-4　两种情况下不同预测周期死亡人数　　单位：人

预测周期	实施国家基本公共卫生服务项目	未实施国家基本公共卫生服务项目	减少死亡人数
10 年	1 519 570	1 809 214	289 644
20 年	3 577 605	4 136 230	558 625
30 年	5 857 687	6 602 179	744 493

本研究只考虑冠心病和脑卒中发病和死亡人数减少的情况。在实施和未实施国家基本公共卫生服务项目两种情况下减少的发病人数被认为是项目实施的另一个效果。通过项目实施，从 2016 年起第 10 年、20 年和 30 年减少的冠心病患者人数分别为 65 093 人、83 165 人和 69 293 人，减少的脑卒中人数分别为 386 888 人、590 021 人和 562 666 人，具体见表 5-5。

表 5-5　实施国家基本公共卫生服务项目减少的冠心病和脑卒中人数预测

单位：人

预测周期	冠心病	脑卒中
10 年	65 093	386 888
20 年	83 165	590 021
30 年	69 293	562 666

马尔可夫模型还分析了每个预测年度的冠心病或脑卒中患者情况，包括年度和年龄分布，并通过对各年度和年龄组患者进行 GDP 或生产力赋值得出经济和社会效益。具体见附表 C4-1~C4-4。

本研究通过 VISES 经济学评价模型测算由于死亡和发病减少带来的经济效益。该模型利用每名劳动者平均生产力估算经济效益。根据我国历史数据预测生产力增长情况，研究通过将每个性别年龄组患者乘以人均 0.5 倍 GDP 计算社会效益。

5.3.3 投资回报率和效益成本比

本研究采用标准经济学模型，通过将上述每年度的数据进行加和计算经济和社会效益，分别按照 0、2%、3% 和 5% 的贴现率计算由于死亡和发病减少带来的 GDP 增加的情况。在上述 4 个贴现率之下，预测的经济效益净现值将分别为 3 305.23（95%*CI*：876.74，5 733.72）、2 107.45（95%*CI*：559.02，3 655.88）、1 698.57（95%*CI*：450.56，2 946.58）和 1 123.10（95%*CI*：297.91，1 948.29）亿元。如果包含社会效益，按照上述 4 个贴现率，总的效益将分别为 6 050.47（95%*CI*：1 604.94，10 496.00）、3 479.56（95%*CI*：922.98，6 036.14）、2 672.97（95%*CI*：709.03，4 636.91）和 1 616.98（95%*CI*：428.92，2 805.04）亿元。在不同国家基本公共卫生服务项目高血压患者管理成本估计值之下，研究计算了效益成本比和内部收益率。如果按照高血压患者管理费用占国家基本公共卫生服务投入的 14.59% 计算，分别按照 0、2%、3% 和 5% 贴现率，效益成本比将分别为 8.9（95%*CI*：2.36，15.44）、6.6（95%*CI*：1.75，11.45）、6.0（95%*CI*：1.59，10.41）和 4.9（95%*CI*：1.30，8.50）；如果包含社会效益，那么效益成本比将分别为 25.1（95%*CI*：6.66，43.54）、17.6（95%*CI*：4.67，30.53）、15.4（95%*CI*：4.08，26.72）和 11.9（95%*CI*：3.16，20.64）。如果仅考虑经济收益，内部收益率为 14.6%（95%*CI*：3.87%，25.33%）；如果包括社会效益，内部收益率则是 20.7%（95%*CI*：6.45%，42.15%）。具体见表 5-6 和表 5-7。

本研究还进行了年龄别分析，结果显示按照分年龄组计算效益成本比和内部收益率将低于全年龄组计算结果。如果利用 2012—2015 年全国高血压调查数据，按照以 3% 贴现率，且高血压患者管理费用占国家基本公共卫生服务项目投入比例为 14.59% 来计算，年龄别分析效益成本比将为 5.9。如果包含社会效益，效益成本比将为 15.1。内部收益率分别为 14.7% 和 20.4%。具体见附件 D。

5.3.4 疾病经济负担分析

本研究利用疾病成本法（WHO-CoI）分析了高血压、冠心病和脑卒中的疾病经济负担。基于 CNHDRC 调查数据中 9 166 名高血压患者、1 047 名冠

表 5-6　不同贴现率下投资回报和成本

单位：亿元

贴现率	投资回报（95%*CI*）		成本（95%*CI*）		
	经济效益净现值	社会效益净现值	10%NBPHS 经费	14.59%NBPHS 经费	18%NBPHS 经费
0	3 305.23（876.74，5 733.72）	6 050.47（1 604.94，10 496.00）	255.26	395.40	443.83
2%	2 107.45（559.02，3 655.88）	3 479.56（922.98，6 036.14）	217.27	336.54	377.20
3%	1 698.57（450.56，2 946.58）	2 672.97（709.03，4 636.91）	194.99	302.04	338.01
5%	1 123.10（297.91，194 829）	1 616.98（42 892，280 504）	158.37	245.32	273.88

表 5-7　不同成本下不同贴现率效益成本比和内部收益率

单位：%（95%*CI*）

成本	不同贴现率效益成本比				内部收益率（95%*CI*）/%
	0（95%*CI*）	2%（95%*CI*）	3%（95%*CI*）	5%（95%*CI*）	
18% 基本公共卫生服务经费作为成本					
GDP-死亡减少/成本	7.2（1.91，12.49）	5.4（1.43，9.37）	4.8（1.27，8.33）	3.9（1.03，6.77）	12.9（3.42，22.38）
GDP-死亡减少加社会效益/成本	20.4（5.41，35.39）	14.3（3.79，24.81）	12.5（3.32，21.68）	9.6（2.55，16.65）	18.8（4.99，32.61）
14.59% 基本公共卫生服务经费作为成本					
GDP-死亡减少/成本	8.9（2.36，15.44）	6.6（1.75，11.45）	6.0（1.59，10.41）	4.9（1.30，8.50）	14.6（3.87，25.33）
GDP-死亡减少加社会效益/成本	25.1（6.66，43.54）	17.6（4.67，30.53）	15.4（4.08，26.72）	11.9（3.16，20.64）	20.7（5.49，35.91）
10% 基本公共卫生服务经费作为成本					
GDP-死亡减少/成本	12.9（3.42，22.38）	9.7（2.57，16.83）	8.7（2.31，15.09）	7.1（1.88，12.32）	17.9（4.75，31.05）
GDP-死亡减少加社会效益/成本	36.7（9.73，63.67）	25.7（6.82，44.58）	22.4（5.94，38.86）	17.3（4.59，30.01）	24.3（6.45，42.15）

心病患者和736名脑卒中患者，分析了患者两周就诊和一年内住院状况。该结果用于分析高血压患者人群的医疗支出，具体见表5-8。

表5-8 2014年CNHDRC调查的高血压患者一年内花费

高血压患者情况	患者数/人	两周就诊花费/元	一年内住院花费/元
高血压控制	7 054	392 167	1 856 960
高血压未控制	2 112	87 945	680 683
冠心病	1 047	118 981	4 457 273
脑卒中	736	113 839	6 338 632

研究计算了血压控制和未控制两组的高血压、冠心病和脑卒中的直接疾病负担，得到三类疾病的年度直接经济负担。血压控制组高血压患者的直接疾病经济负担高于血压未控制组。研究假设两组患者冠心病和脑卒中的年度疾病经济负担没有差别，基于2014年国家卫生健康委卫生发展研究中心的调查，据测算血压控制高血压患者、血压未控制高血压患者、冠心病和脑卒中患者年度直接经济负担分别为1 708.72元，1 404.95元，7 211.82元和12 633.76元。研究通过马尔可夫模型，预测了从2016年开始未来30年间高血压、高血压合并冠心病、高血压合并脑卒中等疾病的发生概率。将上述结果每人年的数据进行加和，结果表明在未实施基本公共卫生服务项目组冠心病和脑卒中患者人数远远多于实施基本公共卫生服务项目组，见表5-9。

通过将高血压、冠心病和脑卒中每人年的疾病经济负担与30年内两组中各类患者人年数相乘，研究得出30年预测期内两组的疾病经济负担。对高血压控制组而言，在不考虑贴现率的情况下，预测的10年、20年和30年高血压、冠心病和脑卒中三类疾病的经济负担分别为2 621.41亿、5 219.13亿和7 380.26亿元；而对高血压未控制组，同样不考虑贴现率，预测的10年、20年和30年高血压、冠心病和脑卒中三类疾病的疾病经济负担分别为2 721.98亿、5 761.72亿和8 472.88亿元。在第30年末，两组疾病经济负担差值为1 114.16亿元。按照高血压患者管理投入359.7亿元计算（14.59%的基本公共卫生服务项目经费），高血压患者管理节省的疾病经济负担是项目投入的3.1倍。本研究疾病经济负担仅仅用来作为分析参考，效益成本比和内部收益率等经济学分析并未纳入疾病经济负担的分析结果，因此没有计算疾病经济负担的95%*CI*。具体结果见表5-10。

表 5-9 每类疾病预测期末（第 30 年）合并患者人年数 单位：人

组别	实施国家基本公共卫生服务项目（高血压控制组）			未实施国家基本公共卫生服务项目（高血压未控制组）		
	高血压	冠心病	脑卒中	高血压	冠心病	脑卒中
男性/岁						
35~44	15 774 791	385 036	494 318	15 236 919	563 014	763 971
45~54	28 925 971	1 042 323	2 618 662	26 704 540	1 402 874	4 050 810
55~64	26 811 417	2 324 601	6 108 210	22 235 813	2 855 632	8 843 384
65~74	11 093 710	1 542 623	3 806 906	8 217 278	1 862 944	5 172 743
75~84	2 829 335	526 010	975 734	1 633 406	674 884	1 385 107
85+	267 002	34 976	69 733	220 257	41 678	85 155
女性/岁						
35~44	9 528 274	89 048	294 487	9 265 155	106 115	497 553
45~54	27 035 525	712 319	2 560 542	25 036 257	810 456	4 103 754
55~64	30 016 795	2 139 024	6 489 494	25 131 870	2 354 465	9 785 280
65~74	14 108 563	1 623 837	4 397 236	10 797 864	1 771 355	6 136 027
75~84	4 322 289	775 930	1 325 807	2 677 173	875 451	2 001 330
85+	569 880	71 819	127 464	442 573	85 147	174 885

注：基于参数可得性和我国人均预期寿命，75~84 岁年龄组的预测年限为 20 年，85 岁及以上年龄组预测年限为 10 年。

表 5-10 两组患者预测期内疾病经济负担 单位：亿元

预测周期	实施国家基本公共卫生服务项目的情况	未实施国家基本公共卫生服务项目的情况	节省的疾病经济负担
10 年	2 621.41	271.98	100.57
20 年	5 219.13	5 761.72	564.13
30 年	7 380.26	8 472.88	1 114.16

5.4 讨论

高血压患者管理的潜在健康和经济效益非常高。据计算，国家基本公共卫生服务项目的干预措施有可能将在未来 30 年减少 74.4 万人死亡。除了健康收益，此项目将产生广泛的经济收益。按照 0、2%、3% 和 5% 的贴现率，按照净现值预测未来 30 年经济效益将分别达到 3 305.23 亿、2 107.45 亿、1 698.57 亿和 1 123.10 亿元；如果考虑社会效益，那么这些收益将达 6 050.47 亿、3 479.56 亿、2 672.97 亿和 1 616.98 亿元。根据高血压患者管理投入的不同估计值，研究分析了效益成本比和内部收益率。按照高血压患者管理投入占国家基本公共卫生服务项目经费的 14.59% 计算，取 3% 的贴现率，效益成本比为 6.0，如果考虑社会效益，则按相同贴现率计算的效益成本比将为 15.4。如果仅考虑经济效益，高血压患者管理的内部收益率为 14.6%，如果加上社会效益，内部收益率将达 20.7%。这些结果高于近期其他慢性病干预投资的结果，例如相似的关于慢性病的投入产出分析显示只考虑经济效益的效益成本比为 5.6，考虑社会效益则为 10.9[44]。这些结果表明，国家基本公共卫生服务项目下由基层医疗服务体系提供的高血压患者健康管理具有较高的投资回报率。

为了解决这种投资可能增加高血压治疗成本的质疑，本研究还计算了高血压、冠心病和脑卒中的直接疾病负担。结果表明，如果不考虑贴现率，高血压患者健康管理将节省 1 114.16 亿元。按照国家基本公共卫生服务项目对高血压患者健康管理投入 359.7 亿元计算（14.59% 的项目经费），节省的直接经济负担是高血压患者管理的 3.1 倍。

本研究分析结果显示社会效益比经济效益还高。主要原因是年轻患者的健康产出低于老年患者人群，如第 3 章讨论，老年群体高血压管理效果更好。经济评估模型显示，年轻人的劳动参与率和生产力远远高于老年患者。如果针对年轻患者采取进一步措施，管理年轻的高血压患者，那么将产生更高的经济效益。

基于前期研究，本章讨论了高血压健康管理经济学评价方法的发展。利用经过充分验证和校准的流行病学参数，本研究构建了以心血管疾病发病和死亡为结果的马尔可夫健康产出模型[38-39]。基于 VISES 经济学评价模型[44-45, 168-169]，开展了经济效益和社会效益分析。总的来说，本研究对我国基层高血压患者管理的经济学评价方法和实践具有一定贡献。

本研究采用的经济学评价模型已经广泛应用于心理健康[169]、心血管疾病[44]、妇幼健康和青少年健康[45, 168]干预等领域。本研究针对我国基层高血压患者健康管理，优化构建的经济学评价模型可能也适用于我国其他健康管理项目或者其他发展中国家。

本研究的分析相对保守，以下几个方面的效益可能被低估。

（1）在马尔可夫模型中，研究只考虑了冠心病和脑卒中，没有考虑其他高血压并发症。例如，多项研究表明肾病是高血压发展到后期的一个较普遍问题[82]。尽管如此，由于高血压肾病的相关流行病学参数不可获得，因此本研究未将肾病纳入分析。

（2）本研究主要基于劳动参与率数据可得性和已有研究，将经济效益分析的年龄界定为70岁及以下[44-45]。但是，世界银行的一项近期研究指出，没有证据表明人们到达一定年龄就肯定不能再产生经济价值，老年人也是家庭生活、社区志愿者和调动其他社会活动的组成部分[181]。随着全球老龄化加剧，我们需要采取更多的措施挖掘和释放老年人的生产力[182]。因此，关于劳动力的估计也偏于保守。

（3）本研究将一个生命年的社会价值赋值为人均0.5倍GDP，这也是相当保守的。文献分析显示，一个生命年的社会价值约为2~4倍GDP[45]。根据已发表的慢性病研究报告，为了区分经济效益和社会效益，本研究将70~80岁人群的一个生命年按照人均0.5倍GDP[44]。尽管如此，随着中国老龄化的加剧，健康预期寿命将进一步延长[170]，更多的人将健康活到80岁以上，意味着将产生更多社会效益。

局限性分析：本研究只是针对高血压患者管理成本和效益的初步分析，不同的研究假设将产生不同的结果。尽管如此，预计到2045年，高血压患者管理的经济效益将是投入的5倍以上。因此，不管研究假设和相关参数如何变化，此类项目的经济效益和社会效益均非常高。

5.5 小结

本研究显示，国家基本公共卫生服务项目中高血压患者管理的潜在健康和经济效益均较高。按照3%的贴现率，如果高血压患者管理的投入占国家基本公共卫生服务项目经费的14.59%，仅考虑经济效益则效益成本比是6.0；如果考虑社会效益，则效益成本比将达15.3。本研究还形成了适合我国基层高血压患者健康管理的经济学评价模型。研究还发现，如果对年轻高血压患者进一步投入，其劳动参与率和生产率将大大提升，进而带来更多经济效益。

6

全书讨论和结论

6.1 整体概述

本研究从增加血压控制患者人数、降低心血管疾病发病率和死亡率以及产生的经济和社会效益等方面，估算了 2009 年至 2015 年国家基本公共卫生服务项目对中国高血压患者的影响。

6.1.1 国家基本公共卫生服务项目下高血压控制

根据 2009 年《中共中央 国务院关于深化医药卫生体制改革的意见》内容分析[183]，2009—2015 年期间，国家基本公共卫生服务项目是中国政府在基层高血压患者健康管理中资金规模最大的投入项目[8, 12, 136]。将该项目看作针对基层医疗卫生服务机构实施高血压患者管理的增量投入，研究尝试分析项目实施之后血压得到有效控制的患者数量的变化。为此，我们建立了 1991—2009 年间的小样本时间序列模型，目的是分析 2009 年之前高血压控制率的变化趋势。

为了获得 2009 年前的全国代表性数据，研究进行了全面的文献回顾，最终选择以 CHNS 数据为主要来源、各类出版物的发表数据为辅助的非连续时间序列数据，并使用拉格朗日插值多项式补齐了 1991—2009 年各年度的高血压控制率数据（详见第 3 章）。基于 1991—2009 年的数据并使用时间序列预测模型，研究预测 2015 年的高血压控制率为 10.46% [95%*CI*（7.33%，13.59%）]。2012—2015 年中国高血压调查（China hypertension survey，CHS）数据显示，2015 年高血压的实际控制率为 14.72%，明显高于预测控制率。因此，国家基本公共卫生服务项目实施后的增量效果为血压控制率增加了 4.26 个百分点。依据 2010 年第六次全国人口普查的人口数据测算，有 9 532 719 名高血压患者的血压得到了有效控制（低于 140/90mmHg）。

此外，本研究对 1991—2015 年期间的人群高血压知晓率、治疗率和控制率进行了年龄别趋势分析。结果显示，65~74 岁年龄组高血压的知晓率和治疗率最高，55~64 岁年龄组的控制率最高。该结果表明，55 岁以上年龄组人群高血压管理效果最佳，而较年轻组患者的管理状态有待改进。进一步分析表明，知晓率不高是年轻高血压患者管理不理想的原因。

尽管研究受一些不确定因素影响，但是研究提供了一种估计我国大型高血压患者管理项目效果的系统分析框架和方法。同时，研究提出的年轻高血压患者管理不佳的问题，为下一阶段国家基本公共卫生服务项目的工作重点提供了决策依据。

6.1.2 长期健康结果估计

根据增加的高血压患者控制人数，我们设置了实施和未实施国家基本公共卫生服务项目两种情境下的长期健康影响，即在实施国家基本公共卫生服务项目情境中，9 532 719 名高血压患者的血压得到有效控制；在未实施项目的情境中，9 532 719 名高血压患者的血压将无法得到有效控制。

利用 2009 年 CHNS 中的高血压患者数据作为代表性数据，研究对两种情境下心血管疾病发病进行多因素风险分析[51，87]。结果发现，在考虑血压水平、糖尿病、血胆固醇、吸烟和 BMI 等因素的情况下，两组心血管疾病最主要的危险因素是血压水平。

为了进行长期预测，论文按照中国心血管疾病决策模型形成了本研究的马尔可夫模型，并进行了数据校准。对于实施国家基本公共卫生服务项目的情境，疾病状态转移参数引用 Gu 等[38] 2015 年发表的相关研究数据；对于未实施项目的情境，疾病状态转移参数根据血压水平对两种情境下每个年龄性别组的心血管疾病风险比进行加权所得[38，113]。

分析两种情境下性别年龄别预测死亡人数，研究发现，如果项目没有实施，心血管疾病的发病和死亡人数将高得多。在预测的30年间，将分别有25 012名、296 258名和744 493名高血压患者免于冠心病、脑卒中和死亡。此外，马尔可夫模型还提供了预测期内每年的高血压患者、冠心病、脑卒中、心血管疾病相关死亡和其他原因死亡的人数。

6.1.3 国家基本公共卫生服务的成本、效益和回报分析

从2009—2015年，国家基本公共卫生服务项目的总投入超过了2 465.7亿元（约366.4亿美元，按1美元兑6.73元人民币的汇率计算）。据估计，用于高血压的管理的经费约占基本公共卫生服务项目总投入的10%~18%（进一步分析采用了3个估计值，即10.0%、14.59%和18.0%）[12，179，180，184]。按照高血压患者管理经费占项目总投入的0%、14.59%和18.00%进行估算，研究得出3个2009—2015年国家基本公共卫生服务项目高血压患者健康管理的投入成本估计值，分别为246.6亿、359.7亿和443.8亿元。

本研究还从社会学的角度进行经济学评估，使用效益成本比指标进行分析。根据VISES提出的健康干预措施经济学评价创新方法[44-45]，研究根据患者死亡减少和发病率降低所带来的劳动参与率提高、GDP增长来估计高血压控制的经济和社会效益，经济效益根据各年龄人群劳动参与率的提高来估计，年龄范围是18~70岁。社会效益估计值为当年人均GDP的一半，年龄范围截至80岁。

在0、2%、3%和5%的贴现率下，预测的经济效益净现值分别为3 305.23亿、2 107.45亿、1 698.57亿和1 123.10亿元；如果加上社会效益，总效益分别为6 050.47亿、3 479.56亿、2 672.97亿和1 616.98亿元。研究还根据高血压管理成本的不同估计值，计算了效益成本比和内部收益率。按照高血压患者健康管理经费占国家基本公共卫生服务项目资金的14.59%测算，采用3%和5%的贴现率，效益成本比高达6.0和4.9；如果包括社会效益，采用相同的贴现率下，效益成本比将达到15.4和11.9；如果只考虑经济效益，内部收益率为14.6%；加考虑社会效益，则内部收益率为20.7%。近期一项关于慢性病防治干预效果研究显示，此类项目的效益成本比为5.6，考虑社会收益则为10.9[44]。与上面的研究相比，国家基本公共卫生服务项目高血压患者管理能够获得更高的投资回报率。

为了分析国家基本公共卫生服务项目是否会增加高血压患者的治疗成本，研究根据相关研究成果[48, 85]和现有数据[52]分析了两种情境下高血压、冠心病和脑卒中的直接疾病负担。结果显示，在不考虑贴现率的情况下，在预测期内项目的实施将节省928.41亿元。按照高血压患者管理经费359.7亿元计算（占国家基本公共卫生服务项目总投入的14.90%），高血压患者管理节省的费用是投入的2.58倍。

6.2 理论和实践价值

本研究构建了国家基本公共卫生服务项目高血压患者健康管理的经济效益评价框架，得到了重要的发现，对政策制定具有较好的启示。

6.2.1 国家基本公共卫生服务高血压患者管理具有较好的投资回报

本研究对国家基本公共卫生服务项目下高血压控制效果进行了评价。结果表明，项目对高血压患者的干预，可以有效改善知晓率、治疗率和控制率，显著降低心血管疾病发病率和死亡率，进而带来社会和经济效益。

与未实施项目情境相比，2009—2015年间，国家基本公共卫生服务项目的实施使得血压得到有效控制的高血压患者增加了9 532 719名。以此为基础，研究预测2016—2045年间将避免744 493名高血压患者死亡。按照3.0%的贴现率计算效益净现值，1元的投入可以产生6.0~15.4元的经济和社会效益。另一项研究（本研究参考了其相关经济指标）显示，我国妇幼保健项目（降消项目）的效益成本比为3.8[45]，项目实施时间是2005—2006年，目的是提高住院分娩人数以降低产妇死亡率。Stenberg等[45]的研究验证了其他研究的结论，包括2012—2015中国高血压调查的研究结果[33]，即高血压水平的改善部分原因是卫生改革和社区高血压管理项目的实施。

本研究分析显示，国家基本公共卫生服务项目具有较高的效益成本比，表明我国基层医疗卫生机构开展慢性病患者管理具有良好效果和效益的投入。同时，此类慢性病患者健康管理可以有效应对心血管疾病的挑战。因此，建议政府进一步增加此类项目的财政投入。

6.2.2 实现政策目标的可靠路径

最新统计数据显示，截至 2017 年底，全国基层医疗卫生机构管理的高血压患者人数已达 1.01 亿人。2012—2015 年中国高血压调查显示，2015 年 35 岁以上的高血压患者为 246 479 307 人。粗略推算，约 41% 的 35 岁以上高血压患者有一定知晓水平，其中 88% 以上的患者可能已经纳入项目管理。然而，这些数据也表明，我国仍有超过一半的高血压患者尚未意识到患病情况，且仍未被纳入管理。

多项研究对国家和地区层面的高血压患者患病率、知晓率、治疗率和控制率进行了研究。例如，Li 等[32]对我国 31 个省（自治区、直辖市）2003—2012 年的研究进行了系统综述，研究发现 2012 年之前有 48 项研究提供了患病率数据，30 项研究提供了知晓率、治疗率和控制率数据。Li 等[32]也发现，20~79 岁高血压患者的知晓率、治疗率和控制率分别为 44.6%、35.2% 和 11.2%。

2017 年 10 月发表在《柳叶刀》上的一项最大样本量方便抽样研究显示，35~75 岁的高血压成年人的知晓率、治疗率和控制率分别为 36.0%、22.9% 和 5.7%[79]。虽然该研究的方便抽样方法影响样本的代表性，但其结果依然揭示了我国高血压患者管理效果不尽如人意。2012—2015 年中国高血压调查结果表明，18 岁以上成年人的高血压患病率、知晓率、治疗率和控制率分别为 23.2%、46.9%、40.7% 和 15.3%[33]。2009 年以后，虽然我国高血压的知晓率、治疗率和控制率有所提高，但与国际水平相比仍有差距[31-32]。国际比较显示，我国高血压管理效果依然存在较大差距。尽管高血压患者健康管理的目的是全面提高知晓率、治疗率和控制率，但从全国层面看三者的水平仍较低[33，79，148，185]。这些分析具有重要的政策指导意义，具体如下。

首先，建议进一步增加国家基本公共卫生服务项目投入，加强高血压患者健康管理。该结论主要基于高血压患者健康管理的成本-效益分析提出。此外，作者和研究团队的研究也证实，高血压患者健康管理是高血压控制的独立因素，即扣除药物依从性后依然具有正向影响[16]。

其次，需要进一步加强我国基层医疗卫生服务体系建设，特别是人力资源和信息系统的能力建设[186]。尽管所有政策措施都很重要，但是有几项措施必须优先考虑，同时必须找出高血压患者管理效果不佳的根本原因。其中之一是“基层医疗卫生服务体系依然薄弱”，具体包括投入不足、缺乏高质量的工作人员以及医疗服务能力不足[12, 66, 75]。

多项研究强调基层医疗卫生服务体系缺乏高质量人才是影响服务能力的重要因素[12, 66]。根据笔者的经验，高质量人力缺乏的根本原因有两个方面。一是基层医疗卫生机构人才队伍支持性政策措施有待进一步完善。2009 年，国家基本公共卫生服务项目开始在全国范围内由基层医疗卫生机构实施。这些服务项目有的在 2009 年之前已经实施，例如疫苗接种和传染病报告；有些是新增项目，如高血压、糖尿病患者健康管理以及老年人健康管理等。然而，基层医疗卫生机构的卫生人员“编制”是根据 2009 年以前的服务数量和功能来确定的[187]。例如，社区卫生服务机构的人员配置标准是在 2006 年发布的，规定了医疗卫生服务功能，明确社区卫生服务机构的人员配置标准为每万服务人口配置 7~8 名社区卫生工作人员[21, 187]。在农村地区，2011 年修订乡镇卫生院人员配置标准，即每 1 000 人口配置 1 名编制人员，并要求每 5 年对编制进行重新核定[22, 187]。农村乡镇卫生院编制标准较高，但是问题在于农村很难招到合格的卫生专业技术人员[12]。同时，由于基层医疗卫生机构的工资普遍低于综合医院，再加上以绩效为导向的薪酬管理体系尚不完善，导致问题更为突出[188]。因此，基层很难吸引临床和公共卫生专业大学毕业生，也很难留住合格的卫生专业技术人才[12]。

慢性病管理需要完善的信息系统收集准确数据、实施有效绩效评估。2017 年，笔者发表在《中国卫生经济》杂志上的一篇文章，以英国质量与成果框架为范例，阐述了完善信息系统对我国基层医疗卫生机构的重要性[189]。

还有一些研究认为，药物可及性和可得性不足也是影响高血压管理效果的重要原因，虽然普通抗高血压药物价格较低，但目前的治疗方法仍然效果不佳[139, 151]。

最近两项研究分析了 12 个高收入国家的高血压知晓率、治疗率和控制率趋势[190]和 44 个中低收入国家的高血压管理状况[63]。这些研究显示，高收入国家的高血压管理效果好于低收入国家。对低收入国家高血压管理效果分析显示，人均 GDP 是高血压控制的关键因素。但是某些中低收入国家高血压控制效果也较好，如拉丁美洲和加勒比地区的国家[62]。中国也属于中低收入国家，因此需要向类似国家学习，改善高血压管理的效果。

另一个问题是我国地区差异明显。已有研究评估了我国不同地区国家基本公共卫生服务项目的高血压控制效果，如针对北京[18]、上海和深圳[191]、甘肃和浙江[65]的相关研究。这些研究显示，国家基本公共卫生服务项目效果存在较显著的地区差异。为了深入分析，笔者利用居民健康询问调查数据（见第5章）进行了全国范围内的区域分析，该研究使用回归分析来估计国家基本公共卫生服务项目提供的管理对高血压控制的影响，以调整其他决定因素的作用[52]。上述研究发现，高血压患者管理效果和地理区域之间存在较强的交互作用。进一步分析表明，基层医疗卫生机构信息化是造成各地区差异的主要因素。

6.2.3 加强对年轻患者的高血压管理

本研究还发现老年高血压患者的管理效果好于年轻患者，年轻患者的疾病管理状况有待改善，与相关研究结果一致[65, 148]。

本研究通过分析性别年龄别高血压患病率、知晓率、治疗率和控制率的发展趋势分析，建立了不同年份研究数据之间的联系。研究发现，基本公共卫生服务项目重点关注老年人，与相关研究结论一致[8]。老年人健康管理效果较好的另一个原因是，国家基本公共卫生服务项目中有多项服务均关注老年人健康管理，包括健康档案和健康教育等。这些项目对高血压有效控制形成叠加效应。然而，深入分析表明，年轻患者的治疗控制率比老年患者要好一些。例如，35~44岁、45~54岁、55~64岁、65~74岁和75岁以上年龄组的患者治疗控制率分别为40.4%、40.0%、38.7%、34.8%和32.6%。这表明，知晓率低是导致年轻高血压患者管理不佳的主要原因。

如第5章所述，实施国家基本公共卫生服务项目的社会效益大于经济效益。其原因之一是项目实施中年轻患者的管理效果不如老年群体。经济学评价模型显示，年轻人的劳动参与率和生产力远高于老年人，而老年人群的收益则主要是社会效益。如果对年轻高血压患者采取更多有效措施，减少更多的过早死亡，经济效益将呈几何级数增加。

6.2.4 循证决策将得到强化

本研究为评估国家和地区层面的卫生健康干预项目投资回报提供了政策工具和分析框架，该方法还可以应用到卫生健康其他领域和项目中。我国已经建立了国家基本公共卫生服务项目的稳定投入机制，每年以人均5元的水平稳步增加。因此，亟须为政策制定者提供可靠的循证依据为增加投入采取进一步的政策措施提供支持。此外，应建立国家基本公共卫生服务项目的动态调整机制。因此，本研究健康影响评价及经济学评价方法为财政投入和社会影响分析提供了良好借鉴。

6.3 研究先进性与局限性分析

6.3.1 研究建立了长期健康结果的综合评价模型

首先，本研究基于数据可得性和评价可行性，建立了对基层医疗卫生机构开展高血压患者健康管理的评价模型。根据高血压患病率、知晓率、治疗率和控制率（包括心血管疾病并发症）等数据，动态评价我国高血压患者健康管理的短期和长期效果。

本研究建立的小样本时间序列模型，在排除社会经济混杂因素影响的前提下，分析国家基本公共卫生服务项目高血压患者健康管理效果。比较而言，以往研究评价干预措施的影响需要采用病例对照或干预对照等成本较高的研究或者设计[167, 192]。在数据有限的条件下，该研究方法使得有效评价卫生健康项目成为可能。

通过构建疾病临床流行病学进展框架和马尔可夫模型，研究还建立了心血管疾病长期健康结果的预测模型。基于 2009 年 CHNS 数据，本研究纳入影响心血管疾病的多项危险因素，包括生物标志物信息等。通过对 2012—2015 年中国高血压调查数据[139]和国家卫生健康委发布的高血压患者管理统计数据的相关分析，本研究按照性别年龄结构分析了高血压患者分布，提升了研究数据的代表性，改善了结果的可靠性。研究团队广泛搜索文献，结果显示本研究是首个针对国家基本公共卫生服务项目高血压患者管理的综合系统经济学评价。

6.3.2 构建了创新型经济学评价模型

许多国家均对高血压患者管理和干预措施进行了经济评价。越南的一项研究使用成本效益框架，从经济学角度对高血压筛查项目的心血管疾病预防效果进行了评估[136]。另一项希腊的研究量化了高血压控制的经济效益，结论是通过控制血压可以有效预防心血管事件并降低发病率，从而节约大量成本[128]。然而，我国依然较缺乏此类证据。本研究还克服了传统经济学评价方法中效益估计的情境（病例对照或干预对照）依赖缺陷[121]。

在以往研究的基础上，我们建立了高血压控制的综合性经济评价框架。我国学者前期的相关研究（2015 年，2008 年）提供了经过校正的流行病学参数，用于估计心血管疾病死亡率和发病率的健康结果[38, 39]。基于 VISES 经济方法[44-45]，本研究开发并验证了社会和效益估计方法学框架。如第 2 章文献综述，近期关于高血压的经济学评价多从医疗角度进行[38, 42]。从这个意义上说，本研究为我国基层医疗卫生机构高血压患者管理的经济评价增加了研究依据。

本研究分析了高血压患者管理的经济和社会效益，不仅包括避免的疾病费用损失和增加的人力资本，还包括个人的社会价值，即每一个生命年相当于 0.5 倍的人均 GDP[44-45]，分析较为系统综合。

6.3.3 本研究的优势

尽管研究模型和估计基于多项假设，但通过采用多因素分析模型对最新流行病学数据和国家代表性数据改善了精确性[38-39]，研究的准确性得到有效提升。因此，研究基于循证证据应用全球流行病学参数，设置了经济学评价的情境。正如方法学部分所强调的，本研究与其他相关研究模型构建方法一致[38, 46, 121]，充分利用了目前国内可用的数据。此外，本研究不仅仅分析死亡减少带来的经济效益，而且确定和估计慢性病发病率降低所带来的经济效益。这项方法同样适用于糖尿病、重型精神疾病甚至是癌症筛查等干预项目。

为了提高研究的准确性，本研究应用了多项国家级具有代表性的系列数据。通过文献综述，研究提取了 1991—2018 年的高血压患病率、知晓率、治疗率和控制率数据，为时间序列分析提供了良好基础。研究基于 2009 年 CHNS 数据库，抽取高血压患者的相关生物标志物信息，分析高血压控制和未控制两种情况下的心血管疾病风险。在马尔可夫模型中，研究采用了近期中国心血管疾病研究经过校准的心血管疾病风险参数[193]。为了提高本研究性别年龄别数据的代表性，研究使用 2012—2015 年中国高血压调查数据和 2010 年人口普查数据改善人口年龄性别分析的代表性。

6.3.4 研究的局限性分析

6.3.4.1 数据可得性

本研究建立了估计卫生健康项目短期和长期健康影响以及经济效益的框

架和路径。由于研究使用了来源于不同调查的数据，所以在计算的精确性方面存在一定的局限性。与大多数经济学评价模型一样，在没有数据的情况下只能采用某种假设。尽管研究对过去 30 年的数据进行了文献综述，但 CHNS 数据依然是本研究数据分析的主要来源。在 2019 年 2 月召开的一次专家研讨会上，有专家指出考虑到调查点的选择和样本量，CHNS 数据可能不如中国高血压调查的数据更具有代表性。

数据使用的另一个局限在于心血管疾病危险因素分析，本研究只能使用 2009 年的数据，数据比较陈旧。虽然 2015 年 CHNS 数据在论文完成前就发表了，但该数据库没有提供相关生物标志物信息，因此不可用。如果能获得 2015 年的数据，本研究的准确性将进一步提高。正如第 4 章所讨论，本研究的另一个局限性是无法获取 75 岁以上人群的心血管疾病风险估计的流行病学参数。

6.3.4.2 建模中的假设可能低估了效益

在马尔可夫建模过程中，心血管疾病被放在马尔可夫链中，我们假设 28 天内致死性心血管疾病在整个估计过程中只发生一次，这可能会低估项目干预的效益，因为心血管疾病急性发作可能会二次或多次出现。此外，我们仅将心血管疾病作为高血压健康结果进行估算，没有考虑肾脏疾病[194]等其他负性结果，这可能会使我们高血压控制的效益进一步被低估。

最后，在社会效益估算中，对一个生命年的社会效益价值仍有争议。本研究所采用的 0.5 倍人均 GDP 值仍是一个保守值，这可能低估产生的社会效益[45]。

6.4 结论和政策建议

首先，本研究的结果对开展进一步深入研究和政策制定具有重要意义。本研究计算了国家基本公共卫生服务项目高血压患者管理将为我国社会节省的经济成本，以货币形式为基层医疗卫生机构慢性病管理提供了效益证据。本研究参考 Stenberg 等研究的经济学评价方法[45]，该方法已经应用于妇女和儿童健康干预项目，显示其投资回报率较高（到 2035 年，以 3% 的贴现率计算，效益成本比为 4.8，总效益成本比为 8.7）。比较而言，国家基本公共卫生服务项目的投资回报率更高，这对该领域的学术研究、政策制定和实施方面都产生了巨大影响。

这项研究丰富了中国高血压患者管理经济学评价证据。通过多个成本和贴现率估计值，研究进行了敏感度分析，该方法同样适用于评估国家基本公共卫生服务其他项目的经济效果，例如我国的癌症筛查和早期干预措施。

其次，这项研究表明，我国在基层医疗卫生机构实施高血压干预具有较高的收益，表明政府有必要继续增加基层高血压患者健康管理的投入。本研究从经济学角度为卫生健康部门提供了评估框架和有效工具，也说明了需要进一步加强干预措施。这项研究的结果有助于对慢性非传染性疾病干预措施进行干预分类，确定优先领域，进而加强财政投入。

对政府的政策建议主要有以下 3 点。

（1）更好地实施国家基本公共卫生服务项目，加大对基层医疗卫生机构的投入，提高卫生人力的数量和质量。

（2）加强信息管理系统，完善基层医疗卫生机构的绩效评价[189]，将信息技术应用于慢性病管理，以提高工作绩效和效率[136]。

（3）下一步，国家基本公共卫生服务项目应加强年轻高血压患者和高危人群管理。作为劳动力的重要组成部分，大多数年轻患者自认为健康状况良好，但事实并非如此。

此外，人们一直呼吁我国需要加强功能社区的基层医疗卫生机构建设，进而为企事业单位员工提供健康管理服务。然而，当前这些机构建设效果欠佳[195-196]。同时，政策制定还应关注流动人口中的年轻患者，加强对这一群体的卫生健康服务提供[160]。

6.5 下一步研究建议

在进行经济学分析时，社会效益不仅由卫生健康部门产生，也会通过经济增长和社会其他方面产生。因此，其中有些收益难以计算。为进一步理解慢性病患者管理投入的潜在社会收益，建议在后续研究中加强地区性分析。

建议从以下方面开展进一步研究：①基于国家层面建立的分析模型，对特定地区进行案例研究；②对基层医疗卫生机构慢性病患者管理进行队列研究，为开展经济学评价提供血压、糖尿病、吸烟状况和其他心血管疾病风险因素的人群信息；③本研究中使用的经济学分析方法可以应用于国家基本公共卫生服务项目的其他内容，如糖尿病患者健康管理、重型精神疾病患者管理以及其他卫生健康干预项目。

参考文献

[1] GERALD B，GU X Y. Health sector reform：lessons from China［J］. Soc Sci Med，1997，45（3）：351-360.

[2] TANG S，MENG Q，CHEN L，et al. Tackling the challenges to health equity in China［J］. Lancet，2008，372（9648）：1493-1501.

[3] YANG G，KONG L，ZHAO W，et al. Emergence of chronic non-communicable diseases in China［J］. Lancet，2008，372（9650）：1697-1705.

[4] Division of Global Health Protection，Global Health，Centers for Disease Control and Prevention. Global Noncommunicable Diseases Fact Sheet［EB/OL］.（2023-2-3）［2023-8-11］https://www.cdc.gov/globalhealth/healthprotection/resources/fact-sheets/global-ncd-fact-sheet.html.

[5] YANG G，WANG Y，ZENG Y，et al. Rapid health transition in China，1990-2010：findings from the Global Burden of Disease Study 2010［J］. Lancet，2013，381（9882）：1987-2015.

[6] 国家心血管病中心. 中国心血管病报告 2013［M］. 北京：中国大百科全书出版社，2013.

[7] 新华社. 我国启动并部署九项国家基本公共卫生服务项目［EB/OL］.（2018-6-6）［2019-7-1］.https://www.gov.cn/jrzg/2009-07/10/content_1362010.htm.

[8] YIP W C，HSIAO W C，CHEN W，et al. Early appraisal of China's huge and complex health-care reforms［J］. Lancet，2012，379（9818）：833-842.

[9] World Bank. Toward a healthy and harmonious life in China：Stemming the rising tide of non-communicable diseases. 2011，Retrieved from http://www-wds.worldbank.org/external/default/WDSContentServer/WDSP/IB/2011/07/25/000333037_20110725011735/Rendered/PDF/634260WP00Box30official0use0only090.pdf

[10] 国家卫生和计划生育委员会. 关于做好 2013 年国家基本公共卫生服务工作的通知

[EB/OL].(2013-6-14) [2018-6-6].www.natcm.gov.cn/yizhengsi/gongzuodongtai/2018-03-24/2794.html

[11] 国家卫生健康委员会，财政部，国家中医药管理局. 关于做好 2018 年国家基本公共卫生服务项目工作的通知（国卫基层发〔2018〕18 号）[EB/OL] .（2018-6-20）[2019-6-6] . www.nhc.qov.cn/cms-search/xxak/getManuscriptXxqk.htm? id=acf4058c09d046b09addad8abd395e20

[12] XIAO N，LONG Q，TANG X，et al. A community-based approach to non-communicable chronic disease management within a context of advancing universal health coverage in China：progress and challenges [J] . BMC Public Health，2014，14 Suppl 2（Suppl 2）：S2.

[13] 国家卫生计生委项目资金监管服务中心. 2013 年基本公共卫生服务绩效评价年度报告 [EB/OL] .（2014-6-1）[2016-7-1]

[14] 中国社区卫生协会. 2015 年国家基本公共卫生服务项目阶段性评估报告 [EB/OL] .（2016-4-2）. [2016-7-1]

[15] TIAN M，WANG H，TONG X，et al. Essential Public Health Services' Accessibility and its Determinants among Adults with Chronic Diseases in China [J] . PLoS One，2015，10 （4）：e0125262.

[16] YIN D，WONG S T，CHEN W，et al. A model to estimate the cost of the National Essential Public Health Services Package in Beijing，China [J] . BMC Health Serv Res，2015，15：222.

[17] WANG H，GUSMANO M K，CAO Q. An evaluation of the policy on community health organizations in China：will the priority of new healthcare reform in China be a success? [J] . Health Policy，2011，99（1）：37-43.

[18] World Bank Group，World Health Organization，Ministry of Finance，et al（2016）. Deepening health reform in China. Growth analysis health measurement project [EB/OL] .（2016-07-22）[2018-6-6] https：//openknowledge.worldbank.org/handle/10986/24720.

[19] HUNG L M，SHI L，WANG H，et al. Chinese primary care providers and motivating factors on performance [J] . Fam Pract，2013，30（5）：576-586.

[20] 国务院办公厅. 关于印发全国医疗卫生服务体系规划纲要（2015—2020 年）的通知（国办发〔2015〕14 号）[EB/OL] .（2015-3-30）[2019-6-17] https：//www.gov.cn/zhengce/content/2015-03/30/content_9560.htm? trs=1.

[21] 中央编办，卫生部、财政部、民政部. 城市社区卫生服务机构设置和编制标准指导意见（中央编办发〔2006〕96 号）[EB/OL] .（2006-8-18）[2018-6-6] . www.nhc.qov.cn/cms-search/xxak/getManuscriptXxqk.htm?id=acf4058c09d046b09addad8abd395e20.

[22] 中央编办、卫生部、财政部《关于印发乡镇卫生院机构编制标准指导意见的通知》

（中央编办发［2011］28号）［EB/OL］.（2011-5-10）［2016-07-01］. https://www.doc88.com/p-9337129116206.html.

［23］LI X，LU J，HU S，et al. The primary health-care system in China［J］. Lancet，2017，390（10112）：2584-2594.

［24］The National Health Commission of China.（2018）. *Report on the progress of the essential public health services in China*. Beijing［EB/OL］.（2018-12-10）［2019-3-30］

［25］中国高血压防治指南修订委员会. 中国高血压防治指南（2018年修订版）［J］. 中国心血管杂志，2019,（24）1：24-56.

［26］WANG J G. Chinese Hypertension Guidelines［J］. Pulse（Basel），2015，3（1）：14-20.

［27］FU W，ZHAO S，ZHANG Y，et al. Research in health policy making in China：out-of-pocket payments in Healthy China 2030［J］. BMJ，2018，360：k234.

［28］财政部，国家发展改革委、民政部、人力资源社会保障部、卫生部. 关于完善政府卫生投入政策的意见（财社〔2009〕66号）［EB/OL］.（2009-7-1）［2018-6-6］. https://www.gov.cn/ztzl/ygzt/content 1661057.htm.

［29］财政部，卫生部. 财政部卫生部关于印发基本公共卫生服务项目补助资金管理办法的通知（财社〔2010〕311号）［EB/OL］.（2010-12-31）［2018-6-6］. https：//wenku.baidu.com/view/bbe7bf0390c69ec3d5bb7565.html? _wkts_=1691731301117&bdQuery=%E8%B4%A2%E6%94%BF%E9%83%A8+%E5%8D%AB%E7%94%9F%E9%83%A8+%E5%9B%BD%E5%AE%B6%E5%9F%BA%E6%9C%AC%E5%85%AC%E5%85%B1%E5%8D%AB%E7%94%9F%E6%9C%8D%E5%8A%A1%E9%A1%B9%E7%9B%AE%E8%B5%84%E9%87%91%E7%AE%A1%E7%90%%.

［30］Department of Health Systems Financing. Geneva：World Health Organization. WHO guide to identifying the economic consequences of disease and injury［EB/OL］.（2020-12-15）［2023-8-11］. https://www.who.int/home/search? indexCatalogue=genericsearchindex1&searchQuery=WHO%20guide%20to%20identifying%20the%20economic%20consequences%20of%20disease%20and%20injury&wordsMode=AnyWord.

［31］BUNDY J D，HE J. Hypertension and Related Cardiovascular Disease Burden in China［J］. Ann Glob Health，2016，82（2）：227-233.

［32］LI D，LV J，LIU F，et al. Hypertension burden and control in mainland China：Analysis of nationwide data 2003-2012［J］. Int J Cardiol，2015，184：637-644.

［33］WANG Z，CHEN Z，ZHANG L，et al. Status of Hypertension in China：Results From the China Hypertension Survey，2012-2015［J］. Circulation，2018，137（22）：2344-2356.

［34］段一萍. 小样本时间序列分析在遭遇段处理中的应用［J］. 兵工自动化，2015，34（9），

92-96.

[35] 任劲涛，朱家海，邵玉梅. 小样本时间序列的数据处理 [J] . 空军工程大学学报（自然科学版），2005，6（3）：71-73.

[36] WU Y，LIU X，LI X，et al. Estimation of 10-year risk of fatal and nonfatal ischemic cardiovascular diseases in Chinese adults [J] . Circulation，2006，114（21）：2217-2225.

[37] ZHANG X F，ATTIA J，D' ESTE C，et al. A risk score predicted coronary heart disease and stroke in a Chinese cohort [J] . J Clin Epidemiol，2005，58（9）：951-958.

[38] GU D，HE J，COXSON P G，et al. The Cost-Effectiveness of Low-Cost Essential Antihypertensive Medicines for Hypertension Control in China：A Modelling Study [J] . PLoS Med，2015，12（8）：e1001860.

[39] GU D，KELLY T N，WU X，et al. Blood pressure and risk of cardiovascular disease in Chinese men and women [J] . Am J Hypertens，2008，21（3）：265-272.

[40] Baan CA，Bos，G，Jacobs-van der Bruggen MAM. Modeling chronic diseases：the diabetes module. [2018-7-1] . https://rivm.openrepository.com/rivm/bitstream/10029/256901/3/260801001.pdf.

[41] MORAN A，GU D，ZHAO D，et al. Future cardiovascular disease in china：markov model and risk factor scenario projections from the coronary heart disease policy model-china [J] . Circ Cardiovasc Qual Outcomes，2010，3（3）：243-252.

[42] XIE X，HE T，KANG J，et al. Cost-effectiveness analysis of intensive hypertension control in China [J] . Prev Med，2018，111：110-114.

[43] 国家卫生和计划生育委员会.2014 中国卫生和计划生育统计年鉴 [M] . 北京：中国协和医科大学出版社，2014.

[44] BERTRAM M Y，SWEENY K，LAUER J A，et al. Investing in non-communicable diseases：an estimation of the return on investment for prevention and treatment services [J] . Lancet，2018，391（10134）：2071-2078.

[45] STENBERG K，AXELSON H，SHEEHAN P，et al. Advancing social and economic development by investing in women' s and children's health：a new Global Investment Framework [J] . Lancet，2014，383（9925）：1333-1354.

[46] United Nations，Department of Economic and Social Affairs，Population Division（2017）. World Population Prospects：The 2017 Revision，DVD Edition.

[47] Organization W H. Package of essential noncommunicable（PEN）disease interventions for primary health care in low-resource settings. [J] .Geneva：World Health Organization，2010.

[48] BURSTEIN R，FLEMING T，HAAGSMA J，et al. Estimating distributions of health

state severity for the global burden of disease study [J] . Popul Health Metr, 2015, 13: 31.

[49] HODGSON T A, MEINERS M R. Cost-of-illness methodology: a guide to current practices and procedures [J] . Milbank Mem Fund Q Health Soc, 1982, 60 (3): 429-462.

[50] POPKIN B M, DU S, ZHAI F, et al. Cohort Profile: The China Health and Nutrition Survey—monitoring and understanding socio-economic and health change in China, 1989-2011 [J] . Int J Epidemiol, 2010, 39 (6): 1435-1440.

[51] GUO J, ZHU Y C, CHEN Y P, et al. The dynamics of hypertension prevalence, awareness, treatment, control and associated factors in Chinese adults: results from CHNS 1991-2011 [J] . J Hypertens, 2015, 33 (8): 1688-1696.

[52] Qin J, ZhangY, Fridman M, Sweeny K, Zhang L, Lin C, et al. (2021) The role of the Basic Public Health Service program in the control of hypertension in China: Results from across-sectional health service interview survey. PLoS ONE 16 (6): e0217185. https://doi.org/10.1371/journal.pone.0217185.

[53] Claxton K, Sculpher M, Culyer A, et al.Discounting and cost-effectiveness in NICE-stepping back to sort out a confusion [J] .Health Economics, 2010, 15 (1): 1-4. DOI: 10.1002/hec.1081.

[54] Jason F. (2023) Net present value (NPV) [EB/OL] . (2023-05-24) [2023-08-11] . https://www.investopedia.com/terms/n/npv.asp.

[55] 卫生部统计信息中心. 2008 年第四次国家卫生服务调查分析报告英文摘要 [EB/OL] . (2010-09-21) [2018-07] . http://www.nhc.gov.cn/mohwsbwstjxxzx/s8211/201009/49166.shtml.

[56] PERMAN G, ROSSI E, WAISMAN G D, et al. Cost-effectiveness of a hypertension management programme in an elderly population: a Markov model [J] . Cost Eff Resour Alloc, 2011, 9 (1): 4.

[57] Georgetown University Health Policy Institute. Disease Management Programs: Improving health while reducing costs? [EB/OL] (2004) [2018-07-01] . https://hpi.georgetown.edu/management/.

[58] SQUIRES H, CHILCOTT J, AKEHURST R, et al. A Framework for Developing the Structure of Public Health Economic Models [J] . Value Health, 2016, 19 (5): 588-601.

[59] TSIACHRISTAS A, CRAMM J M, NIEBOER A, et al. Broader economic evaluation of disease management programs using multi-criteria decision analysis [J] . Int J Technol Assess Health Care, 2013, 29 (3): 301-308.

[60] SCULPHER M J, PANG F S, MANCA A, et al. Generalisability in economic evaluation studies in healthcare: a review and case studies [J]. Health Technol Assess, 2004, 8 (49): iii-iv, 1-192.

[61] World Health Organization. Noncommunicable diseases: hypertension [EB/OL]. (2015-06-29) [2018-12-01]. https://www.who.int/features/qa/82/en/.

[62] GELDSETZER P, MANNE-GOEHLER J, MARCUS M E, et al. The state of hypertension care in 44 low-income and middle-income countries: a cross-sectional study of nationally representative individual-level data from 1 · 1 million adults [J]. Lancet, 2019, 394 (10199): 652-662.

[63] JOFFRES M, FALASCHETTI E, GILLESPIE C, et al. Hypertension prevalence, awareness, treatment and control in national surveys from England, the USA and Canada, and correlation with stroke and ischaemic heart disease mortality: a cross-sectional study [J]. BMJ Open, 2013, 3 (8): e003423.

[64] Unger T, Borghi C, Charchar F, et al. 2020 International Society of Hypertension global hypertension practice guidelines [J]. Journal of Hypertension 38 (6): 982-1004.

[65] WANG J, ZHANG L, WANG F, et al. Prevalence, awareness, treatment, and control of hypertension in China: results from a national survey [J]. Am J Hypertens, 2014, 27 (11): 1355-1361.

[66] HOU Z, MENG Q, ZHANG Y. Hypertension Prevalence, Awareness, Treatment, and Control Following China's Healthcare Reform [J]. Am J Hypertens, 2016, 29 (4): 428-431.

[67] GAKIDOU E, AFSHIN A, ABAJOBIR A A, et al. (2017). Global, regional, and national comparative risk assessment of 84 behavioural, environmental and occupational, and metabolic risks or clusters of risks, 1990-2016: a systematic analysis for the Global Burden of Disease Study 2016 [J]. The Lancet, 2017, 390 (10100): 1345-1422.

[68] W, J, PUGH. (1996). HEALTH AND NUMBERS-BASIC BIOSTATISTICAL METHODS[J].Statistics in Medicine, 1996.DOI: 10.1002/(SICI)1097-0258(19960730) 15: 14<1603: : AID-SIM344>3.

[69] SAMET J, WIPFLI H, PLATZ E, et al. "Morbidity rate." In a Dictionary of Epidemiology (5th ed.) [M]. Oxford: Oxford University Press, 189.

[70] JENG J S, LEE T K, CHANG Y C, et al. Subtypes and case-fatality rates of stroke: a hospital-based stroke registry in Taiwan (SCAN-Ⅳ) [J]. J Neurol Sci, 1998, 156 (2): 220-226.

[71] HARRINGTON R A. Case fatality rate [EB/OL]. (2017-) [2018-9-12]. https://www.britannica.com/science/case-fatality-rate.

[72] STARE J, MAUCORT-BOULCH D. Odds ratio, hazard ratio and relative risk [J] . Metodoloski Zvezki, 2016, 13 (1): 59-67.

[73] KOTCHEN T A, HAJJAR I. Trends in Prevalence, Awareness, in the United States, 1988-2000 [J] . JAMA, 2003, 290 (2): 199-206.

[74] LU J, LU Y, WANG X, et al. (2017) . Prevalence, awareness, treatment, and control of hypertension in China: data from 1.7 million adults in a population-based screening study(China PEACE Million Persons Project) [J]. Lancet,2017,390(10112): 2549-2558. http://dx.doi.org/10.1016/S0140-6736 (17) 32478-32479.

[75] BAI Y, ZHAO Y, WANG G, et al. Cost-effectiveness of a hypertension control intervention in three community health centers in China [J] . J Prim Care Community Health, 2013, 4 (3): 195-201.

[76] GOODING H C, MCGINTY S, RICHMOND T K, et al. Hypertension awareness and control among young adults in the national longitudinal study of adolescent health [J] . J Gen Intern Med, 2014, 29 (8): 1098-1104.

[77] CHEN W W, GAO R L, LIU L S, et al. China cardiovascular diseases report 2015: a summary [J] . J Geriatr Cardiol, 2017, 14 (1): 1-10.

[78] WANG J, NING X, YANG L, et al. Trends of hypertension prevalence, awareness, treatment and control in rural areas of northern China during 1991-2011 [J] . J Hum Hypertens, 2014, 28 (1): 25-31.

[79] SU M, ZHANG Q, BAI X, et al. Availability, cost, and prescription patterns of antihypertensive medications in primary health care in China: a nationwide cross-sectional survey [J] . Lancet, 2017, 390 (10112): 2559-2568.

[80] BAJOREK B V, LEMAY K S, MAGIN P J, et al. Management of hypertension in an Australian community pharmacy setting-patients' beliefs and perspectives [J] . Int J Pharm Pract, 2017, 25 (4): 263-273.

[81] JAMES P A, OPARIL S, CARTER B L, et al. 2014 evidence-based guideline for the management of high blood pressure in adults: report from the panel members appointed to the Eighth Joint National Committee (JNC 8) [J] . JAMA, 2014, 311 (5): 507-520.

[82] GU J, ZHANG X J, WANG T H, et al. Hypertension knowledge, awareness, and self-management behaviors affect hypertension control: a community-based study in Xuhui District, Shanghai, China [J] . Cardiology, 2014, 127 (2): 96-104.

[83] XU J, PAN R, PONG R W, et al. Different Models of Hospital-Community Health Centre Collaboration in Selected Cities in China: A Cross-Sectional Comparative Study [J]. Int J Integr Care, 2016, 16 (1): 8.

[84] TU Q, XIAO L D, ULLAH S, et al. Hypertension management for community-dwelling

older people with diabetes in Nanchang，China：study protocol for a cluster randomized controlled trial［J］. Trials，2018，19（1）：385.

［85］秦江梅，张艳春，张丽芳，等. 典型城市居民慢性病患病率及患者疾病负担分析［J］. 中国公共卫生，2014，30（1）：5-7.

［86］GAO Y，CHEN G，TIAN H，et al. Prevalence of hypertension in china：a cross-sectional study［J］. PLoS One，2013，8（6）：e65938.

［87］XI B，LIANG Y，REILLY K H，et al. Trends in prevalence，awareness，treatment，and control of hypertension among Chinese adults 1991-2009［J］. Int J Cardiol，2012，158（2）：326-329.

［88］Peter T. Preventing the cardiovascular complications of hypertension［J］.European Heart Journal Supplements，2004（suppl_H）：h37-h42.DOI：10.1093/eurheartj/6.suppl_h.h37.

［89］HAMILTON M，THOMPSON E M，WISNIEWSKI T K. THE ROLE OF BLOOD-PRESSURE CONTROL IN PREVENTING COMPLICATIONS OF HYPERTENSION［J］. Lancet，1964，1（7327）：235-238.

［90］LEWINGTON S，CLARKE R，QIZILBASH N，et al. Age-specific relevance of usual blood pressure to vascular mortality：a meta-analysis of individual data for one million adults in 61 prospective studies［J］. Lancet，2002，360（9349）：1903-1913.

［91］LEWINGTON S，LACEY B，CLARKE R，et al. The Burden of Hypertension and Associated Risk for Cardiovascular Mortality in China［J］. JAMA Intern Med，2016，176（4）：524-532.

［92］TURNBULL F，NEAL B，NINOMIYA T，et al. Effects of different regimens to lower blood pressure on major cardiovascular events in older and younger adults：meta-analysis of randomised trials［J］. BMJ，2008，336（7653）：1121-1123.

［93］Tadege GM（2017）Survival Analysis of Time to Cardiovascular Disease Complication of Hypertensive Patients at Felege Hiwot Referal Hospital in Bahir-Dar，Ethiopia：A Retrospective Cohort Study. J Biom Biostat 8：369. doi：10.4172/2155-6180.1000369.

［94］Mamun A A，Williams G M，Peeters A，et al.（2020）. Risk factors and compression of cardiovascular morbidity：a life history analysis of the 46-year follow-ups of the Framingham Heart Study［C］//World Congress on Heart Disease.Medimond，International Proceedings Division，2006.DOI：http://espace.library.uq.edu.au/view/UQ：177652.

［95］D'AGOSTINO R B，LEE M L，BELANGER A J，et al. Relation of pooled logistic regression to time dependent Cox regression analysis：the Framingham Heart Study［J］. Stat Med，1990，9（12）：1501-1515.

［96］BENJAMIN E J，LEVY D，VAZIRI S M，et al. Independent risk factors for atrial fibrillation in a population-based cohort. The Framingham Heart Study [J] . JAMA, 1994, 271 (11): 840-844.

[97] SINGER D E, NATHAN D M, ANDERSON K M, et al. Association of HbA1c with prevalent cardiovascular disease in the original cohort of the Framingham Heart Study [J]. Diabetes, 1992, 41 (2): 202-208.

[98] HARRIS T, COOK E F, GARRISON R, et al. Body mass index and mortality among nonsmoking older persons. The Framingham Heart Study [J] . JAMA, 1988, 259 (10): 1520-1524.

[99] PREIS S R, HWANG S J, COADY S, et al. Trends in all-cause and cardiovascular disease mortality among women and men with and without diabetes mellitus in the Framingham Heart Study, 1950 to 2005 [J] . Circulation, 2009, 119 (13): 1728-1735.

[100] VISRODIA K, SINGH S, KRISHNAMOORTHI R, et al. Systematic review with meta-analysis: prevalent vs. incident oesophageal adenocarcinoma and high-grade dysplasia in Barrett's oesophagus [J] . Aliment Pharmacol Ther, 2016, 44 (8): 775-784.

[101] D'AGOSTINO RB Sr, VASAN R S, PENCINA M J, et al. General cardiovascular risk profile for use in primary care: the Framingham Heart Study [J] . Circulation, 2008, 117 (6): 743-753.

[102] KUULASMAA K, TUNSTALL-PEDOE H, DOBSON A, et al. Estimation of contribution of changes in classic risk factors to trends in coronary-event rates across the WHO MONICA Project populations [J] . Lancet, 2000, 355 (9205): 675-687.

[103] YANG X, LI J, HU D, et al. Predicting the 10-Year Risks of Atherosclerotic Cardiovascular Disease in Chinese Population: The China-PAR Project (Prediction for ASCVD Risk in China) [J] . Circulation, 2016, 134 (19): 1430-1440.

[104] LAW M R, WALD N J, MORRIS J K, et al. Value of low dose combination treatment with blood pressure lowering drugs: analysis of 354 randomised trials [J] . BMJ, 2003, 326 (7404): 1427.

[105] UNAL B, CAPEWELL S, CRITCHLEY J A. Coronary heart disease policy models: a systematic review [J] . BMC Public Health, 2006, 6: 213.

[106] CHAN F, ADAMO S, COXSON P, et al. Projected impact of urbanization on cardiovascular disease in China [J] . Int J Public Health, 2012, 57 (5): 849-854.

[107] CHENG J, ZHAO D, ZENG Z, et al. The impact of demographic and risk factor changes on coronary heart disease deaths in Beijing, 1999-2010 [J] . BMC Public Health, 2009, 9: 30.

[108] 张旭光. 基于 Markov 模型中国中老年人血脂异常筛检经济学评价 [D]. 北京：北京大学医学部，2015.

[109] BARTON P，BRYAN S，ROBINSON S. Modelling in the economic evaluation of health care：selecting the appropriate approach [J]. J Health Serv Res Policy，2004，9 (2)：110-118.

[110] WEINSTEIN M C，COXSON P G，WILLIAMS L W，et al. Forecasting coronary heart disease incidence，mortality，and cost：the Coronary Heart Disease Policy Model [J]. Am J Public Health，1987，77 (11)：1417-1426.

[111] LIGHTWOOD J M，COXSON P G，BIBBINS-DOMINGO K，et al. Coronary heart disease attributable to passive smoking：CHD Policy Model [J]. Am J Prev Med，2009，36 (1)：13-20.

[112] KONFINO J，MEKONNEN T A，COXSON P G，et al. Projected impact of a sodium consumption reduction initiative in Argentina：an analysis from the CVD policy model-Argentina [J]. PLoS One，2013，8 (9)：e73824.

[113] MORAN A，ZHAO D，GU D，et al. The future impact of population growth and aging on coronary heart disease in China：projections from the Coronary Heart Disease Policy Model-China [J]. BMC Public Health，2008，8：394.

[114] CHAN F，Adamo S，Coxson P，et al. Projected impact of urbanization on cardiovascular disease in china [J]. Int J Public Health，2012，57：849-854.

[115] Gagniuc，Paul A. (2017). Markov Chains (From Theory to Implementation and Experimentation) || Absorbing Markov Chains [M].John Wiley & Sons，Inc. 2017.

[116] SONNENBERG F A，BECK J R. Markov models in medical decision making：a practical guide [J]. Med Decis Making，1993，13 (4)：322-338.

[117] HOANG V P，SHANAHAN M，SHUKLA N，et al. A systematic review of modelling approaches in economic evaluations of health interventions for drug and alcohol problems [J]. BMC Health Serv Res，2016，16：127.

[118] World Health Organization. International Statistical Classification of Diseases and Related Health Problems (ICD) [EB/OL]. (2019-5) [2022-12-02]. https://www.who.int/classifications/icd/en/.

[119] MYERS R P，LEUNG Y，SHAHEEN A A，et al. Validation of ICD-9-CM/ICD-10 coding algorithms for the identification of patients with acetaminophen overdose and hepatotoxicity using administrative data [J]. BMC Health Serv Res，2007，7：159.

[120] DRUMMOND M F，SCULPHER M J，TORRANCE G W，et al. Methods for the economic evaluation of health care programmes [M]. 3rd ed. Oxford：Oxford University Press，2005.

[121] DRUMMOND M F，SCULPHER M J，CLAXTON K，et al. Methods for the economic evaluation of health care programmes [M] .4th ed. Oxford：Oxford University Press，2015.

[122] ZHANG D，WANG G，JOO H. A Systematic Review of Economic Evidence on Community Hypertension Interventions [J] . Am J Prev Med，2017，53（6S2）：S121-S130.

[123] HUANG Y，REN J. Cost-benefit analysis of a community-based stroke prevention program in Bao Shan District，Shanghai，China [J] .（2010）.International Journal of Collaborative Research on Internal Medicine & Public Health，2010，2（9）：307-316.

[124] HUANG Y，WANG S，CAI X，et al. Prehypertension and incidence of cardiovascular disease：a meta-analysis [J] . BMC Med，2013，11：177.

[125] MURPHY K，TOPEL R. The value of health and longevity [J] . J Polit Econ，2006，114：871-904.

[126] DUKPA W，TEERAWATTANANON Y，RATTANAVIPAPONG W，et al. Is diabetes and hypertension screening worthwhile in resource-limited settings? An economic evaluation based on a pilot of a Package of Essential Non-communicable disease interventions in Bhutan [J] . Health Policy Plan，2015，30（8）：1032-1043.

[127] NUGENT R，BROWER E，CRAVIOTO A，et al. A cost-benefit analysis of a National Hypertension Treatment Program in Bangladesh [J] . Prev Med，2017，105S：S56-S61.

[128] ATHANASAKIS K，KYRIOPOULOS I I，BOUBOUCHAIROPOULOU N，et al. Quantifying the economic benefits of prevention in a healthcare setting with severe financial constraints：the case of hypertension control [J] . Clin Exp Hypertens，2015，37（5）：375-380.

[129] STEVANOVIć J，O'PRINSEN A C，VERHEGGEN B G，et al. Economic evaluation of primary prevention of cardiovascular diseases in mild hypertension：a scenario analysis for the Netherlands [J] . Clin Ther，2014，36（3）：368-384.e5.

[130] 田惠光，郭则宇，宋桂德，等. 1991—1996 年天津市慢性病综合干预项目成本-效用和成本-效益分析 [J] . 中国慢性病预防与控制，2000，8（5）：196-197，221.

[131] 梁晓华. 高血压社区健康管理卫生经济学评价及糖尿病手机管理效果评价研究 [D] . 北京：北京协和医学院研究生院，2011.

[132] LIANG X，CHEN J，LIU Y，et al. The effect of hypertension and diabetes management in Southwest China：a before-and after-intervention study [J] . PLoS One，2014，9（3）：e91801.

[133] 李锐，王振果，俞顺章.Monte Carlo 模型在糖尿病筛查成本效益分析中的应用 [J] .

中国公共卫生管理，2003（03）：240-242.

［134］唐顺忠. 社区干预管理模式下高血压患者的疗效与成本效益分析［J］. 医学与社会，2011，24（5）：66-68.

［135］MUKHOPADHYAY K，THOMASSIN P J. Economic impact of adopting a healthy diet in Canada［J］. J Public Health（Oxf），2012，20（6）：639-652.

［136］世界银行，世界卫生组织.（2019）. 深化中国医药卫生体制改革—建设基于价值的优质服务提供体系［M］. 北京：中国财政经济出版社，2019.

［137］NGUYEN T P，WRIGHT E P，NGUYEN T T，et al. Cost-Effectiveness Analysis of Screening for and Managing Identified Hypertension for Cardiovascular Disease Prevention in Vietnam［J］. PLoS One，2016，11（5）：e0155699.

［138］HE J，MUNTNER P，CHEN J，et al. Factors associated with hypertension control in the general population of the United States［J］. Arch Intern Med，2002，162（9）：1051-1058.

［139］WANG Z，WANG X，CHEN Z，et al. Hypertension control in community health centers across China：analysis of antihypertensive drug treatment patterns［J］. Am J Hypertens，2014，27（2）：252-259.

［140］WONG M C，WANG H H，WONG S Y，et al. Performance comparison among the major healthcare financing systems in six cities of the Pearl River Delta region，mainland China［J］. PLoS One，2012，7（9）：e46309.

［141］WANG Z，WU Y，ZHAO L，et al. Trends in prevalence，awareness，treatment and control of hypertension in the middle-aged population of China，1992-1998［J］. Hypertens Res，2004，27（10）：703-709.

［142］WU Y，HUXLEY R，LI L，et al. Prevalence，awareness，treatment，and control of hypertension in China：data from the China National Nutrition and Health Survey 2002［J］. Circulation，2008，118（25）：2679-2686.

［143］GU D，REYNOLDS K，WU X，et al. Prevalence，awareness，treatment，and control of hypertension in china［J］. Hypertension，2002，40（6）：920-927.

［144］LI W，GU H，TEO K K，et al. Hypertension prevalence，awareness，treatment，and control in 115 rural and urban communities involving 47 000 people from China［J］. J Hypertens，2016，34（1）：39-46.

［145］LLOYD-SHERLOCK P，BEARD J，MINICUCI N，et al. Hypertension among older adults in low-and middle-income countries：prevalence，awareness and control［J］. Int J Epidemiol，2014，43（1）：116-128.

［146］王立明，李智. 2010 年慢性非传染性疾病流行病学调查［J］. 中国社区医师综合版，2011，27（32）：323-323.

[147] 国家卫生计生委疾病预防控制局. 中国居民营养与慢性病状况报告[M]. 北京：人民卫生出版社，2015：50-55.

[148] LI Y，YANG L，WANG L，et al. Burden of hypertension in China：A nationally representative survey of 174，621 adults[J]. Int J Cardiol，2017，227：516-523.

[149] LI H，LIU F，XI B. Control of hypertension in China：challenging[J]. Int J Cardiol，2014，174（3）：797.

[150] WANG J，ZHANG L. Response to "hypertension control prevalence estimates should account for age"[J]. Am J Hypertens，2014，27（11）：1427.

[151] LI H，LIU F，XI B. Control of hypertension in China：challenging[J]. Int J Cardiol，2014，174（3）：797.

[152] JIANG B，LIU H，RU X，et al. Hypertension detection，management，control and associated factors among residents accessing community health services in Beijing[J]. Sci Rep，2014，4：4845.

[153] WANG X，LI W，LI X，et al. Effects and cost-effectiveness of a guideline-oriented primary healthcare hypertension management program in Beijing，China：results from a 1-year controlled trial[J]. Hypertens Res，2013，36（4）：313-321.

[154] 赵芳，郑建中，陈博文，等. 成都市玉林社区高血压患者契约式管理效果分析[J]. 中华流行病学杂志，2003（10）：45-48.

[155]《中国高血压基层管理指南》修订委员会. 中国高血压基层管理指南（2014年修订版）[J]. 中华健康管理学杂志，2015，9（1）：10-30.

[156] HESKETH T，ZHOU X. Hypertension in China：the gap between policy and practice[J]. Lancet，2017，390（10112）：2529-2530.

[157] WU J X，HE L Y. Urban-rural gap and poverty traps in China：a prefecture level analysis. Applied Economics，2018，50（30），3300-3314.

[158] ZHAI S，WANG P，DONG Q，et al. A study on the equality and benefit of China's national health care system[J]. Int J Equity Health，2017，16（1）：155.

[159] TANG，X，YANG，J，LI，W，et al.（2013）. Urban and rural differences of blood pressure and hypertension control in Chinese communities：pure china study[J]. J Am Coll Cardiol，61（10 suppl. 1）：E1350.

[160] ZHU Y. China's floating population and their settlement intention in the cities：beyond the Hukou reform. Habitat International，2007，31（1）：65-76.

[161] YANG X，LI J，HU D，et al. Predicting the 10-year risks of atherosclerotic cardiovascular disease in Chinese population：The China-PAR Project（Prediction for ASCVD Risk in China）[J]. Circulation，2016，134（19）：1430-1440.

[162] 张艳春，刘昉，蒲琳，等. 基于模型分析的社区高血压患者健康管理效果研究[J].

中国全科医学，2018，21（17）：2082-2086，2090.

［163］SESSO H D，CHEN R S，L'ITALIEN G J，et al. Blood pressure lowering and life expectancy based on a Markov model of cardiovascular events［J］. Hypertension，2003，42（5）：885-890.

［164］李斌. 国务院关于深化医药卫生体制改革工作进展情况的报告—2015 年 12 月 22 日在第十二届全国人民代表大会常务委员会第十八次会议上［J］. 中华人民共和国全国人民代表大会常务委员会公报，2016（1）：4.

［165］WU C Y，HU H Y，CHOU Y J，et al. High Blood Pressure and All-Cause and Cardiovascular Disease Mortalities in Community-Dwelling Older Adults［J］. Medicine（Baltimore），2015，94（47）：e2160.

［166］STANDFIELD L，COMANS T，SCUFFHAM P. Markov modeling and discrete event simulation in health care：a systematic comparison［J］. Int J Technol Assess Health Care，2014，30（2）：165-172.

［167］PENALOZA-RAMOS M C，JOWETT S，MANT J，et al. Cost-effectiveness of self-management of blood pressure in hypertensive patients over 70 years with suboptimal control and established cardiovascular disease or additional cardiovascular risk diseases（TASMIN-SR）［J］. Eur J Prev Cardiol，2016，23（9）：902-912.

［168］SHEEHAN P，SWEENY K，RASMUSSEN B，et al. Building the foundations for sustainable development：a case for global investment in the capabilities of adolescents［J］. Lancet，2017，390（10104）：1792-1806.

［169］CHISHOLM D，SWEENY K，SHEEHAN P，et al. Scaling-up treatment of depression and anxiety：a global return on investment analysis［J］. Lancet Psychiatry，2016，3（5）：415-424.

［170］SWEENY K，FRIEDMAN H S，SHEEHAN P，et al. A Health System-Based Investment Case for Adolescent Health［J］. J Adolesc Health，2019，65（1S）：S8-S15.

［171］刘国光，胡绍文，吴杰. 中国药物经济学评价指南［J］. 中国药物经济学报，2011（3）：6-48.

［172］LUHNEN M，PREDIGER B，NEUGEBAUER E，et al. Systematic reviews of health economic evaluations：a protocol for a systematic review of characteristics and methods applied［J］. Syst Rev，2017，6（1）：238.

［173］DEHMER S P，BAKER-GOERING M M，MACIOSEK M V，et al. Modeled Health and Economic Impact of Team-Based Care for Hypertension［J］. Am J Prev Med，2016，50（5 Suppl 1）：S34-S44.

［174］International Lablor Organization. ILOSTATS Data［EB/OL］.（2019）［2020-7-1］.

https://ilostat.ilo.org/data/.

［175］World Bank，World Development Indicators［EB/OL］.（2019）［2020-7-1］. https://datacatalog.worldbank.org/dataset/world-development-indicators.

［176］JAMES S L，ABATE D，ABATE K H，et al. Global，regional，and national incidence，prevalence，and years lived with disability for 354 Diseases and Injuries for 195 countries and territories，1990-2017：a systematic analysis for the Global Burden of Disease Study 2017［J］. The Lancet，2018，392（10159）：1789-1858.

［177］JO C. Cost-of-illness studies：concepts，scopes，and methods［J］. Clin Mol Hepatol，2014，20（4）：327-337.

［178］国家卫生健康委员会妇幼健康司.《关于做好2017年国家基本公共卫生服务项目工作的通知》政策解读［EB/OL］.（2017年09月05日）［2018年07月01日］. http://www.nhc.gov.cn/jws/s3577/201709/9cb26d17f691491bb3bb0f139bbf3ff1.shtml.

［179］赵志广，陈虾，周彦等. 基于工作量的社区基本公共卫生服务经费分配比例测算［J］. 中国全科医学，2015，18（10）：1124-1128.

［180］程锦泉，卢祖洵，赵志广，等. 社区基本公共卫生服务成本概述［J］. 中国全科医学，2015（18）10：1115-1119.

［181］Flochel T，Ikeda Y，Moroz H，et al.Macroeconomic Implications of Aging in East Asia Pacific［J］.World Bank Other Operational Studies，2015.

［182］MURRUGARRA，E.（2011）. Employability and productivity among older workers：A policy framework and evidence from Latin America. *SP Discussion Paper*，（1113），1-64. http://documents.shihang.org/curated/zh/582931468276366754/pdf/632300NWP0111300public00BOX361509B.pdf.

［183］中共中央 国务院. 关于深化医药卫生体制改革的意见［EB/OL］.（2009-3-17）［2019-6-6］. https://www.gov.cn/jrzg/2009-04/06/content 1278721.htm.

［184］侯万里，赵志广，夏挺松，等. 社区基本公共卫生服务经费预测研究［J］. 中华全科医学，2016，14（6）：879-882.

［185］SHEN Y，WANG X，WANG Z，et al. Prevalence，awareness，treatment，and control of hypertension among Chinese working population：results of a workplace-based study［J］. J Am Soc Hypertens，2018，12（4）：311-322.e2.

［186］HUANG K，SONG Y T，HE Y H，et al. Health system strengthening and hypertension management in China［J］. Glob Health Res Policy，2016，1：13.

［187］Xu，G.（2010）. Staffing standard in public institution：Orientation，mechanism and coping strategies. *Journal of Renmin University of China*，（5），143-150.

［188］秦江梅，张丽芳，林春梅，等. 新医改以来我国基层卫生人力发展规模及配置现状研究［J］. 中国全科医学，2016，19（4）：378-382.

[189] 张艳春，秦江梅，张丽芳，等. 英国质量产出框架对我国家庭医生签约服务激励机制的启示［J］. 中国卫生经济，2017，36（18）：116-119.

[190] ZHOU B，DANAEI G，STEVENS G A，et al. Long-term and recent trends in hypertension awareness，treatment，and control in 12 high-income countries：an analysis of 123 nationally representative surveys. The Lancet，2019，6736（19）：1-13.

[191] LI H，WEI X，WONG M C，et al. A comparison of the quality of hypertension management in primary care between Shanghai and Shenzhen：a cohort study of 3 196 patients［J］. Medicine（Baltimore），2015，94（5）：e455.

[192] HUSEREAU D，DRUMMOND M，PETROU S，et al. Consolidated Health Economic Evaluation Reporting Standards（CHEERS）statement［J］. Eur J Health Econ，2013，14（3）：367-372.

[193] 国家基本公共卫生服务项目基层高血压管理办公室、基层高血压管理专家委员会. 国家基层高血压防治管理指南［J］. 中国循环杂志，2017，32（11）：1041-1048.

[194] PEñALOZA-RAMOS M C，JOWETT S，SUTTON A J，et al. The Importance of Model Structure in the Cost-Effectiveness Analysis of Primary Care Interventions for the Management of Hypertension［J］. Value Health，2018，21（3）：351-363.

[195] 刘向红，杜娟，郭爱民，等. 北京德胜功能社区 18~60 岁在职人群社区卫生服务需求和就医行为及影响因素研究［J］. 中国全科医学，2013，16（39）：3982-3986.

[196] 王芳，李永斌，丁雪，等. 功能社区卫生服务发展现状与问题分析［J］. 中国卫生事业管理，2012，29（12）：894-896.

附录　关键内容分析过程与相关数据

附录 A　第三章主要过程性数据

表 A1　1991—2015 年我国不同年龄组高血压患病率、知晓率、治疗率和控制率

单位：%

分组	1991	1993	1997	2000	2004	2006	2009	2011	2015
患病率									
18~24	2.44	4.21	4.70	3.65	4.50	3.71	3.80	2.37	4.00
25~34	3.74	5.92	6.59	6.35	6.94	5.80	7.84	5.95	6.10
35~44	9.50	9.87	12.14	12.93	13.67	13.41	14.82	12.11	15.90
45~54	16.95	18.06	22.12	22.33	22.92	22.16	28.66	26.48	29.60
55~64	32.84	33.43	36.61	36.71	36.36	33.55	38.88	38.76	44.60
65~74	45.56	44.53	51.97	50.74	49.64	45.83	53.56	49.20	55.70
75+	52.44	51.97	53.53	53.58	56.39	53.05	58.35	54.74	60.20
知晓率									
18~24	8.82	7.84	6.12	3.03	0	11.11	0	7.14	5.70
25~34	22.97	7.92	7.87	11.40	9.47	11.94	9.72	9.64	14.70
35~44	23.04	15.46	9.78	18.95	20.08	20.43	22.36	37.81	31.70
45~54	27.18	28.00	20.85	35.37	34.02	38.02	39.78	51.07	47.00
55~64	36.08	41.12	22.86	38.97	44.47	53.02	48.50	60.41	53.90
65~74	30.08	36.25	32.97	44.39	48.25	55.18	55.52	65.32	58.60
75+	19.49	22.69	25.69	32.56	42.91	49.04	51.38	68.15	57.30

续表

分组	1991	1993	1997	2000	2004	2006	2009	2011	2015
治疗率									
18~24	0	3.92	2.04	0	0	0	0	0	3.40
25~34	9.46	2.97	3.15	4.39	3.16	4.48	6.94	2.41	8.40
35~44	8.90	5.15	5.78	9.82	13.64	15.05	15.85	24.38	24.50
45~54	14.56	13.33	12.39	21.89	22.54	26.59	28.10	40.64	40.30
55~64	23.58	27.51	15.83	26.77	33.58	39.50	40.63	51.12	48.10
65~74	18.70	22.50	24.59	35.20	36.29	43.97	48.34	56.75	52.80
75+	13.56	16.81	15.28	21.51	35.22	40.23	44.00	60.42	52.10
控制率									
18~24	0	3.92	0	0	0	0	0	0	0.60
25~34	4.05	1.98	0	1.75	1.05	1.49	2.78	0.00	3.30
35~44	2.62	1.55	2.67	2.81	4.17	3.58	5.69	7.07	9.90
45~54	2.43	2.67	2.82	4.21	6.97	7.91	8.03	14.84	16.10
55~64	4.55	5.62	2.51	6.00	9.38	10.50	12.02	20.91	18.60
65~74	2.44	2.50	4.59	8.74	10.52	12.47	12.96	21.04	18.40
75+	2.54	2.52	3.47	4.65	8.50	8.05	8.92	19.67	17.00

注：知晓率、治疗率和控制率的分母均为患病人群。

数据来源：1991—2011 年数据来源于国家健康与营养调查；2015 年数据来源于中国高血压调查 Z. Wang et al.（2018）。

```
R Console
+   #combin the exrpession
+   m <- paste(m,"*",y)
+   r <- paste(m,collapse="+")
+
+   #combin the function
+   fbody <- paste("{ return(",r,")}")
+   f <- function(a) {}
+
+   #fill the function's body
+   body(f) <- parse(text=fbody)
+
+   return(f)
+ }
> a = c(1,3,7,10)
> b = c(2.87,2.73,2.95,4.55)
> f <- LagrangePolynomial(a,b)
> f(5)
[1] 2.672222
> a = c(7,10,14,16)
> b = c(2.95,4.55,6.95,7.41)
> f <- LagrangePolynomial(a,b)
> f(12)
[1] 5.870106
>
```

图 A1　拉格朗日插值法 R 语言程序截屏图

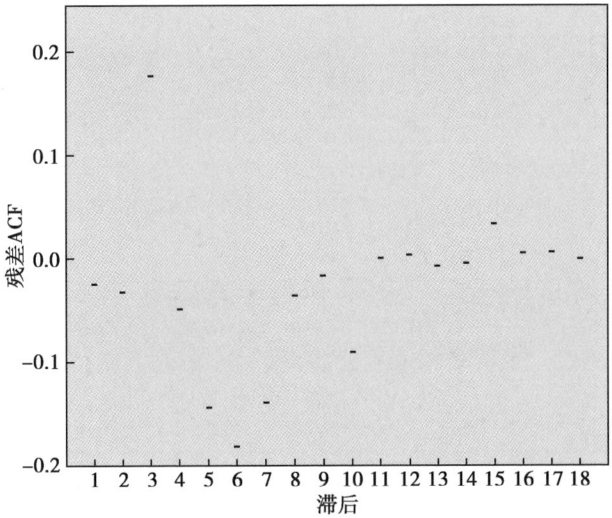

图 A2　1991—2009 年我国高血压控制率时间序列模型残差 ACF（自相关函数）图

表 A2　1991—2018 年我国高血压患病率、知晓率、治疗率和控制率相关文章信息摘录

作者	研究时间/年	地区	抽样方法	城乡（U=城市；R=农村）	年龄范围/岁
Jiang et al.，2014	2008	北京	整群	U	≥50
Chen et al.，2014	2009	重庆	整群	U	≥18
Wang et al.，2014	2007—2010	全国	分层整群	U	18~79
Li et al.，2015	2010—2011	上海与深圳	多阶段随机抽样	U	≥18
Gu et al.，2014	2011	Xuhui，上海市徐汇区	整群	U	≥35
Zhang et al.，2014	2011	Yulin CHSC（成都）	整群	U	≥35
Hou et al.，2016	2008，2012	全国，浙江与甘肃	CHARLS	U、R	≥45
Zhang et al.，2018	2011，2013	全国	CHARLS	U、R	≥45

续表

作者	研究时间/年	地区	抽样方法	城乡（U=城市；R=农村）	年龄范围/岁
Tian et al.，2015	2013	全国	多阶段分层随机抽样	U、R	≥35
Wang et al.，2013	2013	北京	病例对照	U、R	≥18

作者	样本量/例	收缩压/舒张压降低值/mmHg	控制率	控制率改进情况	随访时间
Jiang et al.，2014	9 397	N/A	规律治疗者控制率为45.8%	N/A	N/A
Chen et al.，2014	6 681	3.5（3.2~3.7）/2.9（2.7~3.2）	N/A	N/A	1年
Wang et al.，2014	249 830	N/A	25.5%	37%，单一用药27.7%，联合用药24.1%	N/A
Li et al.，2015	3 196	N/A	83.2% 76.3%	N/A	2年
Gu et al.，2014	3 328		36.1%		
Zhang et al.，2014	3 191	（147±17）*vs.*（133±8）；（83±11）*vs.*（75±6）	32% *vs.* 85%	53%	（33±25）个月
Hou et al.，2016	1 961，1 836	N/A	21.7%、36.4%	14.7%	N/A
Zhang et al.，2018	4 958	N/A	27.3%、35.5%	7.9%	N/A
Tian et al.，2015	2 173	N/A	33.65%	N/A	N/A
Wang et al.，2013	436	N/A	城市：42.1% *vs.* 34.3%； 农村：30.7% *vs.* 10.0%； 城市：70.7% *vs.* 40.0%； 农村：72.9% *vs.* 27.9%	7.8%-城市 20.7%-农村 30.7%-城市 45%-农村	随访3个月 随访1年

注：N/A代表不适用或不可得。

附录 B　第四章主要过程性数据

表 B1　按照血压是否控制对 CHNS 2009 年高血压患者分组，各年龄组特征和危险因素（男性）

年龄组	分组	例数	年龄/岁（$\bar{x}\pm s$）	收缩压/mmHg（$\bar{x}\pm s$）	舒张压/mmHg（$\bar{x}\pm s$）	总胆固醇/（mmol·L^{-1}）（$\bar{x}\pm s$）	高密度脂蛋白胆固醇/（mmol·L^{-1}）（$\bar{x}\pm s$）	BMI/（kg·m^{-2}）（$\bar{x}\pm s$）	糖尿病/例（%）	吸烟/例（%）
35~44	G1	10	41.86 ± 1.66	127 ± 6	83 ± 4	4.97 ± 0.71	1.24 ± 0.32	24.9 ± 1.85	2/10（20.0）	8/10
	G2	22	41.09 ± 2.48	147 ± 15	101 ± 10	5.18 ± 1.10	1.16 ± 0.44	27.3 ± 3.12	4（18.2）	11（50.0）
t（χ^2）值			0.895	4.13	5.49	0.55	−0.55	2.11	0.015	2.57
P 值			0.378	<0.01	<0.01	0.59	0.59	0.04	0.903	0.14

年龄组	分组	例数	年龄/岁（$\bar{x}\pm s$）	收缩压/mmHg（$\bar{x}\pm s$）	舒张压/mmHg（$\bar{x}\pm s$）	总胆固醇/（mmol·L^{-1}）（$\bar{x}\pm s$）	高密度脂蛋白胆固醇/（mmol·L^{-1}）（$\bar{x}\pm s$）	BMI/（kg·m^{-2}）（$\bar{x}\pm s$）	糖尿病/例（%）	吸烟/例（%）
45~54	G1	28	49.24 ± 3.41	127 ± 11	84 ± 6	4.84 ± 0.96	1.14（1.02~1.40）*	25.7 ± 3.82	6（21.4）	18（64.3）
	G2	66	50.29 ± 2.97	149 ± 14	100 ± 11	5.21 ± 0.98	1.25（1.06~1.51）*	26.1 ± 3.25	13（19.7）	37（56.1）
t（χ^2）值			−1.501	7.12	7.23	1.68	−1.62*（Z 值）	0.54	0.037	0.55
P 值			0.137	<0.01	<0.01	0.10	0.11*	0.59	0.848	0.50

续表

年龄组	分组	例数	年龄/岁（$\bar{x}\pm s$）	收缩压/mmHg（$\bar{x}\pm s$）	舒张压/mmHg（$\bar{x}\pm s$）	总胆固醇/（mmol·L^{-1}）（$\bar{x}\pm s$）	高密度脂蛋白胆固醇/（mmol·L^{-1}）（$\bar{x}\pm s$）	BMI/（kg·m^{-2}）（$\bar{x}\pm s$）	糖尿病/例（%）	吸烟/例（%）
55~64	G1	35	60.03 ± 3.01	129 ± 11	83 ± 6	5.12 ± 0.91	1.24 ± 0.31	25.0 ± 2.66	9（25.7）	15（42.9）
	G2	91	60.24 ± 2.92	152 ± 18	97 ± 13	4.97 ± 0.85	1.27 ± 0.37	24.7 ± 3.11	17（18.7）	44（48.4）
t（χ^2）值			−0.369	7.12	6.40	−0.88	0.54	−0.46	0.763	0.31
P 值			0.713	<0.01	<0.01	0.38	0.59	0.65	0.382	0.69
年龄组	分组	例数	年龄/岁（$\bar{x}\pm s$）	收缩压/mmHg（$\bar{x}\pm s$）	舒张压/mmHg（$\bar{x}\pm s$）	总胆固醇/（mmol·L^{-1}）（$\bar{x}\pm s$）	高密度脂蛋白胆固醇/（mmol·L^{-1}）（$\bar{x}\pm s$）	BMI/（kg·m^{-2}）（$\bar{x}\pm s$）	糖尿病/例（%）	吸烟/例（%）
65~74	G1	42	69.23 ± 3.03	127 ± 10	80 ± 7	4.61 ± 0.85	1.28 ± 0.34	23.4 ± 3.55	6（14.3）	20（47.6）
	G2	91	69.13 ± 2.78	157 ± 15	91 ± 11	5.10 ± 0.94	1.31 ± 0.38	23.4 ± 3.76	20（22.0）	32（35.2）
t（χ^2）值			0.196	11.48	5.87	2.35	0.43	3.25	1.081	1.87
P 值			0.845	<0.01	<0.01	0.02	0.67	0.00	0.298	0.19
年龄组	分组	例数	年龄/岁（$\bar{x}\pm s$）	收缩压/mmHg（$\bar{x}\pm s$）	舒张压/mmHg（$\bar{x}\pm s$）	总胆固醇/（mmol·L^{-1}）（$\bar{x}\pm s$）	高密度脂蛋白胆固醇/（mmol·L^{-1}）（$\bar{x}\pm s$）	BMI/（kg·m^{-2}）（$\bar{x}\pm s$）	糖尿病/例（%）	吸烟/例（%）
75~84	G1	16	78.57 ± 2.63	126 ± 9	77 ± 9	4.61 ± 0.89	1.30 ± 0.34	23.3 ± 3.47	3（18.8）	6（37.5）
	G2	42	78.89 ± 2.49	160 ± 19	92 ± 11	5.00 ± 0.79	1.31 ± 0.39	23.4 ± 3.77	10（23.8）	12（28.6）
t（χ^2）值			−0.429	6.56	4.80	1.63	0.08	0.09	0.171	0.43
P 值			0.669	<0.01	<0.01	0.11	0.94	0.93	0.680	0.54

续表

年龄组	分组	例数	年龄/岁（$\bar{x}\pm s$）	收缩压/mmHg（$\bar{x}\pm s$）	舒张压/mmHg（$\bar{x}\pm s$）	总胆固醇/（mmol·L^{-1}）（$\bar{x}\pm s$）	高密度脂蛋白胆固醇/（mmol·L^{-1}）（$\bar{x}\pm s$）	BMI/（kg·m^{-2}）（$\bar{x}\pm s$）	糖尿病/例（%）	吸烟/例（%）
85+	G1	2	87.65 ± 1.48	127.00 ± 5.19	65.83 ± 6.84	4.85 ± 2.22	1.36 ± 0.58	20.97 ± 0.40	0	0
	G2	3	89.17 ± 3.20	156.67 ± 6.11	89.78 ± 8.39	4.70 ± 1.03	1.55 ± 0.23	23.77 ± 3.63	0	0
t 值			–0.604	U 检验	U 检验	U 检验	U 检验	U 检验	N/A	N/A
P 值			0.589	0.400	0.400	0.800	1.000	0.400	N/A	N/A

注：针对年龄、血压、总胆固醇和高密度脂蛋白胆固醇，开展独立样本 *t* 检验；针对糖尿病患病情况和吸烟状况，开展 χ^2 检验。* 针对非正态分布数据，研究用了非参数检验，括号里面列的是四分位数。*U* 检验是 Mann-Whitney *U* 检验。

表 B2　按照血压是否控制对 CHNS 2009 年高血压患者分组，各年龄组特征和危险因素（女性）

年龄组	分组	例数	年龄/岁（$\bar{x}\pm s$）	收缩压/mmHg（$\bar{x}\pm s$）	舒张压/mmHg（$\bar{x}\pm s$）	总胆固醇/（mmol·L^{-1}）（$\bar{x}\pm s$）	高密度脂蛋白胆固醇/（mmol·L^{-1}）（$\bar{x}\pm s$）	BMI/（kg·m^{-2}）（$\bar{x}\pm s$）	糖尿病/例（%）	吸烟/例（%）
35~44	G1	7	42.49 ± 2.02	131 ± 10	86 ± 4	5.14 ± 1.26	1.31 ± 0.25	24.5 ± 3.36	1（14.3）	0
	G2	22	40.54 ± 2.82	155 ± 29	102 ± 11	4.65 ± 0.85	1.30 ± 0.23	26.1 ± 4.41	2（9.1）	〔1（4.5）〕
t（χ^2）值			1.683	2.14	3.51	–1.19	–0.11	0.90	0.155	0.33
P 值			0.104	0.05	0.003	0.25	0.91	0.38	0.694	1.00

续表

年龄组	分组	例数	年龄/岁（$\bar{x}\pm s$）	收缩压/mmHg（$\bar{x}\pm s$）	舒张压/mmHg（$\bar{x}\pm s$）	总胆固醇/（mmol·L^{-1}）（$\bar{x}\pm s$）	高密度脂蛋白胆固醇/（mmol·L^{-1}）（$\bar{x}\pm s$）	BMI/（kg·m^{-2}）（$\bar{x}\pm s$）	糖尿病/例（%）	吸烟/例（%）
45~54	G1	43	50.92 ± 2.82	125 ± 10	82 ± 6	5.30 ± 1.23	1.53（1.24~1.76）*	24.9 ± 3.37	10（23.3）	0
	G2	59	51.03 ± 2.87	152 ± 15	97 ± 11	5.22 ± 1.12	1.34（1.12~1.52）*	26.6 ± 3.74	9（15.3）	7（11.9）
t（χ^2）值			−0.188	10.29	7.94	−0.35	−2.58（Z值）	2.45	1.051	5.48
P值			0.852	0.000	0.000	0.73	0.01	0.02	0.305	0.02
年龄组	分组	例数	年龄/岁（$\bar{x}\pm s$）	收缩压/mmHg（$\bar{x}\pm s$）	舒张压/mmHg（$\bar{x}\pm s$）	总胆固醇/（mmol·L^{-1}）（$\bar{x}\pm s$）	高密度脂蛋白胆固醇/（mmol·L^{-1}）（$\bar{x}\pm s$）	BMI/（kg·m^{-2}）（$\bar{x}\pm s$）	糖尿病/例（%）	吸烟/例（%）
55~64	G1	51	60.27 ± 2.86	127 ± 11	81 ± 6	5.24 ± 0.99	1.40 ± 0.51	25.3 ± 3.03	11（21.6）	1（2.0）
	G2	128	60.23 ± 2.72	156 ± 15	96 ± 8	5.48 ± 0.97	1.33 ± 0.31	25.7 ± 3.46	32（25.0）	11（8.6）
t（χ^2）值			0.074	12.36	11.93	1.52	−1.10	0.66	0.235	2.57
P值			0.941	0.000	0.000	0.13	0.27	0.51	0.628	0.18
年龄组	分组	例数	年龄/岁（$\bar{x}\pm s$）	收缩压/mmHg（$\bar{x}\pm s$）	舒张压/mmHg（$\bar{x}\pm s$）	总胆固醇/（mmol·L^{-1}）（$\bar{x}\pm s$）	高密度脂蛋白胆固醇/（mmol·L^{-1}）（$\bar{x}\pm s$）	BMI/（kg·m^{-2}）（$\bar{x}\pm s$）	糖尿病/例（%）	吸烟/例（%）
65~74	G1	63	70.04 ± 2.94	131 ± 8	79 ± 8	5.24 ± 0.99	1.38 ± 0.37	25.2 ± 3.41	22（34.9）	〔1（1.6）〕
	G2	109	70.31 ± 2.89	156 ± 15	90 ± 11	5.27 ± 1.02	1.44 ± 0.30	24.7 ± 4.25	29（26.6）	〔11(10.1)〕
t（χ^2）值			−0.578	12.05	6.93	0.18	1.10	−0.90	1.323	4.45
P值			0.546	0.000	0.000	0.86	0.27	0.37	0.250	0.06

续表

年龄组	分组	例数	年龄/岁（$\bar{x}\pm s$）	收缩压/mmHg（$\bar{x}\pm s$）	舒张压/mmHg（$\bar{x}\pm s$）	总胆固醇/（mmol·L^{-1}）（$\bar{x}\pm s$）	高密度脂蛋白胆固醇/（mmol·L^{-1}）（$\bar{x}\pm s$）	BMI/（kg·m^{-2}）（$\bar{x}\pm s$）	糖尿病/例（%）	吸烟/例（%）
75~84	G1	22	78.30 ± 2.26	126 ± 13	79 ± 9	4.87 ± 0.88	1.40 ± 0.35	24.3 ± 4.52	7（31.8）	0
	G2	60	79.24 ± 2.75	164 ± 24	87 ± 11	5.51 ± 0.88	1.46 ± 0.35	23.5 ± 4.32	15（25.0）	〔5（8.3）〕
t（χ^2）值			−1.431	7.72	3.30	2.94	0.72	−0.76	0.381	1.95
P 值			0.156	0.000	0.003	0.004	0.48	0.45	0.537	0.32
年龄组	分组	例数	年龄/岁（$\bar{x}\pm s$）	收缩压/mmHg（$\bar{x}\pm s$）	舒张压/mmHg（$\bar{x}\pm s$）	总胆固醇/（mmol·L^{-1}）（$\bar{x}\pm s$）	高密度脂蛋白胆固醇/（mmol·L^{-1}）（$\bar{x}\pm s$）	BMI/（kg·m^{-2}）（$\bar{x}\pm s$）	糖尿病/例（%）	吸烟/例（%）
85+	G1	1	86.50	137.67	75.00	4.04	1.78	19.33	0	0
	G2	4	85.80 ± 0.81	164.08 ± 5.87	87.33 ± 6.37	4.68 ± 1.31	1.38 ± 0.30	23.91 ± 3.39	0	0.25
t 值			0.771	U 检验	U 检验	U 检验	U 检验	U 检验	N/A	N/A
P 值			0.497	0.200	0.200	1.000	0.800	0.800	N/A	N/A

注：针对年龄、血压、总胆固醇和高密度脂蛋白胆固醇，开展独立样本 t 检验；针对糖尿病患病情况和吸烟状况，开展 χ^2 检验。

* 针对非正态分布数据，研究用了非参数检验，括号里面列的是四分位数。

U 检验是 Mann-Whitney U 检验。

表 B3 性别年龄别城乡人口结构与死亡率

分组	死亡率/100 000		人口结构占比/%	
	城市	农村	城市	农村
男性				
35~	116.12	166.82	2.72	4.08
40~	220.52	268.42	2.61	4.64
45~	274.92	349.22	2.25	3.93
50~	531.18	627.51	1.65	3.05
55~	755.40	830.51	1.49	3.37
60~	1 227.23	1 368.67	1.01	2.53
65~	1 984.41	2 305.59	0.67	1.79
70~	3 169.18	3 725.56	0.57	1.38
75~	5 167.37	6 138.59	0.41	0.94
80~	9 052.67	10 598.65	0.21	0.49
85+	18 323.58	19 594.67	0.11	0.23
女性				
35~	48.04	67.15	2.56	3.92
40~	96.84	109.39	2.43	4.56
45~	118.50	149.91	2.07	3.91
50~	234.83	293.95	1.57	2.92
55~	324.37	393.48	1.50	3.25
60~	606.47	721.00	1.03	2.39
65~	1 064.47	1 296.45	0.71	1.71
70~	1 882.75	2 290.84	0.61	1.36
75~	3 509.27	3 945.77	0.44	1.07
80~	6 721.27	7 423.16	0.24	0.66
85+	15 318.04	15 928.79	0.15	0.42

资料来源：2014 年中国卫生和计划生育统计年鉴。

表 B4　两组患者马尔可夫模型预测参数

分组	性别年龄别高血压患者人口结构/%	冠心病					脑卒中					非心血管疾病死亡率/100 000
		前期冠心病患病率/%*	G1 组冠心病发病率/100 000	G2 组冠心病发病率/100 000	28 天病死率（占比）	冠心病病死率（占比）	前期脑卒中患病率/%*	G1 组脑卒中发病率/100 000	G2 组脑卒中发病率/100 000	28 天病死率（占比）	脑卒中病死率（占比）	
男性												
35~44	9.36	0.6	130	215	0.12	0.02	1.3	24	49	0.25	0.02	149
45~54	7.13	1.2	135	223	0.21	0.03	3.2	145	298	0.18	0.02	305
55~64	5.23	3.4	220	363	0.29	0.03	8.8	670	1 378	0.12	0.02	696
65~74	2.71	4.7	500	825	0.33	0.05	14.2	1 250	2 571	0.20	0.04	1 741
75~84	1.28	6.0	2 010	4 641	0.48	0.18	15.0	2 510	8 314	0.45	0.11	4 142
85+*	0.21	6.0	2 010	3 317	0.48	0.65	15.0	2 510	5 163	0.45	0.28	10 806
女性												
35~44	8.92	0.4	19	26	0.18	0.00	0.9	23	39	0.18	0.01	67
45~54	6.8	1.3	49	69	0.23	0.02	2.4	180	376	0.14	0.01	141
55~64	5.13	3.1	141	198	0.27	0.01	6.0	800	1 670	0.15	0.02	333
65~74	2.75	4.0	310	432	0.43	0.04	10.0	1 500	2 515	0.20	0.04	946
75~84	1.48	6.0	1 900	3 276	0.51	0.17	12.0	2 500	7 799	0.45	0.11	2 670
85+*	0.34	6.0	1 900	3 248	0.51	0.55	12.0	2 500	6 263	0.45	0.30	8 335

注：* 由于 85 岁及以上年龄组参数不可得，所以用 75~84 岁年龄组参数替代；85 岁及以上年龄组冠心病和脑卒中死亡率数据来源于 2013 年中国卫生统计年鉴，取城乡性别-年龄别疾病死亡率，人口结构来源于 2010 年人口普查数据。

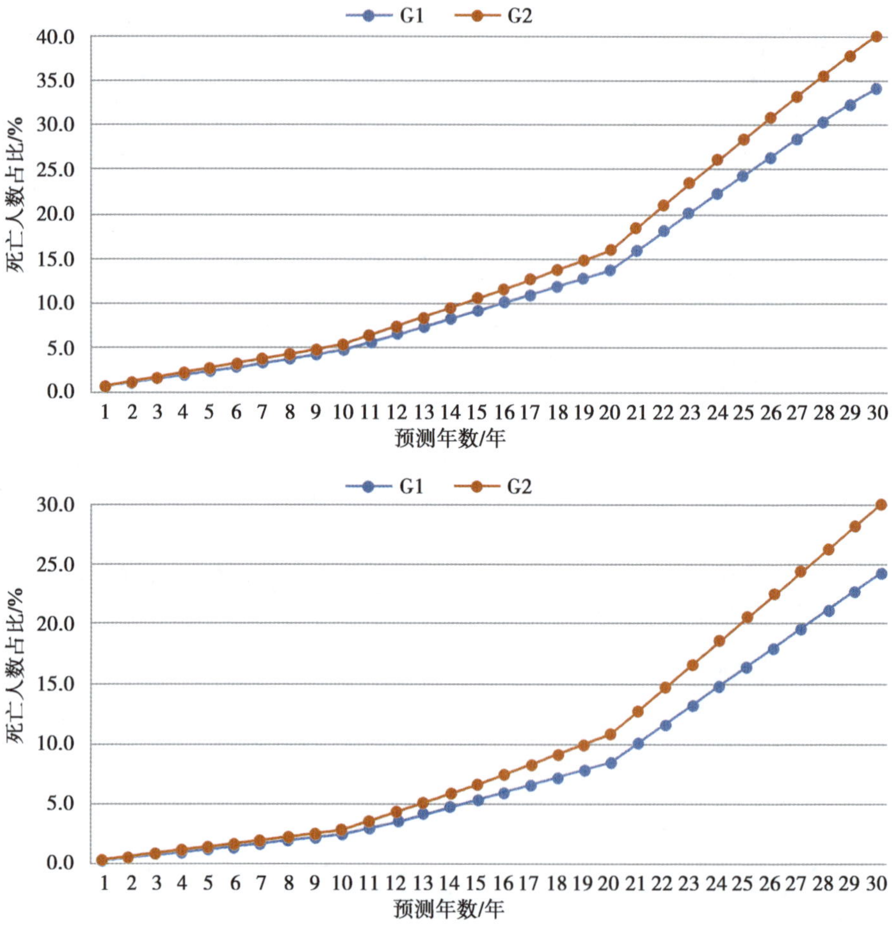

图 B1　45~54 岁年龄组 G1 和 G2 死亡人数占比（男性，上图；女性，下图）

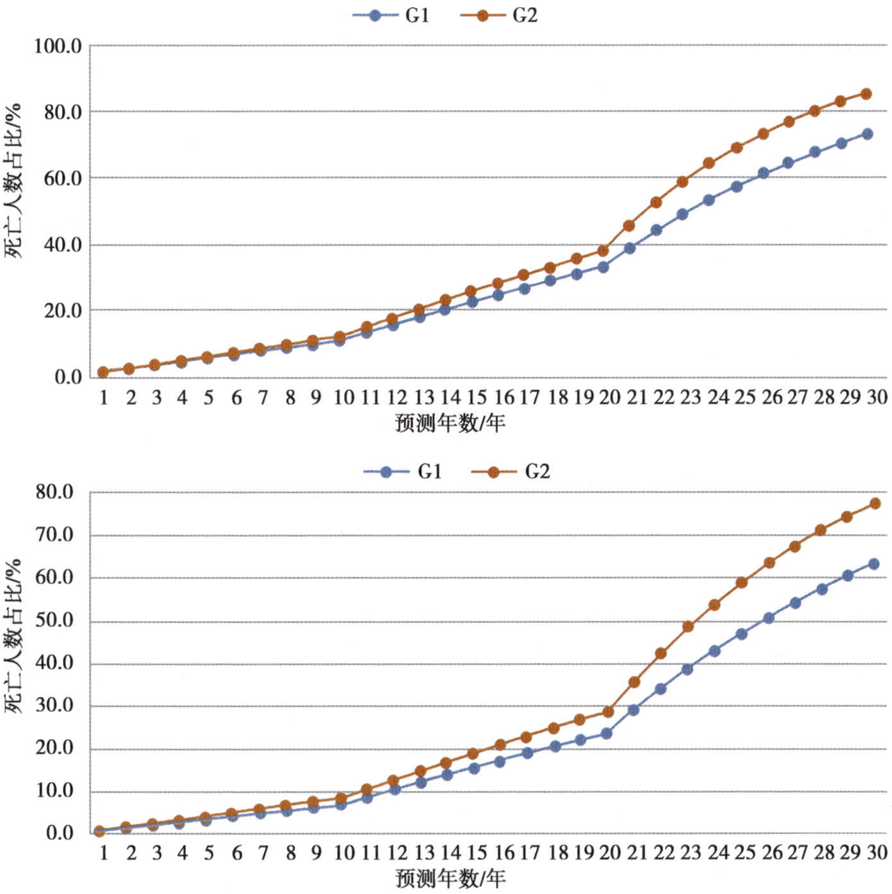

图 B2　55~64 岁年龄组 G1 和 G2 死亡人数占比（男性，上图；女性，下图）

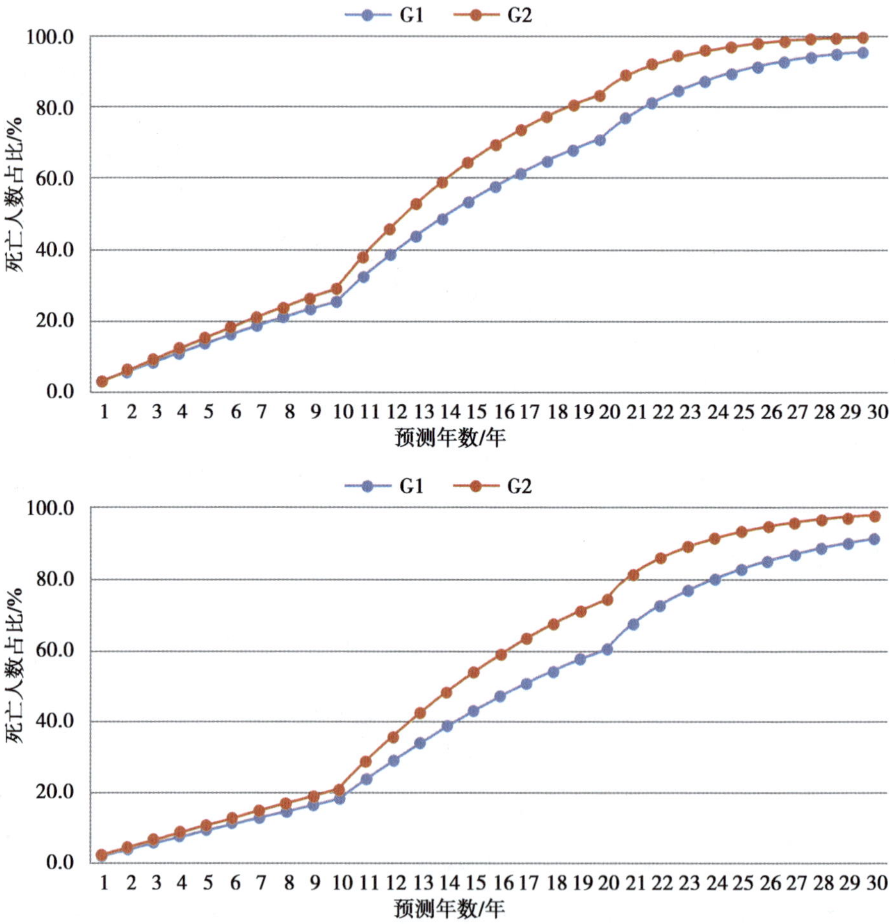

图 B3　65~74 岁年龄组 G1 和 G2 死亡人数占比（男性，上图；女性，下图）

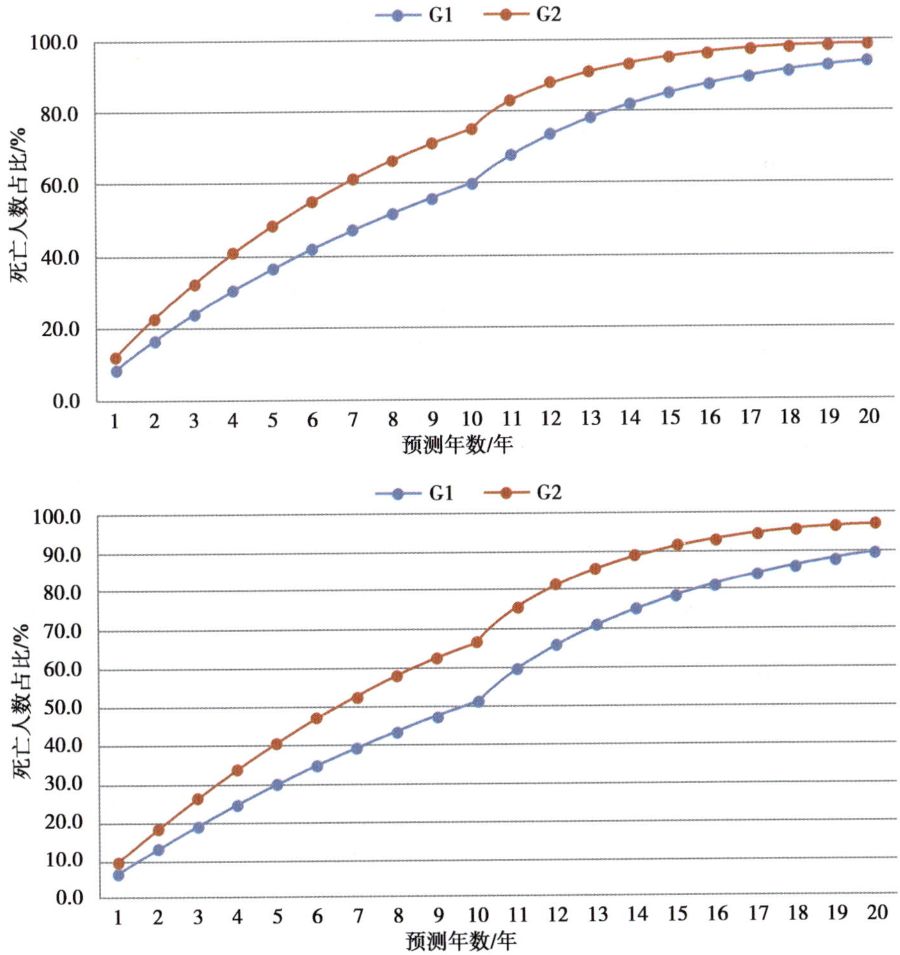

图 B4　75~84 岁年龄组 G1 和 G2 死亡人数占比（男性，上图；女性，下图）

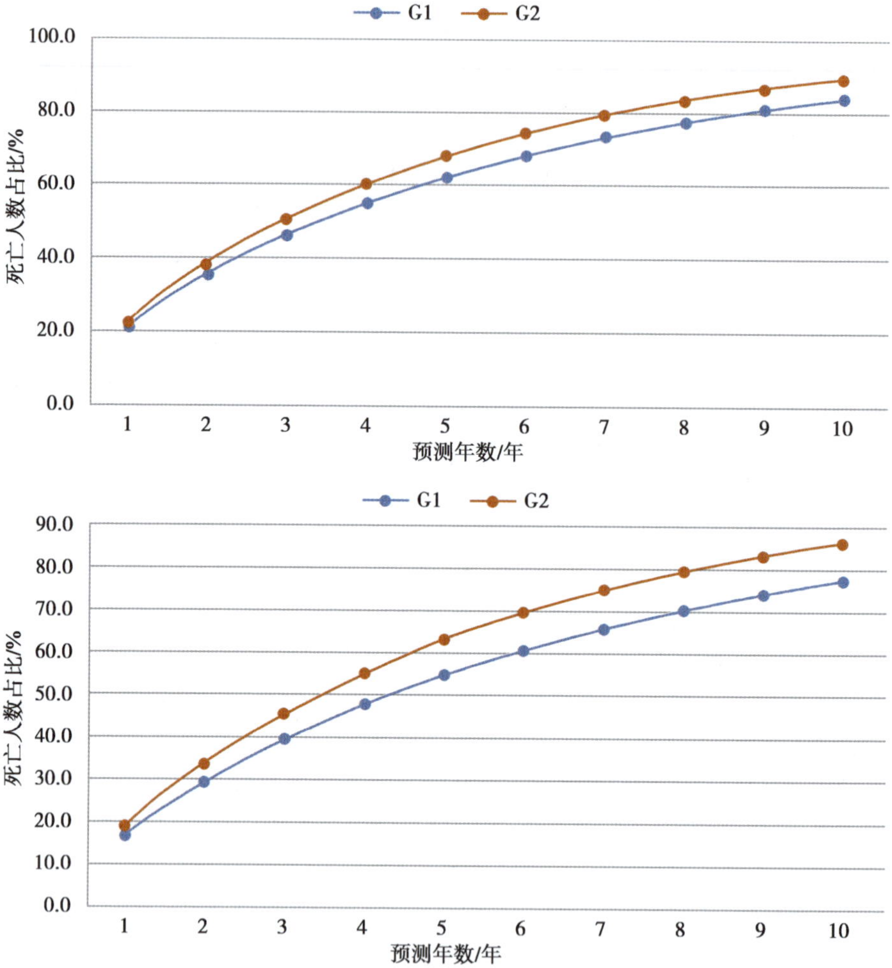

图 B5　84+岁年龄组 G1 和 G2 死亡人数占比（男性，上图；女性，下图）

附录 C　第五章主要过程性数据

在表 C1 中，高血压指单纯高血压，冠心病指高血压合并冠心病，脑卒中指高血压合并脑卒中。

表 C1　两组高血压患者性别年龄别 30 年预测期末累计患病概率　　单位：人年

分组	项目实施情境（血压得到控制）			项目未实施情境（血压未得到控制）		
	单纯高血压	冠心病	脑卒中	单纯高血压	冠心病	脑卒中
男性/岁						
35~44	38 995 672	27 995	1 383 296	37 275 289	57 935	2 354 312
45~54	78 488 850	70 185	5 150 234	73 006 122	153 108	8 442 201
55~64	62 237 009	74 190	9 025 025	57 005 290	152 649	11 803 038
65~74	23 815 907	33 350	4 940 132	21 392 395	69 469	6 020 998
75~84	2 854 003	5 164	604 500	2 568 392	10 365	705 204
85+	19 126	44	4 028	18 115	79	4 401
女性/岁						
35~44	28 232 339	9 984	605 057	27 124 297	33 404	1 297 875
45~54	69 464 945	61 294	3 769 957	62 434 246	161 475	8 068 701
55~64	75 686 346	122 564	10 214 433	61 836 177	283 756	17 756 172
65~74	27 049 344	64 610	6 100 186	20 073 023	135 737	9 370 996
75~84	4 193 453	11 759	937 886	2 942 426	28 158	1 402 902
85+	29 168	87	5 621	23 291	240	7 896

注：考虑到参数不可获得和我国人口平均预期寿命，75~84 岁和 85 岁及以上年龄组患者的预测期限分别为 20 年和 10 年。

表 C2　基于 CHNS 2015 年调查估算各性别年龄组高血压患者平均年龄

分组	例数	平均值	标准差	分组	例数	平均值	标准差
男性/岁				女性/岁			
35~44	39	41.10	2.761	35~44	36	41.06	2.540
45~54	154	50.06	2.705	45~54	168	50.61	2.606
55~64	296	60.10	2.715	55~64	331	60.34	2.674
65~74	310	69.06	2.824	65~74	337	68.89	2.720
75~84	104	78.23	2.735	75~84	150	78.68	2.781
85+	15	87.33	2.127	85+	17	87.53	21.25

注：* 考虑到参数不可获得和我国人口平均预期寿命，75~84 岁和 85 岁及以上年龄组患者的预测期限分别为 20 年和 10 年。

表 C3-1　项目实施和未实施两种情境下各年龄组预测年份死亡差异和年龄（男性）

预测年份	35~44 岁年龄组		45~54 岁年龄组		55~64 岁年龄组		65~74 岁年龄组		75~84 岁年龄组		85 岁~年龄组	
	年龄	人数	年龄	人数	年龄	人数	年龄	人数	年龄	人数	年龄	人数
2016	42	94	51	533	61	1 698	70	2 956	79	13 547	88	1 086
2017	43	102	52	578	62	1 810	71	3 085	80	12 203	89	1 220
2018	44	110	53	620	63	1 913	72	3 176	81	10 603	90	977
2019	45	118	54	661	64	2 006	73	3 233	82	8 911	91	675
2020	46	125	55	700	65	2 090	74	3 260	83	7 237	92	403
2021	47	132	56	737	66	2 166	75	3 260	84	5 650	93	180
2022	48	139	57	772	67	2 233	76	3 237	85	4 193	94	9
2023	49	146	58	805	68	2 292	77	3 194	86	2 888	95	–116
2024	50	153	59	836	69	2 344	78	3 133	87	1 743	96	–203
2025	51	159	60	866	70	2 390	79	3 058	88	758	97	–259
2026	52	379	61	1 663	71	5 921	80	22 089	89	–1 378		
2027	53	395	62	1 735	72	5 865	81	18 769	90	–5 064		
2028	54	411	63	1 800	73	5 775	82	15 453	91	–6 099		
2029	55	425	64	1 858	74	5 656	83	12 289	92	–6 184		
2030	56	439	65	1 909	75	5 512	84	9 368	93	–5 880		
2031	57	452	66	1 954	76	5 346	85	6 738	94	–5 410		
2032	58	464	67	1 993	77	5 163	86	4 420	95	–4 882		
2033	59	476	68	2 027	78	4 966	87	2 415	96	–4 349		
2034	60	487	69	2 055	79	4 756	88	710	97	–3 840		
2035	61	497	70	2 078	80	4 538	89	–715	98	–3 368		
2036	62	851	71	4 963	81	30 424	90	–5 625				
2037	63	881	72	4 874	82	25 215	91	–10 257				
2038	64	908	73	4 762	83	20 212	92	–11 421				
2039	65	931	74	4 630	84	15 569	93	–11 260				
2040	66	952	75	4 482	85	11 373	94	–10 541				
2041	67	970	76	4 320	86	7 661	95	–9 594				
2042	68	985	77	4 146	87	4 438	96	–8 583				
2043	69	997	78	3 963	88	1 690	97	–7 590				
2044	70	1 008	79	3 774	89	–616	98	–6 658				
2045	71	1 016	80	3 579	90	–2 515	99	–5 807				

注：计算过程中负值按照 0 处理。

表 C3-2 项目实施和未实施两种情境下各年龄组预测年份死亡差异和年龄（女性）

预测年份	35~44 岁年龄组		45~54 岁年龄组		55~64 岁年龄组		65~74 岁年龄组		75~84 岁年龄组		85 岁~年龄组	
	年龄	人数	年龄	人数	年龄	人数	年龄	人数	年龄	人数	年龄	人数
2016	42	14	52	332	61	2 043	70	2 307	80	14 376	89	2 662
2017	43	14	53	353	62	2 205	71	2 451	81	13 441	90	2 942
2018	44	15	54	374	63	2 355	72	2 569	82	12 233	91	2 551
2019	45	15	55	394	64	2 493	73	2 663	83	10 871	92	1 956
2020	46	16	56	413	65	2 621	74	2 736	84	9 445	93	1 352
2021	47	16	57	432	66	2 738	75	2 788	85	8 017	94	814
2022	48	17	58	450	67	2 845	76	2 823	86	6 634	95	367
2023	49	17	59	468	68	2 943	77	2 841	87	5 326	96	14
2024	50	18	60	486	69	3 031	78	2 844	88	4 111	97	−254
2025	51	18	61	503	70	3 111	79	2 834	89	3 002	98	−450
2026	52	113	62	1 744	71	5 313	80	22 187	90	2 262		
2027	53	120	63	1 843	72	5 274	81	19 909	91	−2 111		
2028	54	126	64	1 935	73	5 216	82	17 477	92	−4 417		
2029	55	132	65	2 020	74	5 141	83	15 013	93	−5 572		
2030	56	138	66	2 097	75	5 051	84	12 603	94	−6 059		
2031	57	144	67	2 167	76	4 946	85	10 306	95	−6 148		
2032	58	150	68	2 230	77	4 831	86	8 161	96	−6 002		
2033	59	155	69	2 288	78	4 704	87	6 192	97	−5 719		
2034	60	161	70	2 339	79	4 569	88	4 409	98	−5 361		
2035	61	166	71	2 384	80	4 427	89	2 816	99	−4 966		
2036	62	562	72	4 017	81	29 393	90	454				
2037	63	594	73	3 958	82	25 698	91	−5 405				
2038	64	623	74	3 887	83	21 988	92	−8 446				
2039	65	649	75	3 807	84	18 383	93	−9 869				
2040	66	673	76	3 717	85	14 964	94	−10 342				
2041	67	695	77	3 620	86	11 784	95	−10 257				
2042	68	715	78	3 516	87	8 874	96	−9 850				
2043	69	733	79	3 407	88	6 246	97	−9 266				
2044	70	749	80	3 292	89	3 904	98	−8 595				
2045	71	763	81	3 174	90	1 842	99	−7 893				

表 C4-1　项目实施和未实施两种情境下各年龄组预测年份冠心病患者差异和年龄（男性）

预测年份	35~44 岁年龄组		45~54 岁年龄组		55~64 岁年龄组		65~74 岁年龄组		75~84 岁年龄组		85 岁~年龄组	
	年龄	人数	年龄	人数	年龄	人数	年龄	人数	年龄	人数	年龄	人数
2016	42	428	51	799	61	1 370	70	1 735	79	4 783	88	405
2017	43	854	52	1 586	62	2 677	71	3 302	80	8 189	89	648
2018	44	1 276	53	2 361	63	3 925	72	4 714	81	10 510	90	777
2019	45	1 695	54	3 123	64	5 114	73	5 981	82	11 981	91	825
2020	46	2 111	55	3 874	65	6 247	74	7 114	83	12 795	92	820
2021	47	2 523	56	4 613	66	7 326	75	8 121	84	13 105	93	781
2022	48	2 933	57	5 341	67	8 353	76	9 013	85	13 035	94	721
2023	49	3 340	58	6 056	68	9 328	77	9 798	86	12 685	95	650
2024	50	3 743	59	6 761	69	10 255	78	10 483	87	12 132	96	575
2025	51	4 144	60	7 454	70	11 134	79	11 077	88	11 440	97	501
2026	52	4 501	61	8 442	71	12 882	80	15 999	89	9 207		
2027	53	4 853	62	9 381	72	14 430	81	19 231	90	7 350		
2028	54	5 199	63	10 274	73	15 794	82	21 148	91	5 814		
2029	55	5 540	64	11 123	74	16 988	83	22 055	92	4 550		
2030	56	5 875	65	11 928	75	18 024	84	22 194	93	3 515		
2031	57	6 204	66	12 692	76	18 914	85	21 762	94	2 672		
2032	58	6 528	67	13 415	77	19 669	86	20 915	95	1 991		
2033	59	6 847	68	14 100	78	20 301	87	19 777	96	1 444		
2034	60	7 161	69	14 746	79	20 818	88	18 445	97	1 009		
2035	61	7 469	70	15 357	80	21 230	89	16 995	98	665		
2036	62	7 896	71	16 540	81	26 675	90	13 384				
2037	63	8 301	72	17 572	82	30 006	91	10 425				
2038	64	8 684	73	18 464	83	31 707	92	8 014				
2039	65	9 047	74	19 227	84	32 170	93	6 059				
2040	66	9 390	75	19 870	85	31 706	94	4 485				
2041	67	9 713	76	20 404	86	30 566	95	3 227				
2042	68	10 018	77	20 836	87	28 946	96	2 228				
2043	69	10 305	78	21 176	88	27 004	97	1 443				
2044	70	10 574	79	21 430	89	24 861	98	832				
2045	71	10 826	80	21 605	90	22 612	99	364				

表 C4-2 项目实施和未实施两种情境下各年龄组预测年份冠心病患者差异和年龄（女性）

预测年份	35~44 岁年龄组		45~54 岁年龄组		55~64 岁年龄组		65~74 岁年龄组		75~84 岁年龄组		85 岁~年龄组	
	年龄	人数	年龄	人数	年龄	人数	年龄	人数	年龄	人数	年龄	人数
2016	42	17	52	156	61	588	70	623	80	3 140	89	739
2017	43	33	53	309	62	1 148	71	1 197	81	5 442	90	1 207
2018	44	50	54	461	63	1 680	72	1 724	82	7 058	91	1 475
2019	45	67	55	610	64	2 185	73	2 208	83	8 114	92	1 599
2020	46	83	56	758	65	2 664	74	2 649	84	8 718	93	1 620
2021	47	100	57	903	66	3 117	75	3 052	85	8 960	94	1 571
2022	48	116	58	1 047	67	3 547	76	3 417	86	8 914	95	1 476
2023	49	132	59	1 189	68	3 952	77	3 747	87	8 644	96	1 353
2024	50	149	60	1 329	69	4 335	78	4 045	88	8 203	97	1 215
2025	51	165	61	1 467	70	4 695	79	4 311	89	7 634	98	1 072
2026	52	214	62	1 850	71	5 220	80	7 539	90	6 354		
2027	53	262	63	2 213	72	5 692	81	9 757	91	5 186		
2028	54	310	64	2 557	73	6 114	82	11 156	92	4 138		
2029	55	357	65	2 884	74	6 489	83	11 894	93	3 210		
2030	56	403	66	3 192	75	6 819	84	12 107	94	2 399		
2031	57	449	67	3 483	76	7 109	85	11 905	95	1 698		
2032	58	494	68	3 757	77	7 359	86	11 383	96	1 101		
2033	59	539	69	4 015	78	7 573	87	10 618	97	597		
2034	60	583	70	4 258	79	7 752	88	9 674	98	178		
2035	61	626	71	4 485	80	7 900	89	8 605	99	−166		
2036	62	746	72	4 805	81	11 029	90	6 754				
2037	63	861	73	5 089	82	12 993	91	5 114				
2038	64	969	74	5 339	83	14 021	92	3 680				
2039	65	1 071	75	5 559	84	14 304	93	2 445				
2040	66	1 168	76	5 748	85	14 001	94	1 393				
2041	67	1 259	77	5 910	86	13 247	95	510				
2042	68	1 345	78	6 046	87	12 152	96	−221				
2043	69	1 426	79	6 158	88	10 808	97	−816				
2044	70	1 502	80	6 247	89	9 290	98	−1 291				
2045	71	1 573	81	6 315	90	7 660	99	−1 662				

表 C4-3　项目实施和未实施两种情境下各年龄组预测年份脑卒中患者差异和年龄（男性）

预测年份	35~44 岁年龄组		45~54 岁年龄组		55~64 岁年龄组		65~74 岁年龄组		75~84 岁年龄组		85 岁~年龄组	
	年龄	人数	年龄	人数	年龄	人数	年龄	人数	年龄	人数	年龄	人数
2016	42	109	51	1 448	61	8 365	70	8 412	79	11 160	88	870
2017	43	216	52	2 875	62	16 389	71	16 072	80	19 352	89	1 408
2018	44	323	53	4 282	63	24 080	72	23 031	81	25 181	90	1 709
2019	45	430	54	5 669	64	31 451	73	29 335	82	29 138	91	1 842
2020	46	535	55	7 035	65	38 510	74	35 030	83	31 626	92	1 860
2021	47	640	56	8 382	66	45 268	75	40 157	84	32 968	93	1 802
2022	48	744	57	9 710	67	51 733	76	44 756	85	33 427	94	1 695
2023	49	848	58	11 018	68	57 916	77	48 864	86	33 214	95	1 561
2024	50	950	59	12 307	69	63 824	78	52 514	87	32 500	96	1 413
2025	51	1 052	60	13 577	70	69 467	79	55 740	88	31 420	97	1 262
2026	52	1 726	61	19 949	71	78 047	80	66 254	89	26 258		
2027	53	2 391	62	26 055	72	85 725	81	73 147	90	21 879		
2028	54	3 045	63	31 901	73	92 565	82	77 203	91	18 177		
2029	55	3 691	64	37 497	74	98 626	83	79 054	92	15 055		
2030	56	4 327	65	42 850	75	103 964	84	79 213	93	12 430		
2031	57	4 953	66	47 969	76	108 630	85	78 093	94	10 230		
2032	58	5 571	67	52 860	77	112 675	86	76 025	95	8 391		
2033	59	6 179	68	57 530	78	116 144	87	73 273	96	6 858		
2034	60	6 779	69	61 987	79	119 080	88	70 048	97	5 583		
2035	61	7 369	70	66 238	80	121 524	89	66 515	98	4 527		
2036	62	10 343	71	72 578	81	131 652	90	55 427				
2037	63	13 191	72	78 220	82	137 307	91	46 092				
2038	64	15 917	73	83 215	83	139 494	92	38 249				
2039	65	18 526	74	87 608	84	139 027	93	31 673				
2040	66	21 020	75	91 443	85	136 559	94	26 170				
2041	67	23 405	76	94 761	86	132 617	95	21 573				
2042	68	25 682	77	97 601	87	127 620	96	17 741				
2043	69	27 856	78	99 998	88	121 901	97	14 554				
2044	70	29 930	79	101 987	89	115 722	98	11 907				
2045	71	31 907	80	103 598	90	109 290	99	9 714				

表 C4-4　项目实施和未实施两种情境下各年龄组预测年份脑卒中患者差异和年龄（女性）

预测年份	35~44 岁年龄组		45~54 岁龄组		55~64 岁年龄组		65~74 岁年龄组		75~84 岁年龄组		85 岁~年龄组	
	年龄	人数	年龄	人数	年龄	人数	年龄	人数	年龄	人数	年龄	人数
2016	42	43	52	1 742	61	10 362	70	7 335	80	13 574	89	2 314
2017	43	87	53	3 467	62	20 359	71	14 163	81	24 308	90	3 861
2018	44	130	54	5 175	63	30 002	72	20 513	82	32 661	91	4 829
2019	45	173	55	6 868	64	39 299	73	26 407	83	39 026	92	5 368
2020	46	216	56	8 543	65	48 260	74	31 870	84	43 735	93	5 591
2021	47	259	57	10 203	66	56 895	75	36 924	85	47 073	94	5 588
2022	48	302	58	11 847	67	65 211	76	41 592	86	49 279	95	5 427
2023	49	344	59	13 474	68	73 218	77	45 893	87	50 556	96	5 160
2024	50	387	60	15 086	69	80 924	78	49 846	88	51 078	97	4 827
2025	51	430	61	16 682	70	88 338	79	53 472	89	50 989	98	4 457
2026	52	982	62	23 693	71	94 939	80	67 971	90	45 492		
2027	53	1 528	63	30 452	72	100 983	81	78 969	91	40 389		
2028	54	2 070	64	36 967	73	106 500	82	87 054	92	35 700		
2029	55	2 606	65	43 243	74	111 518	83	92 723	93	31 427		
2030	56	3 137	66	49 287	75	116 065	84	96 399	94	27 563		
2031	57	3 663	67	55 106	76	120 167	85	98 441	95	24 089		
2032	58	4 184	68	60 706	77	123 849	86	99 152	96	20 983		
2033	59	4 699	69	66 092	78	127 136	87	98 787	97	18 219		
2034	60	5 210	70	71 271	79	130 049	88	97 563	98	15 772		
2035	61	5 716	71	76 248	80	132 611	89	95 661	99	13 612		
2036	62	7 938	72	80 438	81	146 777	90	84 513				
2037	63	10 081	73	84 250	82	156 836	91	74 418				
2038	64	12 146	74	87 705	83	163 499	92	65 329				
2039	65	14 135	75	90 824	84	167 371	93	57 187				
2040	66	16 051	76	93 625	85	168 964	94	49 925				
2041	67	17 895	77	96 125	86	168 709	95	43 475				
2042	68	19 669	78	98 343	87	166 971	96	37 766				
2043	69	21 376	79	100 295	88	164 057	97	32 729				
2044	70	23 016	80	101 995	89	160 225	98	28 299				
2045	71	24 593	81	103 460	90	155 690	99	24 415				

附录 D　性别年龄别高血压控制状况和投入产出与成本效益再分析

1. 1991—2009 年高血压控制率趋势分析

应用拉格朗日插值法，将 1991—2009 年各年龄组数值进行插值完善，结果见表 D1。

表 D1　按照拉格朗日插值法完善的 1991—2009 年各个年龄组血压控制率数据

单位：%

年份	控制率				
	35~44 岁	45~54 岁	55~64 岁	65~74 岁	75+岁
1991	2.62	2.43	4.55	2.44	2.54
1992	1.86	2.60	5.58	2.41	2.48
1993	1.55	2.67	5.62	2.50	2.52
1994	1.59	2.68	5.00	2.74	2.65
1995	1.87	2.67	4.06	3.14	2.86
1996	2.26	2.70	3.12	3.75	3.14
1997	2.67	2.82	2.51	4.59	3.47
1998	2.71	3.19	3.41	5.96	3.77
1999	2.75	3.66	4.63	7.39	4.15
2000	2.81	4.21	6.00	8.74	4.65
2001	3.22	4.90	6.98	9.29	5.74
2002	3.65	5.61	7.88	9.67	6.87
2003	4.00	6.32	8.68	10.03	7.85
2004	4.17	6.97	9.38	10.52	9.38
2005	3.81	7.50	7.78	11.55	8.30
2006	3.58	7.91	10.50	12.47	8.50
2007	3.68	8.15	10.55	13.13	7.93
2008	4.32	8.21	11.01	13.34	8.16
2009	5.69	8.03	12.02	12.96	8.92

由于趋势分析的数据少于 20，所以研究使用了小样本时间序列分析，小样本不连续数据使用拉格朗日插值法进行完善，形成连续性数据。利用 SPSS 22.0 统计软件，进行了时间序列预测分析。根据专家模型法和模型数据，利用差分自回归移动平均（autoregressive integrated moving average，ARIMA）模型（35~44 岁年龄组和 65~74 岁年龄组，2、0、1；其他年龄组 1、0、1）进行线性趋势预测分析，结果见表 D2。

残差自相关函数（auto-correlation function，ACF）结果显示，数据呈现随机分布，没有离群值（异常值），表明模型具有较好的拟合优度（附录 B）。

表 D2　不同年龄组高血压控制率时间序列预测分析模型数据与结果

Control-模型-1	预测目标数	模型拟合		Ljung-Box Q（18）			异常值（离群值）/个数
		静态 R^2 值	R^2 值	统计值	自由度	P 值	
35~44	1	0.736	0.955	3.410	3	0.333	0
45~54	1	0.984	0.984	39.293	16	0.001	0
55~64	1	0.882	0.882	11.618	16	0.770	0
65~74	1	0.995	0.995	26.241	15	0.036	0
75+	1	0.949	0.949	18.986	16	0.269	0

利用 1991—2009 年数据建立的模型得出 2010—2015 年高血压控制率的预测值，包括预测区间上限值和下限值。按照 1991—2009 年的趋势估计，2015 年 35~44 岁年龄组高血压患者血压控制率将是 11.64%［95%*CI*（8.34%，14.93%）］；45~54 岁将是 10.39%［95%*CI*（8.99%，11.79%）］；55~64 岁将是 13.79%［95%*CI*（10.28%，17.29%）］；65~74 岁将是 17.60%［95%*CI*（15.57%，19.64%）］；75 岁及以上将是 12.04%［ 95%*CI*（10.11%，13.96%）］。详见表 D3 和图 D1~D5。

表 D3　2010—2015 年基于预测模型得到不同年龄组高血压控制率预测值

单位：%

年龄组	模型结果	2010 年	2011 年	2012 年	2013 年	2014 年	2015 年
35~44	预测值	7.34	8.82	9.88	10.54	11.03	11.64
	UCL	6.85	7.58	7.84	7.86	7.94	8.34
	LCL	7.83	10.06	11.91	13.21	14.11	14.93

续表

年龄组	模型结果	2010 年	2011 年	2012 年	2013 年	2014 年	2015 年
45~54	预测值	8.11	8.58	9.04	9.50	9.95	10.39
	UCL	7.71	7.75	7.98	8.29	8.63	8.99
	LCL	8.51	9.41	10.10	10.71	11.27	11.79
55~64	预测值	12.25	12.47	12.74	13.06	13.41	13.79
	UCL	9.98	9.52	9.50	9.67	9.95	10.28
	LCL	14.52	15.41	15.99	16.45	16.88	17.29
65~74	预测值	12.74	13.01	13.79	14.96	16.31	17.60
	UCL	12.14	11.77	12.06	12.99	14.28	15.57
	LCL	13.33	14.25	15.52	16.94	18.34	19.64
75+	预测值	9.56	10.12	10.63	11.11	11.58	12.04
	UCL	8.26	8.41	8.79	9.22	9.66	10.11
	LCL	10.87	11.82	12.47	13.01	13.50	13.96

注：UCL 表示预测值区间上限值；LCL 表示预测值区间下限值。

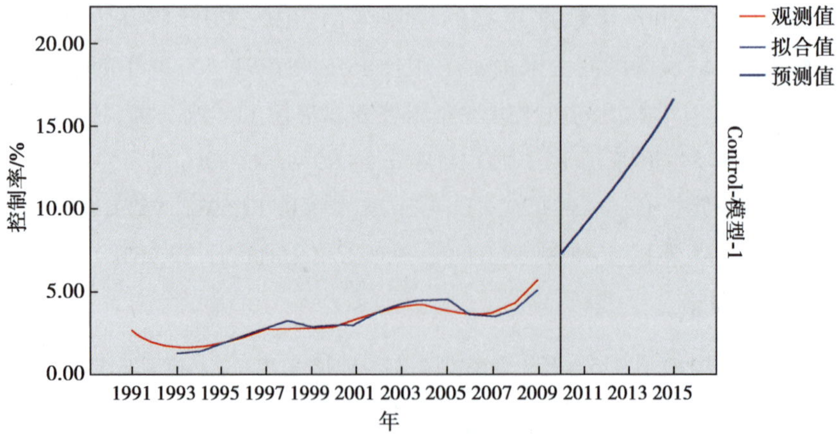

图 D1　2010—2015 年 35~44 岁年龄组高血压患者血压控制率预测示意图（基于 1991—2009 年数据）

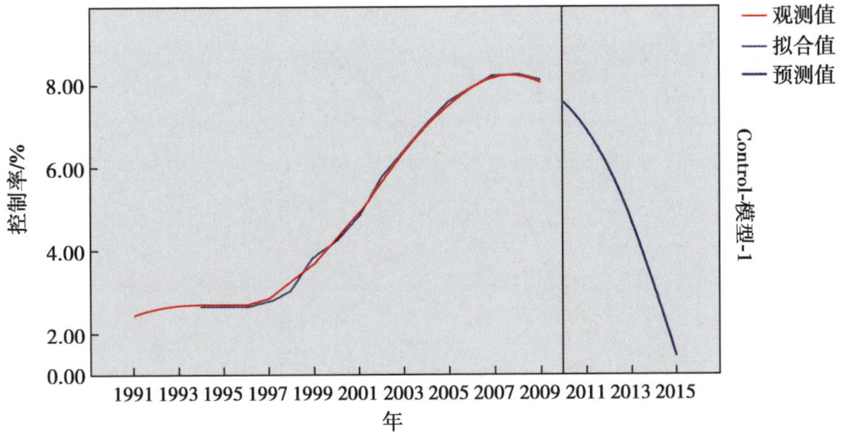

图 D2　2010—2015 年 45~54 岁年龄组高血压患者血压控制率预测示意图（基于 1991—2009 年数据）

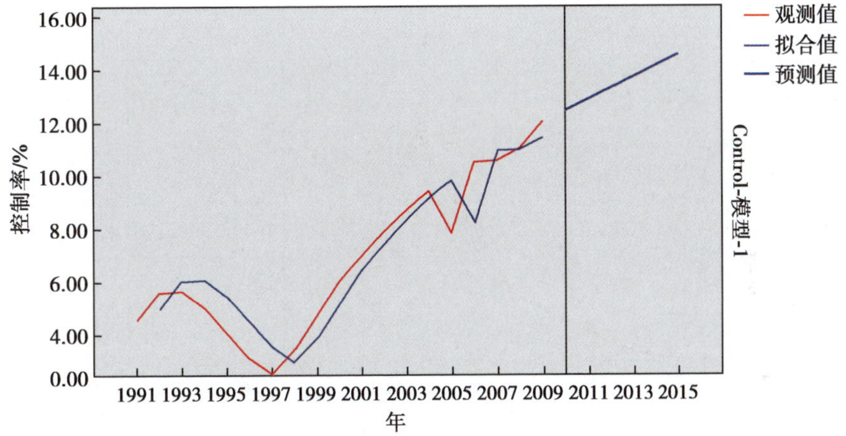

图 D3　2010—2015 年 55~64 岁年龄组高血压患者血压控制率预测示意图（基于 1991—2009 年数据）

2. 国家基本公共卫生服务项目高血压控制率的估计

根据 2012—2015 年中国高血压调查数据，35 岁及以上成人高血压患病率是 32.62%（Z. Wang et al.，2018）。表 D3 分别列出 2015 年高血压患者血压控制率的预测值和实际值。基于同样的人口数据和方法，据估算，2009—2015 年国家基本公共卫生服务项目的实施，对 35~44 岁年龄组、45~54 岁年龄组、55~64 岁年龄组、65~74 岁年龄组和 75 岁及以上年龄组的男性成人高血压

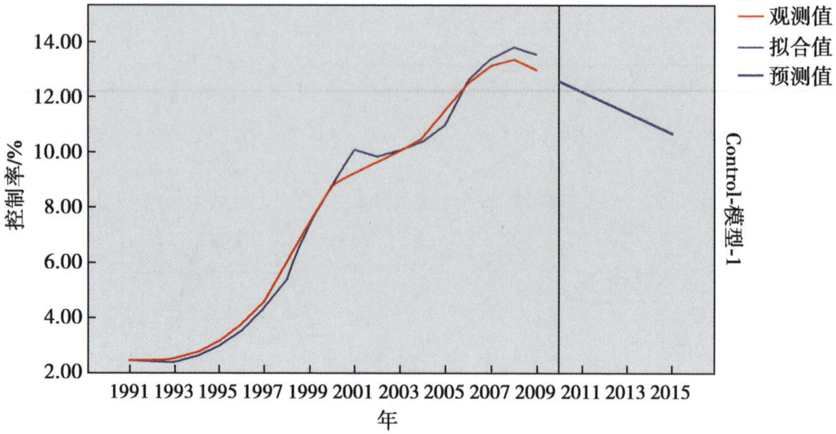

图 D4　2010—2015 年 65~74 岁年龄组高血压患者血压控制率预测示意图（基于 1991—2009 年数据）

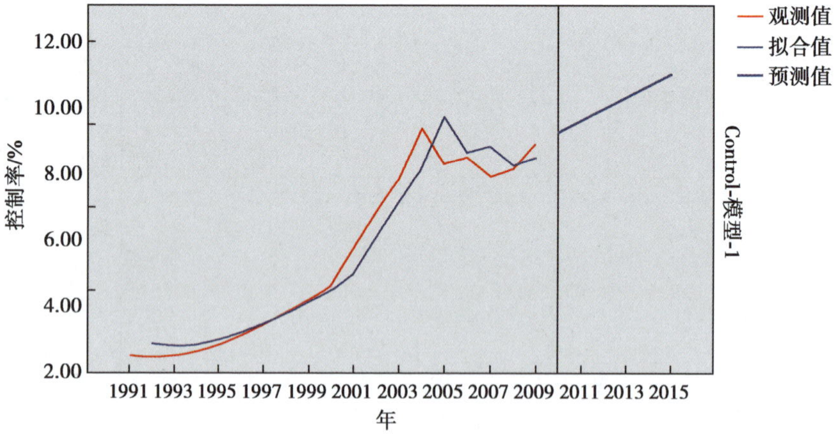

图 D5　2010—2015 年 75 岁及以上年龄组高血压患者血压控制率预测示意图（基于 1991—2009 年数据）

患者血压控制人数将分别增加 0、1 635 397、1 564 164、170 388 和 617 939 人，女性分别增加 0、1 568 221、1 523 002、169 167 和 761 170 人。国家基本公共卫生服务项目实施增加的血压控制总人数为 8 009 449（1 581 856，13 065 018）人。详见表 D4。

3. 心血管疾病患者和死亡人数减少分年龄估计值

在项目实施情境下，与项目未实施情境相比，在 10 年预测期末减少的冠

表 D4　国家基本公共卫生服务项目实施高血压控制人数估计值
（中国高血压调查 2012—2015 年）

分组	人口数	患病率/%	高血压控制值实际值/%	高血压控制值预测值/%	增加的高血压控制人数/例（95%*CI*）
男性/岁					
35~44	127 459 929	15.90	9.90	11.64	0* （–1 019 386，316 152）
45~54	96 759 903	29.60	16.10	10.39	1 635 397 （1 234 424，2 036 370）
55~64	72 912 562	44.60	18.60	13.79	1 564 164 （425 999，2 705 581）
65~74	38 237 979	55.70	18.40	17.6	170 388 （–264 102，602 749）
75+	20 695 107	60.20	17.00	12.04	617 939 （378 737，858 388）
女性/岁					
35~44	122 114 836	15.90	9.90	5.1	0** （–976 638，302 894）
45~54	92 785 346	29.60	16.10	10.39	1 568 221 （1 183 718，1 953 723）
55~64	70 993 810	44.60	18.60	13.79	1 523 002 （414 788，2 634 382）
65~74	37 963 871	55.70	18.40	17.6	169 167 （–262 209，598 428）
75+	25 491 986	60.20	17.00	12.04	761 170 （466 524，1 057 351）
合计	705 415 330	N/A	N/A	N/A	8 009 449 （1 581 856，13 065 018）

注：N/A 表示不适用；* 实际值为–352 631，为了让其符合现实负值均改为 0；** 实际值为–337 843，为了让其符合现实负值均改为 0。

心病、脑卒中和死亡人数分别为 34 198、262 071 和 284 796 人；在 20 年预测期末，减少的冠心病、脑卒中和死亡人数分别为 41 632、380 448 和 355 955 人；在 30 年预测期末，减少的冠心病、脑卒中和死亡人数分别为 23 476、306 955 和 697 204 人。具体结果见表 D5~D7。在表 D7 中，30 年预测期末时

表 D5　10 年预测结果

分组	项目实施情境			项目未实施情境			减少的心血管疾病和死亡人数		
	冠心病	脑卒中	死亡	冠心病	脑卒中	死亡	冠心病	脑卒中	死亡
男性/岁									
35~44	0	0	0	0	0	0	0	0	0
45~54	28 028	58 081	74 940	36 894	74 975	84 533	8 866	16 895	9 593
55~64	54 048	175 359	164 325	63 991	241 358	185 745	9 942	65 999	21 420
65~74	6 787	23 312	43 431	8 284	31 636	48 917	1 498	8 325	5 486
75~84	14 880	38 654	367 123	19 243	62 137	461 696	4 363	23 482	94 573
85+	0	0	0	0	0	0	0	0	0
女性/岁									
35~44	0	0	0	0	0	0	0	0	0
45~54	22 406	54 314	36 259	24 454	77 383	42 386	2 048	23 069	6 127
55~64	52 134	150 108	102 949	56 438	229 354	129 034	4 304	79 246	26 085
65~74	5 883	22 877	30 395	6 460	30 180	34 721	578	7 303	4 326
75~84	21 925	52 314	387 116	24 525	90 065	504 302	2 599	37 751	117 186
85+	0	0	0	0	0	0	0	0	0
合计	206 091	575 018	1 206 538	240 289	837 089	1 491 334	34 198	262 071	284 796

表 D6　20 年预测结果

分组	项目实施情境			项目未实施情境			减少的心血管疾病和死亡人数		
	冠心病	脑卒中	死亡	冠心病	脑卒中	死亡	冠心病	脑卒中	死亡
男性/岁									
35~44	0	0	0	0	0	0	0	0	0
45~54	37 774	117 997	223 107	53 930	198 647	258 446	16 156	80 650	35 339
55~64	50 749	180 250	512 768	65 212	276 766	588 904	14 463	96 517	76 136
65~74	2 908	8 579	119 758	3 377	13 368	141 137	469	4 788	21 379
75~84	648	2 350	577 566	269	1 608	607 277	−378	−741	29 711
85+	0	0	0	0	0	0	0	0	0
女性/岁									
35~44	0	0	0	0	0	0	0	0	0
45~54	31 915	125 437	130 749	37 784	223 040	167 533	5 869	97 603	36 783
55~64	46 528	196 755	358 829	52 158	292 013	433 827	5 630	95 258	74 998
65~74	3 626	10 721	101 975	3 766	17 627	125 479	140	6 905	23 504
75~84	1 418	4 434	678 536	701	3 902	736 641	−717	−532	58 105
85+	0	0	0	0	0	0	0	0	0
合计	175 566	646 523	2 703 289	217 197	1 026 971	3 059 245	41 632	380 448	355 955

表 D7　30 年预测结果

分组	项目实施情境			项目未实施情境			减少的心血管疾病和死亡人数		
	冠心病	脑卒中	死亡	冠心病	脑卒中	死亡	冠心病	脑卒中	死亡
男性/岁									
35~44	0	0	0	0	0	0	0	0	0
45~54	44 586	152 647	557 423	61 918	258 449	651 470	17 332	105 801	94 047
55~64	24 109	69 487	1 139 026	26 293	109 558	1 331 195	2 185	40 071	192 168
65~74	128	472	162 371	45	289	168 586	−84	−183	6 215
75~84	648	2 350	577 566	269	1 608	607 277	−378	−741	29 711
85+	0	0	0	0	0	0	0	0	0
女性/岁									
35~44	0	0	0	0	0	0	0	0	0
45~54	35 127	186 822	378 264	41 445	292 405	468 063	6 318	105 583	89 798
55~64	30 054	90 911	959 687	29 015	148 021	1 176 142	−1 039	57 110	216 455
65~74	250	794	154 590	110	640	165 295	−140	−154	10 705
75~84	1 418	4 434	678 536	701	3 902	736 641	−717	−532	58 105
85+	0	0	0	0	0	0	0	0	0
合计	136 320	507 917	4 607 465	159 796	814 872	5 304 669	23 476	306 955	697 204

较大年龄组有一些负值（65~74 岁和 75~84 岁年龄组）。这是因为在项目未实施情境下，更多高血压患者死于心血管疾病，因此患者总人数减少，特别是脑卒中患者。该结果也进一步验证了第 4 章的分析结果。

4. 效益成本比和投资回报率再分析

在正文中，按照中国高血压调查 2012—2015 年数据进行全年龄组分析。按照 3% 的贴现率，高血压患者管理成本占国家基本公共卫生服务项目经费的 14.59%，只考虑经济效益，效益成本比为 6.0。如果包括社会效益，效益成本比为 15.4。内部收益率分别为 14.6% 和 20.7%。

此处，按照中国高血压调查 2012—2015 年数据进行分年龄组分析。按照 3% 的贴现率，高血压患者管理成本占国家基本公共卫生服务项目经费的 14.59%，只考虑经济效益，效益成本比为 5.9。如果包括社会效益，效益成本比为 15.1。内部收益率分别为 14.7% 和 20.4%。详见表 D8 和 D9。

表 D8　不同贴现率下成本和投资回报率数据　　单位：百万元

	0	2%	3%	5%
投资回报率/亿元（95%*CI*）				
GDP- 避免死亡，净现值	321 976（63 590，525 207）	206 498（40 783，336 840）	166 880（32 959，272 215）	110 882（21 899，180 871）
社会效益，净现值	597 498（118 005，974 639）	343 187（67 779，559 807）	263 261（51 994，429 432）	158 597（31 323，258 704）
成本/亿元				
10% 的基本公共卫生服务项目经费	25 526	21 727	19 499	15 837
14.59% 的基本公共卫生服务项目经费	37 243	31 699	28 449	23 107
18% 的基本公共卫生服务项目经费	45 947	39 108	35 099	28 507

表 D9　不同贴现率下效益成本比和内部收益率

单位：%（95%*CI*）

效益成本比	0	2%	3%	5%	内部收益率
按照 18% 的基本公共卫生服务项目经费计算成本					
GDP-避免死亡/成本	7.0（1.38，11.42）	5.3（1.05，8.65）	4.8（0.95，7.83）	3.9（0.77，6.36）	12.9（2.5，21.0）
GDP-死亡避免+社会效益/成本	20.0（3.95，32.62）	14.1（2.78，23.00）	12.3（2.43，20.06）	9.5（1.88，15.50）	18.6（3.7，30.3）
按照 14.59% 的基本公共卫生服务项目经费计算成本					
GDP-避免死亡/成本	8.6（1.70，14.03）	6.5（1.28，10.60）	5.9（1.17，9.62）	4.8（0.95，7.83）	14.7（2.9，24.0）
GDP-死亡避免+社会效益/成本	24.7（4.88，40.29）	17.3（3.42，28.22）	15.1（2.98，24.63）	11.7（2.31，19.09）	20.4（4.0，33.3）
按照 10% 的基本公共卫生服务项目经费计算成本					
GDP-避免死亡/成本	12.6（2.49，20.55）	9.5（1.88，15.50）	8.6（1.70，14.03）	7.0（1.38，11.42）	18.0（3.6，29.4）
GDP-死亡避免+社会效益/成本	36.0（7.11，58.72）	25.3（5.00，41.27）	22.1（4.36，36.05）	17.0（3.36，27.73）	24.0（4.7，39.1）

致　谢

本书完全基于主编 2015—2020 年在澳大利亚维多利亚大学所做的博士论文编译完成。作为主编，我想借此机会为本书编撰致谢如下。

首先，感谢我的主导师——Peter J. Sheehan 教授，他敏锐的洞察力和解决关键问题的能力令人印象深刻。其次，感谢联合导师——Kim Sweeny 博士和秦江梅教授，他们在论文撰写过程中提供了卓具建设性的指导意见和无时无刻的鼓励和帮助。Kim Sweeny 博士是一位优秀的导师，他在经济学和数学建模方面造诣颇深，而且擅长研究论文写作。我永远不会忘记，与 Kim Sweeny 博士一起反复修改完善我的博士论文的时光。秦江梅教授是一位多学科专家，多年来致力于我国卫生政策相关研究，在基层卫生研究方面卓有建树。作为我的直接领导，秦教授不仅为研究提供了关键技术支持，而且创造了重要的工作条件和环境。再次，感谢维多利亚大学战略经济研究中心的 Bruce Rasmussen 主任和 Margarita Kumnick 女士在博士研究期间给予我的支持和帮助。

傅卫主任和张振忠教授，先后作为国家卫生健康委卫生发展研究中心的领导，为我的博士学习和工作提供了重要支持。特别感谢国家卫生健康委卫生发展研究中心的付强主任和甘戈副主任，他们的鼓励和支持为本书的出版提供了必要条件。

在博士研究期间，国家卫生健康委员会办公厅的刘利群副主任、基层卫生健康司的鄂啟顺二级巡视员和陈凯处长，为完善本研究基层卫生改革政策建议提供了指导。本研究多处引用了顾东风院士的相关研究方法与结果，借此对顾院士表示感谢。同时，2018 年时任国家卫生健康委基层卫生健康司基本公卫处处长张并立、北京大学医学部的陈育德教授和武阳丰教授为研究方法和论文完善提供了重要专家建议。

感谢我的同事张丽芳研究员和林春梅助理研究员，在研究过程中提供了精神支持，对中文书稿的编辑作出重要贡献。

孙方红女士及其爱人钟建军先生、女儿单美月女士在我的博士研究期间提供了生活上的帮助和支持。我的爱人柏永生先生、女儿柏一雯作为家庭成员后盾，为研究提供了莫大的精神支持和鼓励；感谢我的父母张清全先生和谢贵明女士，让孩子完成博士论文是我父母的梦想之一。

我深感荣幸结识到上述优秀的导师、领导、老师、同事和家人，你们无私和慷慨的帮助是完成本书的动力和基石。

1 Recapitulate

1.1 Background

Before China adopted the socialist market economy (SME) in the 1980s, its primary healthcare system had led the world in improving the life expectancies of its citizens. Unfortunately, this system encountered many problems, including the reduction of government investment in healthcare, decentralization of public health services and the weakening role of primary healthcare in public health [1-2]. Meanwhile, with the rapid development of society, the prevalence of high risk behaviours, including unhealthy diets, physical inactivity and smoking, accelerated to an unprecedented degree [3]. As a result, the leading cause of mortality in China shifted relatively quickly from infectious diseases and perinatal conditions to non-communicable diseases and injuries [3], also known as non-communicable diseases (NCDs). NCDs mainly include cardiovascular disease (CVD), heart attack and stroke, chronic respiratory diseases (such as chronic obstructed pulmonary disease and asthma), diabetes and cancer [4].

By 2010, there had been 1.7 million deaths in China resulting from stroke, 948, 700 from ischemic heart disease (IHD) and 934, 000 deaths attributed to chronic obstructive pulmonary disease [3, 5]. As estimated by the 2013 *Report of CVD* in China, 70% of strokes and 50% of myocardial infarctions, as the main CVDs, were caused by high blood pressure (BP) [6]. Yang et al. also reported that 24% of Chinese population aged 15+ years were diagnosed with hypertension in 2012 (i.e., 270 million hypertensive patients)[6]. Another risk factor for patients with CVD was diabetes, which was prevalent among 11.6% of Chinese adults in 2010[5].

In recognition of the failure of the prevailing health system, and in order to curb the rapid increase of CVD, the Chinese Central Government introduced a new healthcare reform plan in 2009 [7]. This was designed to improve the primary healthcare system in both essential medical care and public health service provision. One important part of the reform was the program entitled the National Basic Public Health Service (NBPHS) to all, which was composed of the major public health service program and the basic public health service program. The basic public health service program, which is often referred to as the National Basic Public Health Service. It is a defined package of basic healthcare services delivered by community health organizations (CHOs) throughout the country[8]. The NBPHS was designed in response to the increasing burden imposed by NCDs, includeing health education and disease management of hypertension and diabetes [9]. In order to implement the policy, the government developed the criteria of service delivery for the NBPHS [10-11]. To finance the NBPHS, in 2009 it was stated that different levels of government would be required to provide an investment of 15 yuan (CNY) per capita each year. This amount has increased regularly by five CNY a year: from 20 CNY in 2011 to 40 CNY in 2015. Xiao et al. [12] estimated that about 18% of the investment was spent on the disease management of patients with hypertension, which was the largest investment in hypertension throughout China's history. What had been gained in terms of social and economic benefit, and whether such a large investment is worthwhile to be continued in a long run, both rely on a comprehensive economic evaluation.

A number of studies in China have attempted to evaluate the NBPHS. For instance, in 2016, an *Annual Report of Essential Public Health Services Performance Evaluation* was published by the Center for Project Supervision and Management, which is affiliated to the Ministry of Health [13]. In 2014, the

Community Health Association of China undertook the assessment of the national basic public health service programs [14]. A more recent study evaluated the accessibility and its determinants of essential public health service among adults with chronic diseases in China, and pointed out that the effectiveness of disease management needed to be improved [15]. Yin et al. [16] calculated the expected cost of a national essential public services package in Beijing by developing a workload-based model. They concluded that the present investment on NBPHS was not enough for what was needed.

Nevertheless, no research conducted has evaluated the economic and social benefits of this large investment. In other words, no economic evaluation has been conducted in a systematic manner. The research presented in this thesis has developed a framework for the economic evaluation of such interventions. It is designed to estimate the benefits and effectiveness of the investment in the NBPHS in terms of reduced costs, and increased productivity and financial benefits. The investment case for the program is estimated in the form of benefit-cost ratios and internal rate of returns.

1.2 Aims of the research

Based on three streams of national data for the years from 2009 to 2015, this research first estimated the health outcomes of such a program for providing basic public health services in China in terms of more patients managed and better control of hypertension. Then the long-term health outcomes were calculated using appropriate techniques (Markov model), linking these outcomes to hypertension. Accordingly, a framework for economic evaluation was developed to assess the economic and selected social benefits arising from the health outcomes in terms of increasing workforce participation, reducing health care costs and providing benefits to the community. Comparing the benefits with the costs, an investment case for the program was generated in terms of benefit-cost ratios or internal rates of return. Within this context, the specific aims of the research were:

1. To analyze the outcomes of the NBPHS in terms of managing more patients

and improving the control rate of hypertension from 2009 to 2015.

2. To develop a Markov model to predict long-term health outcomes from improved hypertension control from 2016 to 2045, in terms of CVDs avoided and deaths averted.

3. To use a cost-benefit analysis framework for disease management of hypertension by CHOs in China and estimate the investment case for the NBPHS expressed in terms of investment metrics (benefit-cost ratios and internal rates of return).

4. To provide policy recommendations for the Chinese government on further investment in chronic disease interventions through the primary healthcare system.

The reasons for selecting the period from 2009 to 2015 are twofold: first, during this period, the NBPHS was a major invaluable policy measure undertaken at the national level for hypertension management in China [8, 12, 17]; second, hypertension management data were available for trend analysis, which is explained in Chapter 3.

1.3 Introduction to the NBPHS

The NBPHS has played a major part in equalizing access to basic public health services by both urban and rural residents. This was one of the four main goals of the new health care reform plan issued in 2009 [18]. The NBPHS is delivered through the basic health care service system, based on a grass-roots health care service network. A set of NBPHS items were identified and defined, which included disease management of hypertension.

1.3.1 Primary healthcare system of China

As indicated above, the NBPHS is designed to be delivered through a grass-roots health care service network, namely the primary healthcare system of China. The quality of healthcare is dependent on the funding and resourcing of primary healthcare facilities.

The primary care system in China was founded on a three-tier health system, consisting of urban community health service facilities (centres or stations), township health centres, and village clinics and other primary care facilities [18-20]. Each tier of the system is mandated to deliver essential healthcare services to the Chinese population, especially the aged and patients with chronic diseases[12]. It was widely researched that no healthcare system can function without quality healthcare professionals. Therefore, this study reviewed policies on human resourcing in primary health care facilities. In 2006, the functions and staffing standards of urban community health service facilities were defined by a related policy document [21]. In 2011, these functions and staffing standards of township hospitals were revised by the National Health and Family Planning Commission[22].

Policy review shows that the NBPHS has been the biggest investment and the most major policy measure on hypertension management in primary health care in China. This study employed trend analysis and policy analysis to control the impact of differences in the timing across space.

To evaluate the impacts of the NBPHS on hypertension, further analysis was conducted to link outcomes with the performance of the primary care facilities, especially in terms of health professionals and expertise. This is explained in Chapter 6.

1.3.2 The NBPHS program

The government funded the services of the NBPHS program and provided it to all residents for free through primary health care institutions [12], regardless of their hukou (a record officially identifying the living area of the residents) [23]. The management of hypertension was one of the NBPHS items within the program.

The intention expressed by the *Opinion on the New Health Reform of China 2009*, was that urban and rural residents should be gradually provided with basic public health services, which consist of disease prevention and control, maternity and childcare, and health education, among other services. The average standard funding per capita for the NBPHS should be no less than 15 CNY. It increased to 25 CNY in 2011, 30 CNY in 2013, 35 CNY in 2014 and 40 CNY in 2015 (Department of Primary Care, n.d.). According to the 2010 Chinese Census, the population of 31 provinces (autonomous regions, municipalities directly under the central government) in China was 1, 332, 810, 869. Therefore, over 246.57 billion CNY (around 36.64 billion USD, at an exchange rate of 6.73 CNY per USD) was invested in this program. An estimation of how much was spent on hypertension is provided in Chapter 5 for the purpose of economic evaluation.

Although the specifications of basic public health services were revised three times, in 2011, 2013 and 2017[24], the specifications for hypertension management did not change much across the three revisions. As the evaluation conducted in this research was based on data from 2009 to 2015, the 2013 version of the service delivery criteria was used to explain the NBPHS program and the content of hypertension control. The 2013 NBPHS specification included 13 types of basic public health services with 43 specific service items with the numbers of types and items increasing from 2011 to 2017. This included the management of health records for urban and rural residents, health education, health management of elderly people, health management of hypertension patients and so forth[10]. All services referred to by these criteria were to be implemented mainly by township hospitals and community health service centres, which were required to shoulder part of the responsibility of service delivery.

1.3.3 Specifications for managing hypertension patients

According to the specifications of public health service delivery developed by the NHFPC, the target population for management of hypertension were adults aged 35 and above[10]. Healthcare delivered through primary healthcare facilities mainly included hypertension screening and management (The National Health and Family Planning Commission of China, 2013). Primary health care facilities were to provide screening to people aged 35 years or above for hypertension, and if diagnosed, the patient would be taken into standard management as follows:

- For permanent residents aged 35 and above, measure their blood pressure on their first visit to primary health care facilities.
- For people with abnormal BP (SBP $\geqslant$ 140 mmHg and/or DBP $\geqslant$ 90 mmHg)

at his or her first visit to a doctor, remove the external factors raising up BP and re-measure the BP. If the BPs measured on 3 different days remained abnormal, the patient would be diagnosed as hypertensive and put on the list of hypertension management under the NBPHS. If necessary, referral was to be made to hospitals for further diagnosis, with follow-up referral results in two weeks.

- For high-risk populations, advices were to be provided on behavioral recommendations.

The specifications stated that regular (at least four times a year) follow-up and evaluations of hypertension should be delivered face-to-face. The services delivered included measuring BP and evaluating emergent conditions, ascertaining the date for the next follow-up, and providing advices on medication according to blood pressure (BP) levels. This was in line with the Chinese hypertension guidelines discussed by Wang[25-26].

In addition, the government determined that community healthcare facilities should provide health examinations for hypertensive patients once a year. This would include measuring body temperature, pulse, breathing, blood pressure, height, weight, waistline, as well as undertaking skin, superficial lymph node, heart, lung and abdomen examinations, and making primary evaluations of oral cavity, vision and physical activity functions. Details are in the health examination table listed in *Residents' Health Reford Management Specifications*[10, 25].

A performance evaluation indicator system was established by the National Health Commission of China, comprising the following indicators:

(1) Hypertension health management rate = Number of hypertension patients managed/Number of hypertension patients within the community × 100%.

(2) Standard management rate of hypertension = Number of hypertension patients meeting a criterion/Number of hypertension patients managed × 100%.

(3) Control rate of hypertension = Number of patients with BP controlled in the latest follow-up/Number of patients managed × 100%.

The evaluation indicator system demonstrated that the goal of hypertension management was hypertension control, and this is used for evaluation of the NBPHS program in this thesis.

1.3.4 The NBPHS funding mechanism and hypertension control

To make an economic evaluation of hypertension management under the NBPHS, it is necessary to understand its funding mechanism and the broader Chinese healthcare financing system.

According to international standards, healthcare in China is financed through three channels: government, society (non-government social insurance, commercial health insurance, and donations) and out-of-pocket payments[27]. Government funds are transferred directly to healthcare facilities and generally used for employment, infrastructure, equipment purchasing and for subsidizing the delivery of public health services. Funds from health insurance and out-of-pocket payments go to medical care facilities upon individuals' healthcare seeking, and are used under a revenue and expenditure balance system according to government regulations [28].

The NBPHS is funded by the government, which considers it a subsidy to primary healthcare facilities[29]. People have access to NBPHS services free of charge [8]. Given that the NBPHS represents a governmental investment into primary care facilities, performance evaluation has been conducted by the government county/district[29]. Following that, in order to make better use of funding and improve the performance of primary healthcare staff, the Ministry of Finance and Ministry of Health jointly released a policy on how to use the NBPHS funds for primary care facilities. These funds can be used for healthcare staff payments and consumable materials related to the NBPHS, but cannot be used for infrastructure, equipment, training and other infrastructure improvement[29].

Theoretically, with the implementation of the NBPHS' disease management program, more patients would have access to services, and as a consequence, better treatment. This would then result in more hypertensive patients seeking medical care, and getting regular treatment and medication, thus leading to an improved hypertension control. Such an investment, therefore, might increase healthcare expenditure from the patient side through health insurance and individual out-of-pocket payments. On the other hand, as a result of the program's hypertension management, treatment might be more efficient and effective, resulting in fewer negative consequences from hypertension, thus potentially saving healthcare expenditure. The funding of the NBPHS is additional to revenues from general health care and it is free for people to receive the care. Figure 1-1 provides a visual representation of the relationships between management and the treatment-related care of hypertension.

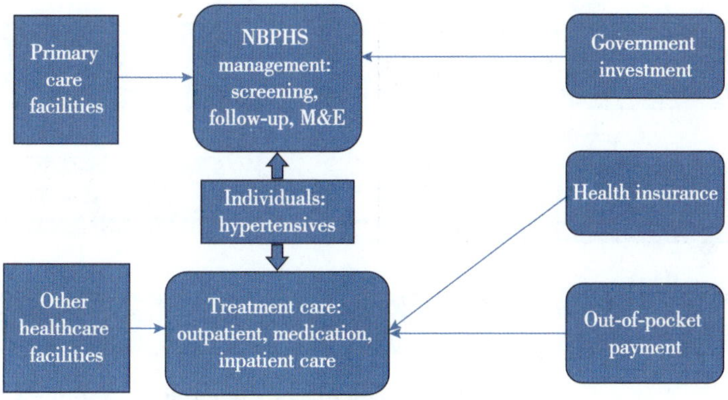

Figure 1-1 Funding mechanism for healthcare services of hypertension management in China

Note: M&E stands for monitoring and evaluation.

To determine whether the NBPHS increases or decreases healthcare expenditure, a cost of illness (CoI) method was employed[30]. This is discussed further in Chapter 5.

1.4 Conceptual framework, methodologies and data sources

1.4.1 Framework and conceptual components of the research

Figure 1-2 is a diagrammatic representation of this research. The left-hand side of this figure shows the general terms of the research, and the right-hand side shows the economic evaluation indicators used.

As the NBPHS program was launched in 2009, this study used the data from that year to reflect the baseline status and the 2015 data to reflect the final status

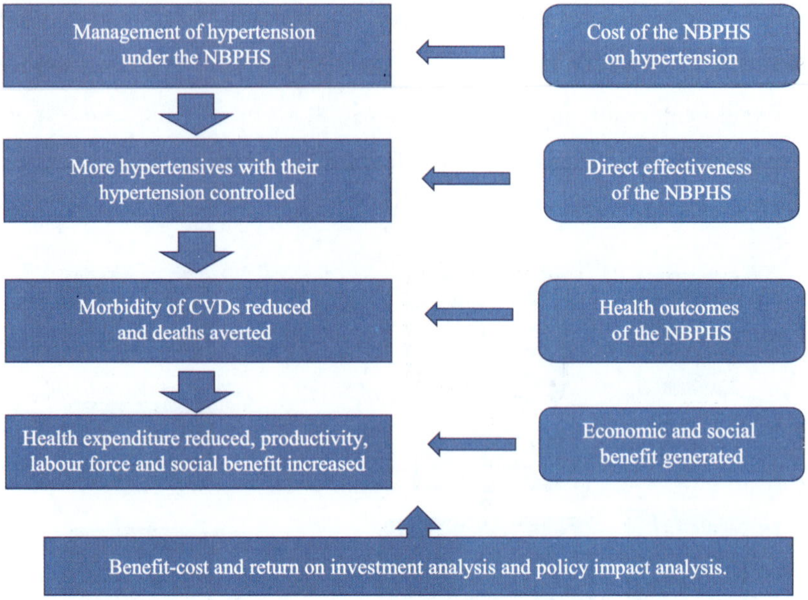

Figure 1-2 Framework of the study

of the program, over a seven-year period. Based on the available data, this thesis comprises four main sections: the role of the NBPHS in terms of managing more people and providing better hypertension control; the long-term benefits arising from hypertension control; the benefits estimation and benefit-cost analysis of the program; and the findings and policy implications.

1.4.2 Components of the study

1.4.2.1 Using a time series model to identify the contribution of the NBPHS

A full literature review was conducted on prevalence, awareness, treatment and control (PATC) of hypertension in China from 1990 to the present. Representative data were identified to analyze the PATC of adults aged 35 years and above at the national level[31-33]. The Lagrange interpolation polynomial technique was employed to complete the missing data from 1991 to 2009[34-35]. Time series predicting analysis was performed with the expert modeler method and the predicted control rate of 2015 was calculated. The difference between the predicted and observed control rate of 2015 was considered to represent the incremental effectiveness of the NBPHS program. A literature review was performed to validate the estimate of trend analysis. In addition, age-specific analysis was made on the PATC of hypertension to analyze the mechanism of the NBPHS in hypertension management. Details are given in Chapter 3.

To conduct a comparative analysis, two scenarios were established in this study. The NBPHS scenario was represented by the incremental number of hypertensive patients under control. This is discussed in Chapter 3. The non-NBPHS scenario was identified as the number of hypertensive patients out of control.

1.4.2.2 Using a Markov model to project long-term health outcomes

According to the studies of Wu et al.[36] and Zhang et al.[37], the fatal or non-fatal outcomes of hypertension were mainly coronary heart disease (CHD) and stroke. Therefore, the significance of controlling hypertension was to prevent the trend of development of these related diseases. The long-term outcomes of the NBPHS program were estimated with a Markov model, as used in previous studies [38-39], in terms of adverse health episodes reduced and lives saved.

The direct health outcomes were identified as hypertension control, and long-term health outcomes were identified as morbidity averted and deaths reduced. These terms are explained as follows:

- "Hypertension control" : the total number of hypertensives with their hypertension controlled from 2009 to 2015. This represents the direct impact on patients.
- "Morbidity reduced" : morbidities of stroke and CHD reduced during the 30-year period are calculated, which are analyzed in Chapter 4.
- "Deaths averted" : this was projected based on mortality from CVDs averted, to reflect long-term health outcomes. Again, this is explained in Chapter 4.

A sample of hypertensives from the China Health and Nutrition Survey (CHNS) 2009 was employed to simulate the two scenarios discussed above. It was discovered that between the two simulated groups, the major risk factor for CVD was the BP level, where blood pressure, diabetes, blood cholesterol, smoking, and body mass index (BMI) were considered[40]. Comparisons were conducted on the difference of the two groups of age-gender specific risk factor distributions.

Statistical analyses were conducted using SPSS 22.0 software.

A Markov model was established according to the CVD policy model-China (CDPM) [38, 41], which had been well developed and calibrated. For the NBPHS scenario, the model parameters used to determine disease transitions were based on a recent published study[38]. For the non-NBPHS scenario, the parameters were weighted by risk ratios of the two scenarios for each age-gender group based on BP and risk of CVD in the Chinese population[39].

In this study, a Markov model was used for the hypertensive population aged 35+ years in China, according to the CDPM [38, 42]. The structure of the Markov model is illustrated in Chapter 4. The patient of either the hypertension-controlled or-uncontrolled group can shift to one of the six health states: hypertension only, acute heart disease, acute stroke, chronic CHD, chronic stroke, and death. It was assumed that there was no remission to a CVD-free state after an incident of CVD. Other health states or diseases were not considered. CHD and stroke were analyzed separately rather than in the form of CHD, stroke or the combination of both. A shift between any two health states was defined as the transition probability, which was derived from Gu et al.'s[38] recent study. Each state and event had an annual probability of transition to a different CVD state. The hypertensive population was stratified by age in 10-year categories and gender.

The initial stroke or CHD event, which include cardiac arrest, myocardial infarction, and angina, and its sequelae for 28 days were described in the CDPM [4, 38]. The cycle of the Markov model was one year. The 28-day case fatality was considered instant death from acute CHD or stroke. One-year case fatalities of CHD and stroke were calculated based on CHD and stroke mortality, and prior-prevalence of CHD and stroke, in line with Gu et al.'s[38] study. The non-CVD mortality equaled the difference between the all-cause death rate of the population[43] and the CHD mortality and stroke mortality.

In this study, the dynamic process of hypertension patients aged 35+ years follows that used in the CDPM[38, 41] and is further explained in Chapter 4.

1.4.2.3 Estimation of economic and social benefits

This study estimated the economic and social impact of health benefits generated from hypertension control, and the reduced morbidity, mortality and other adverse health episodes. Economic and social benefits in monetary terms were modelled from the following aspects:

- Direct costs of illness avoided from hypertension control by the individuals and families concerned, including medical and other costs related to the illness, carer costs, costs on transport, and immediate loss of income.
- Benefits of higher gross domestic product (GDP) originated from improved health, including effects attributed to increased labour supply from morbidity and mortality averted, and productivity increased because fewer employees worked while ill.
- Social benefits were estimated in terms of the disease control impact to the community by estimating the value of a statistical life year in terms of per capita GDP beyond the economic benefit. According to recent studies, this equals 0.5 times the GDP per capita[44, 45].

A benefit-cost metric was employed for economic evaluation in this study from a societal perspective by estimating labour force and GDP increases from morbidity averted and lives saved. The benefits consist of both economic and social benefits.

The economic benefits from increased workforce participation for the working population was estimated with a maximum age of 65 years. Social benefits were considered equal to 0.5 GDP per capita estimated with a maximum age of 80 years.

Economic benefits: The economic modelling of mortality followed a cohort from 2016 to 2045 to determine rates of death and incidents. The economic impact from avoided mortality was calculated based on the labour force participation of every age-gender group and year category. The contribution to economic output was estimated by multiplying the number of people in each age-gender group by a productivity rate that varies with age and year. Each subsequent year, as they aged, the age-specific participation rate was applied to that cohort to calculate the labour force for that cohort in that year. Account was also taken of average death rates by age. The labour force in any year was obtained by adding together all the cohorts up to that year. The participation rates used were grouped by age and gender categories of the International Labor Organization (ILO) [46]. GDP per labour force was based on statistical data from 2017. The labour force by gender and age was accessed through the ILO (Bertram et al., 2018). Population and death rate data were extracted from the United Nations (UN) for 2017[46]. For each age-gender group, for the cohort of hypertensives whose lives were saved in a particular year, average ages were calculated based on the CHNS 2009 12 age-gender categories (male/female, 35-, 45-, 55-, 65-, 75-and 85+). The population structure was also taken from the UN population report [46]. The persons are the sum of all persons of working age who were employed and those who were unemployed.

Social benefits: The social and economic components of the value of a life year saved were distinguished, as their effects may vary in different investment analyses. In light of the discussion above, in this study, we consider the total value of a life year under these two components as equal to 0.5 times GDP per capita, which was at the lower bound of the range employed in previous studies. This was made up of a social value equal to half of the sample GDP per capita, and hence common across countries, and the economic benefits of increased labour force participation calculated as national values[45]. These assumptions varied in sensitivity analyses.

Benefit estimation from morbidity averted: In this study, morbidities only include CHD and stroke, as they are the main health consequences identified in the model and in previous studies[47]. The benefit estimation from morbidities averted was based on the numbers of deaths averted, according to the severity of diseases (Burstein et al., 2015).

Direct cost of illness (CoI) avoided: This was calculated for hypertension, CHD, and stroke, according to the method provided by the WHO guide[30]. Direct costs measured the value of medical care used to prevent, diagnose, and treat a particular disease, also known as the total direct costs[49]. Expenses related to caring for a sick family member were not included, as this is difficult to measure.

1.4.2.4 Calculation of benefit-cost ratio and internal rate of return

To evaluate the benefits and costs of the NBPHS program, this study calculated the net social benefit, benefit-cost ratio and internal rate of return for such an investment.

1.4.3 Data source

Three streams of data from the Chinese government and published literature were used, as follows:

- The first stream of data was gathered from a literature review. As indicated earlier, a systematic review was conducted on hypertension PATC from 1990 to the present, through which representative data were extracted to analyze the PATC of adults aged 35 years and above at the national level[50].
- The second stream of data was from the CHNS conducted in 2009. A total of 9, 552 participants were included in the analysis and 1, 025 participants were hypertensives who had been diagnosed by health professionals. The measurements and definitions of hypertension, awareness, treatment and control are in line with previous studies[51]. Of the hypertensives, 1, 017 were aged 35 years and above. Their data were adopted in this study and categorized into the hypertension-controlled group and the hypertension-uncontrolled group, where uncontrolled hypertension was defined as SBP/DBP≥140/90mmHg.
- The third data source was a household interview survey conducted by the China National Health Development Research Center in 2014, across 17 provinces in China. Sample households were selected under a multi-stage stratified clustering method, covered 20, 777 households with 62, 097 respondents in total. Among these, 9, 607 hypertensives were identified[52]. This survey was used for analyzing the CoI associated with hypertension, CHD and stroke in the hypertension-controlled group and hypertension-uncontrolled group.
- The fourth data source was the China Hypertension Survey (CHS) 2012-2015, which was conducted under a stratified multi-stage random sampling method. It obtained a nation-wide representative sample of 451, 755 people aged over 18 years from 31 provinces (autonomous regions, municipalities directly under the central government) in China from October 2012 to December 2015. The study results were published in 2018[33]. The age-gender structure was weighted according to the 2010 Chinese Census population data.

Based on the above data and conceptual framework, a literature review was undertaken focused on all the research processes, and quantitative methods were adopted, including comparative analysis, trend analysis and modelling analysis.

1.4.4 Calculating the benefits, benefit-cost ratio and internal rate of return

Based on the costs and benefits data collected, a benefit-cost ratio and rate of return on investment were calculated. In the selection of discount rates, this research is mainly concerned with the maximization of the present value of health. An appropriate discount rate was employed based on the theoretical framework provided by [53] with reference to the discount rates used, such as 0, 2%, 3%, and 5%. Sensitivity analysis was employed to justify the research results with estimations of different projected data.

Net present value (NPV) was employed to estimate both the economic and social benefits of the program generated from hypertension control. NPV is the difference between the present value of cash inflows and cash outflows during a defined period [54]. NPV is used in capital budgeting and investment planning for estimating the outcome of an investment[54], which will be described in Chapter 5.

1.5 Structure of the book

The thesis is composed of six chapters. Chapter 1 provides an introduction to the thesis, presenting the background and rationale of the study, its research objectives, the general conceptual framework and the methodologies employed. Chapter 2 presents the literature review focused on hypertension, the relationship between hypertension and CVDs, the long-term health outcome estimations of healthcare, and the economic evaluation of hypertension management. This review also outlines the process used in selecting an appropriate methodology for this study. Chapter 3 examines the effectiveness of the NBPHS in terms of hypertension control by establishing a trend analysis model. Chapter 4 describes the performance of a health outcome estimation of the NBPHS from the perspective of CVDs avoided or postponed, or death averted. This chapter also outlines the development of a Markov model based on a CDPM. Chapter 5 clarifies the cost of hypertension management under the NBPHS. It also outlines the process of economic evaluation of the NBPHS based on the research findings presented in Chapter 4, applying an innovative cost-benefit framework. Chapter 6 presents a discussion of the policy implications of the research results, including the steps that the Chinese government can take to address the findings. This final chapter also outlines the study's contributions to knowledge, its research significance, as well as its limitations (specifically in terms of the methodology and data accessibility).

2

Hypertension and its consequences, health outcome quantification, and economic evaluations

2.1 Introduction

The NBPHS was launched nation-wide in China in 2009. Before 2009, patients with any diseases, including chronic conditions, tended to visit 'big hospitals' [18]. This limited the accessibility, availability and quality of healthcare for chronic diseases [55]. To combat the problem and strengthen primary health care delivery, a new health care reform was launched[17]. The NBPHS was established in this context. Another objective in implementing the NBPHS was to facilitate tiered health care delivery for chronic disease interventions and guide patients into using primary healthcare [7, 15]. This study aims to evaluate the program in terms of quantity, quality, impact and economic outcomes, to see whether the above policy goals have been achieved.

As described in Chapter 1, hypertension management under the NBPHS involves a multi-intervention approach composed of hypertensive screening processes, evidence-based guidelines of practice, collaborative practice models, education for patient self-management, measurement and evaluations of process and outcome, and routine feedback[56]. The NBPHS is designed to improve the health of patients and to save health care service costs related to avoidable complications, including emergency room visits and hospitalizations. This clearly denotes its economic significance [57].

However, research on the economic benefits of prevention and public health programs has been limited, as traditional methods of economic evaluation are not always appropriate[58]. In addition, hypertension is a risk factor for CVDs and is also related to other risk factors, such as age, gender, BMI, smoking, diabetes, and cholesterol[37]. This makes it even more complex to conduct an economic evaluation of hypertension management.

To address this challenge, health economists have tried to provide a general framework for economic evaluations of healthcare programs. Tsiachristas et al.[59] developed a general decision analysis model. This established five objectives of disease management programs, as follows: a) improvement of the process of care delivery; b) improvements in patient lifestyles and self-management behavior; c) improvements of biomedical, physiological and clinical health outcomes; d) gains of quality of life; and e) total health outcomes. Sculpher et al.[60] emphasized that economic evaluations should use patient-level data and decision analytic modelling.

Economic evaluation requires that a money value be assigned to all or part of the disease management process and it should link investment with outcomes. Considering this, this review aimed to develop a research agenda for this study based on the following.

- First, as the target disease is hypertension, this study set out to review hypertension and its consequences.
- Secondly, the study sought to review changes in the process of care delivery for the management of hypertension under the NBPHS. A further step was to link the changes in care delivery with changes in patient lifestyles or self-management behavior, including awareness, treatment and control. This aligns with parts a) and b) of the Tsiachristas et al.[59] study, discussed above.
- Thirdly, aiming at quantifying part c) of the Tsiachristas et al.[59] study,

this research sought to review how to estimate clinical health outcomes while taking into consideration other epidemiological factors using risk prediction models.

- Fourthly, this research sought to further quantify health outcomes from the Tsiachristas et al.[59] study, and how to transform clinical outcomes into long-term health outcomes.

- Lastly, as the final health outcomes would be translated into economic terms, the study sought to review commonly used economic evaluation frameworks with the intention of selecting the most appropriate one for this study.

These components form the framework of the literature review presented in this chapter, as illustrated in Figure 2-1.

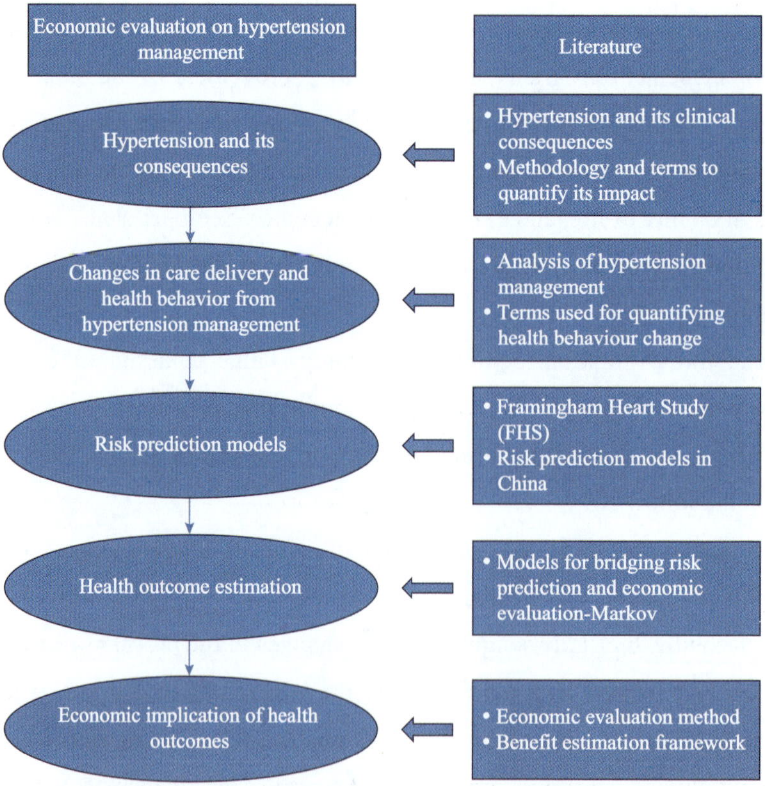

Figure 2-1 Structural components of the literature review

2.2 Hypertension and its consequences

2.2.1 Hypertension and CVD

Blood pressure (BP) is expressed by systolic pressure divided by diastolic pressure and is expressed by millimeters of mercury (mmHg) above the surrounding atmospheric pressure[61]. Hypertension (or high blood pressure) is usually defined as either systolic BP (SBP) equivalent to or over 140 mmHg, or diastolic BP (DBP) equal to or over 90 mmHg.

In population surveys, hypertension is measured directly by using a BP monitor or is self-reported typically when the person is asked if they have previously been diagnosed as hypertensives by a physician or are currently under medication for hypertension [61-62]. This definition is recommended by the WHO and the International Society of Hypertension[61-64], and is widely used in the NBPHS[62, 65].

Treated hypertension is defined as currently taking anti-hypertensive medication among hypertensive patients. Controlled hypertension is considered as an average SBP of less than 140 mmHg and an average DBP of less than 90 mmHg over two (or three) measurements in people with hypertension [33, 66].

Hypertension can lead to many adverse events for health. *The Global Burden of Disease study* in 2016 found that high BP was the most important risk factor globally for the burden of disease for women and the second most important (after smoking) for men[67], mainly because of its role in IHD and stroke.

2.2.2 Terms used in the study of hypertension and its consequences

This economic evaluation of the NBPHS draws upon a range of sources using several epidemiological terms. Definitions of some of these are presented below.

- Prevalence is the proportion of a population that has a condition at a specific time, but it is influenced by both the rate at which new cases are occurring and the duration of the disease[68].

• Incidence is generated by dividing the number of new patients with a disease during a defined period (usually a year) by the number of the population considered, who do not suffer from the disease initially[68].

Prevalence is a term for description of the extent of a disease in a population, while incidence is used to express the rate of developing new cases of disease. Also, prevalence is affected by the duration people live with a disease, something incidence usually does not consider[68].

In describing the change of hypertension, prevalence is used to set up a context for the whole analysis and to estimate the number of hypertensive patients for estimates. Incidence is used to describe the new diseases attributable to hypertension, mainly CVDs, which are described later in this chapter.

Hypertension is an important cause of the mortality and morbidity resulting from CVD. CVD in China has a high case fatality [31]. The definitions of, and relationships between, these terms are explained as follows:

• Morbidity is another term for illness. Morbidities are not deaths. A person can have several co-morbidities simultaneously. Prevalence is used to measure the level of morbidity in a population.

• Mortality is a term for death. Mortality rate is a measure of the number of deaths in a population, divided by the size of the population, during a unit of time. The mortality rate is often described in units of deaths per 1, 000 people annually. It is totally different from morbidity, and from the incidence rate [69].

• Case fatality, also called case fatality rate or case fatality ratio, is the share of people who die from a particular disease compared to the total number of patients diagnosed with the disease in a defined period. The case fatality rate is often used for prognosis, and a comparatively high rate indicates a relatively poor outcome[70-71].

These terms are used and explained further in the modelling undertaken for this study (see Chapter 4).

A number of epidemiological terms are commonly used to describe hypertension as a risk factor of CVD. These are as follows:

• Relative risk (RR) or ratio of risk. For comparison of risks among groups,

RR is a statistic of choice. In epidemiology, RR is the ratio of the probability of an outcome in an exposed group to the probability of that in an unexposed group [72]. It is computed as:

RR = [A/(A + B)] ÷ [C/(C + D)] = A(C + D)/C(A + B)

- The odds ratio (OR) is the ratio of the probability of an event occurring in a group and is a comparison of odds. It is calculated as follows:

OR = (A/B) ÷ (C/D) = AD/BC

where:

A = the number of people who get a certain ill condition in the exposed group;

B = the number of people who do not get the ill condition in the exposed group;

C = the number of people who get a certain ill condition in the unexposed group;

D = the number of people who do not get the ill condition in the unexposed group.

Therefore, A/(A+B) is the incidence in the exposed group, and C/(C+D) is the incidence of the unexposed group. OR and RR measure the association between the exposure and the outcome.

OR can be used to compare the risk of CVDs in different hypertensive patient groups, for example, those with different BP levels.

- The hazard ratio (HR) is similar in concept to the RR and is used if the risk is not constant regarding time. Data collected at different times is employed and in the context of survival over time, it is often employed. For example, given an HR of 0.5, the RR of dying in one group is half the risk of dying in the other group[72]. The HR is often estimated as the coefficients of Cox proportional hazard regression models, as hazard is connected to the survival function.

In summary, regarding hypertension and its complications: (a) prevalence can be used to describe both risk factors, including hypertension and complications, which are mainly CVDs; (b) incidence and morbidity are mainly used for CVDs as complications; (c) mortality and case fatality are used for the ending point of risk factors or complications; and (d) the HR is used to describe the strength of risk factors and their quantitative relationship with CVDs.

The following three terms are commonly used in analyzing health status changes for hypertension and many studies have been conducted on these topics.

- Awareness means being aware that you have hypertension. When derived from surveys, it is commonly defined by the answer "Yes" to the interview question "Have you ever been diagnosed by a physician or a health professional as a hypertensive (high blood pressure)?" [73]
- Treatment means undertaking some treatment for hypertension, such as a change in diet or physical activity and taking anti-hypertensive medication. In surveys, it is defined as self-reported use of anti-hypertensive medications.
- Control of hypertension means that the hypertension is at some defined level or lower, typically if the SBP/DBP is less than 140/90 mmHg[61, 74].

The prevalence of hypertension has been increasing in recent years in China[16, 52, 75-76]. The CHS 2012-2015 reported that 23.2% of the Chinese adult population, aged above 18 years, had hypertension and another 41.3% had pre-hypertension [33]. The survey on the Status of Nutrition and Health of the Chinese[77] revealed that prevalence of hypertension among adults aged≥18 years old was 25.2% in 2012. However, the awareness, treatment and control rates are at a very low level[76, 78].

By using the above terms, health behaviour changes can be quantified.

Recent studies have better explained the relationship between blood pressure, morbidity and mortality related to CVDs in China[31]. Increases in SBP were related to a greater risk of CVD compared to corresponding increases in DBP. As reported by D. Gu et al.[39], compared to those with BP <110/75 mmHg, the relative risks of CVD incidence were 1.09, 1.25, 1.49, 2.15, 3.01, and 4.16 for those with systolic/diastolic BP of 110-119/75-79, 120-129/80-84, 130-139/85-89, 140-159/90-99, 160-179/100-109, and ≥180/110 mmHg. Therefore, the goal of hypertension management is to lower blood pressure, get hypertension controlled, and finally, reduce cardiovascular morbidity and mortality.

An economic evaluation of different measures in hypertension interventions could help determine the impact of each measure in reducing the burden of disease. Several efforts have been made to evaluate interventions on hypertension in China[38, 79].

In 2015, the impact of anti-hypertensive drugs with a cost-effectiveness analysis was evaluated[38]. This study concluded that expanded hypertension treatment from low-cost medication was borderline cost-effective. In 2018, Xie et al. [42] conducted an economic evaluation on intensive hypertension management in China, concluding that it was more cost-effective than standard hypertension control. However, evidence of economic evaluation on hypertension management is scarce [59].

2.3 The role of the NBPHS in the management and control of hypertension

Guidelines of hypertension management have clearly stated that lowering BP and controlling hypertension is the key to reduce CVDs [33, 80-81]. The authors of these guidelines have also reviewed the evidence for treatments for lowering hypertension and set out recommendations for this, including improving lifestyle factors, comprising diet and physical activity, as well as anti-hypertensive medications. The implementation of these recommendations has increased the awareness of the role of hypertension in advanced economies, and has been important in improving hypertension control and reducing the death rate from CVDs[81]. Hypertension management under the NBPHS represents the implementation of these health intervention guidelines.

Detailed guidelines have been issued by the National Health and Family Planning Commission on how the NBPHS should be implemented by CHOs [24]. According to the specifications for hypertension management in the NBPHS program:

(1) Community health service facilities are obligated to conduct screening of hypertension; with all patients aged 35 years and above required to be screened by measuring their BP upon their first contact with general practitioners (GPs) or other doctors in primary care facilities. The results of the screening are conveyed to the patients, which may result in a major increase in the level of awareness of hypertension.

(2) If the patient is diagnosed with hypertension, primary care doctors are

required to conduct regular visits (four times a year) to those patients. They record what medications are being taken, and give professional help if necessary, including supervision and advices on medication[82].

(3) In cases of deterioration, GPs are obligated to refer patients to an appropriate hospital for further treatment. This facilitates timely treatment with appropriate care [83].

(4) The NBPHS program provides better access to GPs[15]. Before the introduction of the NBPHS program, Chinese patients tended to visit doctors in hospitals, where available time is limited for each patient. In addition, the in-hospital treatment mainly focuses on medication without considering non-pharmacological interventions[84].

Theoretically, hypertension management can be improved in terms of awareness, treatment and control. This has been confirmed in the evidence of several studies [15, 66, 86]. Many studies on the rates of awareness, management and control of hypertension have been conducted in China in recent years based on large sample surveys. The most recent was conducted in 2017[74], based on a survey of 1.7 million community-dwelling adults focused on an analysis of hypertension prevalence, awareness, treatment and control. Several other studies were also based on cross-sectional surveys[25, 33, 86].

However, none of the abovementioned studies explored the dynamic progress of hypertension interventions. Two other studies did conduct dynamic trend analysis of hypertension prevalence, awareness, treatment and control. Both used the CHNS conducted in 2013 and 2015[49, 87]. But, while these studies provided a good basis for the development of hypertension interventions, neither of them evaluated the effectiveness of the program. Without a random control trial study aimed at evaluating programs, it is very difficult to quantify the impact of awareness.

Based on data accessed through the literature review, this study analyzed the role of the NBPHS using trend analysis, with 2009 as a point of division. As stated in the above studies, awareness and treatment are structural indicators for hypertension, and control is the goal of hypertension interventions to prevent deterioration. Therefore, the focus of this study was on the analysis of hypertension control. Details of this analysis are presented in Chapter 3.

2.4 How to quantify the risk of CVDs for hypertension

Research efforts to understand the role of hypertension as a risk factor can be dated back to the 1920s. Paullin et al.[88] reviewed 500 patients in the US and concluded that hypertension consequences could be categorized into seven groups, related to the heart, arteries, central nervous system, eyes, lungs, kidneys and other organs. They also demonstrated that cardiac hypertrophy is the first complication of hypertension, which was evident in 66.4% (332/500) of the patients reviewed. Hamilton et al. [89] conducted a study of the relationship between hypertension and stroke, and found that BP control could significantly reduce complications in males and stroke in females.

A meta-analysis proved that for adults aged 40-69 years, each difference of 20 mmHg in the usual SBP (which is equivalent to 10 mmHg usual DBP) accounts for over a twofold difference in the stroke mortality, and with twice differences in case-fatalities from IHD and other vascular causes[90, 91]. Randomized clinical trials have proved that lowering SBP by 10 mmHg, lowers the risk of stroke and IHD by about one-fourth [92]. In China, evidence confirms that there is an obvious increase in the relative risk of CVD incidence as BP increases[39, 93].

2.4.1 International studies on risk equations

Cox regression models are commonly used for risk estimation of CVDs, and the most well-known study is the Framingham Heart Study (FHS) in the US[94]. This study began in 1948, with the main purpose of identifying the common factors or characteristics that contribute to CVD. The study involved a large group of participants who had not yet developed overt symptoms of CVD. The key outcome from the FHS was that the major risk factors of CVD were identified, which included hypertension, high blood cholesterol, diabetes, obesity, smoking, and physical inactivity. The study also provided evidence of the effects of related factors, including blood triglyceride and high-density lipoprotein (HDL) cholesterol levels, as well as age, gender, and psychosocial issues. The FHS is widely used and cited all over the world, generating over 1, 200 articles in top medical journals in the past half century.

Different methodologies have been employed in the estimation of parameters of risk factors[95]. The first methodology is logistic regression, which was used in Benjamin, Levy, Vaziri, D'Agostino and Belanger's[96] study. They used gender-specific multiple logistic regression models to select independent risk factors for atrial fibrillation, with OR and RR used for risk factors. Other studies using this same approach are those of Singer, Nathan, Anderson, Wilson and Evans [97] and Harris et al.[98]. The second method used is Cox regression, with HR used to express the relative risk of the factors analyzed[99], as this can better express the risk relationships by taking time into account.

In 2007, the World Health Organization and the International Society of Hypertension (WHO/ISH) generated a risk prediction chart for estimating the 10-year risk of fatal or non-fatal CVD by gender, age, SBP, smoking status, total blood cholesterol and diabetes mellitus (DM) for each WHO region (China belongs to the WHO West Pacific Region). The WHO/ISH risk prediction chart provided a visual and direct method for the public to acquaint themselves with CVD risks all over the world. This represents a world-wide application of FHS risk equations.

2.4.2 Risk prediction models developed in China

In terms of the consequences of CVD, early studies, especially for the western population, considered CHD to be the main complication. However, it is evident that CVDs should include not only CHD but also stroke, and strokes account for more deaths than CHD[36-37]. Many longitudinal studies such as the FHS and MONICA the MONICA is a project which aimed to evaluate trends of cardiovascular mortality and morbidity, and the relationship between these trends and changes in risk factor levels and/or medical care[100], among others, have been undertaken in a range of countries to quantify the importance of the various risk factors that contribute to IHD and stroke. Meta-analyses and critical reviews of these and other studies have been undertaken by researchers[101-102]. In recent years, models used for predicting risks have been further developed, with more factors taken into account and time used as a dynamic factor[38, 103]. Models used for risk prediction of CVDs in the Chinese population have also been developed. These are discussed as follows.

In 2005, Zhang et al.[37] developed a risk prediction score of CVD based on a Chinese cohort. It used age, SBP, total cholesterol (TC), BMI and smoking as covariates and considered CHD, ischemic/hemorrhagic stroke as dependent variables. Their study concluded that the risk stratification rules derived from Caucasian cohorts overestimated the Oriental people's CHD risk. As a result, they derived a stratification rule for CHD, ischemic and hemorrhagic stroke for Chinese men.

In 2006, Wu et al.[36] generated a gender-specific optimal 10-year risk prediction model for ischemic CVDs (ICVDs: including ischemic stroke and coronary events) in the Chinese population. They used Cox-proportional hazard regression, with data from the US-People's Republic of China(PRC) *Collaborative Study of Cardiovascular and Cardiopulmonary Epidemiology* (the USA-PRC Study). This demonstrated the relationship between ICVDs and risk factors, composed of age, SBP, total cholesterol, BMI, current smoking status, and DM in both men and women.

In 2016, Gu et al.[38] generated a 10-year risk prediction equation for atherosclerotic CVD (ASCVD) from four contemporary Chinese cohorts. In this study, they used the following risk factors: age, region, urban and rural, current smoking status, waist circumference, SBP, DBP, anti-hypertensive treatment within two weeks, total cholesterol, high density lipoprotein cholesterol (HDL-C), DM, and family history. They then predicted ASCVD for 10 years[103]. This study was based on a large sample size and focused on all ASCVD, defined as non-fatal acute myocardial infarction or CHD death or fatal or non-fatal stroke.

The study by Wu et al. [36] provided a simplified risk score system that could easily transform risk scores of ICVDs into 10-year risk probabilities. The study by Gu et al.[38] developed a risk prediction model for the Chinese general population and calibrated parameters in line with statistical data from China and the WHO. A similar application was performed in a 2016 study for the Chinese population[103].

The above studies provided a basis for long-term risk prediction tools.

Based on the 2015 study parameters, this study sought to develop a long-term health outcome estimation model with the CHNS data to perform risk predictions of CVDs. This is discussed further in Chapter 4.

2.5 Estimating health outcomes from hypertension control

Moran et al. [43] reported that modest decreases in SBP could result in a significant impact on the progression of CVDs in the Chinese population. Considering hypertension to be a main risk factor, the WHO/ISH formulated CVD risk prediction charts for implementation all around the world [64]. Lowering SBP by 10 mmHg or the DBP by 5 mmHg reduced the risk of stroke by about 35% and that of IHD events by about 25% at the age of 65[39, 90]. An analysis of 354 randomized trials revealed that three anti-hypertension drugs at half of the standard dose were estimated to lower SBP by 20 mmHg or DBP by 11 mmHg, which would result in a 63% reduction in stroke risk or a 46% reduction in IHD risk[104].

It was estimated that uncontrolled hypertension accounted for 750, 000 CVD deaths a year. Given that the prevalence of hypertension could be reduced by 25%, 130, 000 CVD deaths could be avert[105]. In China, it was reported that anti-hypertensive intervention could avert the risk of stroke by 35% to 40%, the risk of myocardial infarction (MI) by 20% to 25%, and that of heart failure by over 50%[6].

While risk equations provided a good tool for linking hypertension as a risk factor to fatal and non-fatal CVDs, most risk predictions were based on a 10-year duration. The commonly used terminologies for hypertension were prevalence, incidence, case fatality, and mortality, which were generally quantified on a one-year basis or an even shorter time.

To estimate life-span analysis, a health outcome predictor based on a longer term should be generated. Therefore, many efforts have been focused on developing models to integrate risk equations and the long-term health outcomes of disease control in and out of China [96]. A systematic review by Unal et al. [105] stated that by 2006, 42 CHD models had been developed and applied to CVD modelling, and six of these were considered major models widely used by researchers[90]. In China, the CDPM model[106], impact model[107], and Markov model[108] have been studied to different extents. As described in Figure 2-2, CVDs, which are mainly composed of CHD and stroke, are caused by many risk factors, including age, gender, hypertension and other related factors. The relationship between risk factors and CVDs is described in HR. CVDs will increase the risk of death, of which probabilities are described in case fatality and morbidity.

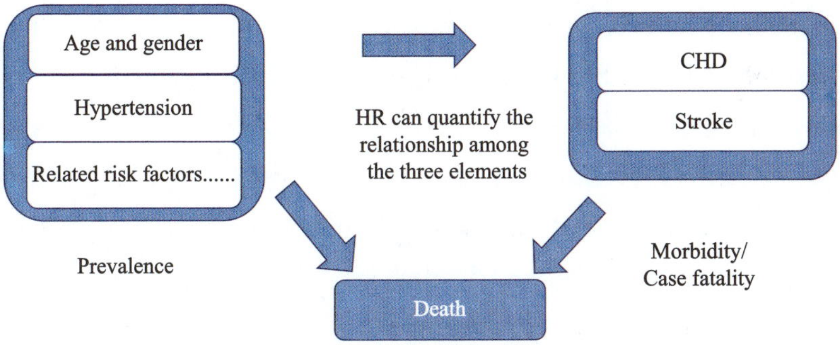

Figure 2-2 Relationships among hypertension, other risk factors and CVDs

2.5.1 Introduction to the CHDP model and its application in this study

Markov models are among the main approaches adopted when modelling economic evaluations in health care [109]. In China, the CHDP (Coronary Heart Disease Policy) model, which is based on the Markov model, is widely used and has been well developed for risk prediction of CVDs [38].

The CHDP model is a state-transition, cell-based model that was developed in the 1980s. It consists of three sub-models[110]: a demographical/epidemiological model; a bridge model; and a disease history model. The model can perform simulation of the effects of an intervention employing different case fatality rates and calculating the effects of long-term (up to 30 years) mortality, morbidity and costs. It has been applied in the US[111], Argentina[112] and China[38, 41].

This model is well developed and applied in China, and is known as the Cardiovascular Disease Policy Model-China model (CDPM). The methodology has been developed since 2008, and the latest study applying it was conducted in 2015. The research progress in China is reviewed as follows.

In 2008, Moran et al.[113] conducted a study on the relationship between population growth and aging, and coronary heart diseases in China, developing the CHDP model for the Chinese population. In the study, China-specific CHD risk factors, incidence, case fatality, and prevalence data were integrated, and a Chinese-cohort-based model were generated, which was calibrated to age-specific Chinese mortality rates. It calculated disability-adjusted life years (DALYs) of CHD with a projected Chinese population aged 35-84 years. Moran et al.'s (2008) results predicated that during the period 2020-2029, there would be 7.8 million excess CHD events (a 69% increase from the 2000-2009 period) and 3.4 million CHD deaths (a 64% increase), together with a 67% annual burden growth of CHD death and disability on adults aged under 65 years.

In 2010, the same research team further developed the CHDP model [41]. In this study, CVDs were projected from 2010 to 2030, including both CHD and stroke, among people aged 35-84 years old. Moran et al. [42] discovered that between 2010 and 2030, aging and population growth would contribute to an increase in CVD by more than half, and that unfavorable trends in BP, total cholesterol, diabetes and BMI would likely accelerate the epidemic.

In 2012, Chan et al. used the CHDP model to project the impact of urbanization on CVD over the period 2010 to 2030. They concluded that urbanization would increase CHD incidence by 73-81 per 100, 000 and stroke incidence slightly [114].

In 2015, Gu et al. led another study, with the model focused on the cost-effectiveness of low-cost essential anti-hypertensive medicines for hypertension control in China[35]. In this study, for the first time, the CHDP model was used for an economic evaluation of hypertension interventions in China and parameters were well calibrated. The authors estimated screening of hypertension, implementation of the essential medicine program, and administration of the hypertension management program. Costs of medication, disease-related expenditure, and quality-adjusted life years (QALYs) from prevention of CVDs or lost from drug side effects were estimated for untreated adults who were to 35-84 years old during 2015-2025.

These applications of the CHDP model provide a good basis for better structuring the process of hypertension in the Chinese setting, using the latest epidemiological parameters for better estimation. Most importantly, the studies provide a method and guide for this study to transform 10-year risk predictions of CVDs into annual risk predictions. This makes it possible to predict long-term health outcomes.

2.5.2 The Markov model and scope of diseases for this study

This study sought to develop a Markov model based on the Gu's study[38]. The Markov model is a stochastic model for simulating randomly changing systems[115]. It is assumed that future states depend only on the current state, not on the events that occurred before them. The Markov model is a convenient way of simulating the prognosis of diseases with ongoing risks[116]. The hypothesis of the model is that the patient is always in one of several defined states of health, named as Markov states. All events related are modelled as transitions from one state to another. In this study, the states for the Markov model consist of hypertension, CVDs, death attributable to CVDs and non-CVD death. The transition from one state to another can be generated from risk equations, as described in Chapter 1. Under each state, a utility can be assigned, where DALYs are commonly used[117]. The contribution of the utility to the overall process depends on the length of time spent in the state.

Epidemiological parameters for the transition of hypertension to CVDs is cited from Gu's study[38], which have been adjusted and calibrated with other statistical data. Risk for those within the NBPHS program was considered the same as for the general population. And the non-NBPHS scenario was simulated using the 2009 CHNS. Then, following Gu et al.'s[38] model, the Markov model was employed to estimate the 30-year health outcomes. The scope of diseases considered in this study follows the Gu et al.study[38], which reviewed the CVDs related to hypertension [106] as listed below:

- Coronary heart disease (CHD): Myocardial infarction, angina and other ischemic heart disease, and a fixed proportion of "ill-defined" CVD coded events.
- Stroke: Defined by ICD-9 codes 430-438 (excluding transient ischemic attack) or ICD-10 I60-I69.

ICD is the international standard for reporting diseases and health conditions[118]. ICD-9, the International Classification of Diseases Ninth Revision, and ICD-10, the Tenth Revision coding systems, are used to identify specific patient cohorts and assess their clinical outcomes with risk adjustment in many cases[119]. Data of CHD, stroke incidence and prevalence were from the China hypertension epidemiology follow-up study (Moran et al., 2010). The CHDP mortality projections were validated with age-specific and overall CHDs and stroke mortality numbers for the years 2000-2010, as studied by the WHO[38, 41].

2.6 Economic evaluation of health programs

2.6.1 Some basics

According to Drummond et al.[119-120], there are four types of health care program economic evaluations: cost-effectiveness analysis (CEA); cost-utility analysis (CUA); cost-benefit analysis (CBA); and cost-minimization analysis (CMA). Drummond et al.[121] further developed the definitions of the above concepts for health programs, as follows:

- CMA: Deals with costs only, which stands for a partial form of economic evaluation.
- CEA: The outcomes of programs are described by the natural effects or physical units, which include "years of life gained" or "cases correctly diagnosed" .
- CUA: A broader form of CBA in which the outcome of programs is adjusted based on health state preference scores or utility weights, often expressed by QALYs gained or disability life years avoided. The most common measure of consequences

in CUAs is QALY.

- CBA: A form of analysis which attempts to value the monetary consequences of programs. It is the broadest form of analysis, with the beneficial consequences of a program ascertained to justify the cost or not.

2.6.2 CBA and valuing the benefit in CBA

As emphasized by the WHO health economic evaluation agenda, the focus on the economic benefit of prevention and public health programs has been limited [59].

A systematic review of economic evidence on community hypertension interventions conducted in 2016[122], indicated that only four studies were conducted from 1995 to late 2015 in China. Of these studies, two employed CEA[38, 75], and the other two conducted CBA[18, 123]. The 2010 study by Y. Huang[124] and Ren[123] involved an evaluation of a community-based stroke prevention program, in which benefit was defined as CoI saved. However, only stroke was considered, which is only one consequence of hypertension, as discussed earlier. In addition, future costs and benefits were not analyzed, and the methodology was not clearly explained for use in economic evaluation. The study conducted by Wang et al.[17] only analyzed cost savings from hypertension management through a one-year follow-up study on 140 hypertensive patients in Beijing. In general, these two cost-benefit studies were not representative in terms of economic evidence for national hypertension management programs in China, and the methodologies used were not comprehensive enough as benchmarked in Drummond et al.'s interpretation of CBA[120].

To improve the methods of economic evaluation in China, this study employed a CBA framework, with benefit defined as assigning money values to the outcomes of healthcare programs[121].

Every life saved is a benefit to the individual, as they enjoy additional years with better quality of life. The community also benefits through a reduction in treatment costs or a gain from individuals, who can contribute to social and economic affairs. There is an extensive range of studies on the value of a life year and the estimation of benefits from healthcare interventions. In the fourth edition of their study of *Methods for the Economic Evaluation of Health Care Programs*, Drummond et al.[121] illustrated that willingness to pay (WTP) is commonly used for benefit estimation. It attempts to measure underlying consumer demand and value the non-marketed social goods, including healthcare programs. However, Drummond et al.[121] also pointed out that each of the methods used, including WTP, has its strengths and weaknesses. The WTP method, although commonly used and well developed, has two major deficiencies: one is hypothetical and the other is that QALYs, once used for benefit estimation through WTP, may not include social benefit[121]. Several studies in the US have estimated that the value of a life year is equal to US$150, 000[125], but other competing views and methods exist.

To solve the above deficiencies, Stenberg et al.[45] developed an innovative metrics for calculating return to investment in women and children's health, which broadened the estimation of the benefits of health programs. In their study, health benefits were considered to be composed of economic benefits and social benefits. The economic benefits were estimated from increased workforce participation for the working age population based on labour force participation rates and productivity for each age-gender group. The social benefits from longer, healthy life expectancy were estimated by assigning a certain proportion of GDP per capita[44-45]. Compared to traditional frameworks of benefit estimation, where WTP was commonly used, this benefit estimation framework addressed the problem of bias in preference-based methodologies and provided a tangible and measurable tool for benefit estimation.

However, the framework has never been used specifically on NCDs in China. Therefore, based on Stenberg et al.'s framework[44-45], this study applied the newly developed benefit estimation model to NCD interventions, specifically hypertension management in China.

2.6.3 International evidence on the economic evaluation of community-based hypertension interventions

Many studies of economic evaluations of hypertension interventions or management at the primary care level have been conducted. This study reviews several of these international studies.

In Bhutan, Dukpa et al.[126] performed an economic evaluation of the WHO package of essential non-communicable (PEN) disease interventions in primary health care settings based on modeling[48]. The models applied consisted of a decision tree and a Markov model. Final outcomes under the decision model were termed lifetime costs and DALYs averted under three scenarios: no screening; current PEN program; and universal screening. The Markov model for hypertension contained four health states: uncontrolled hypertension, controlled hypertension, stroke and death. The age range of the adult cohort was 40 years or older and the length of each cycle was one year. DALYs were calculated using WHO standard methods. Dukpa et al.'s[126] study concluded that a screening program conducted by the primary care facilities represented a good value for money.

In Bangladesh, a CBA of the national hypertension treatment program was conducted from a societal perspective, and the results showed the return on investment of providing BP lowering drugs to 60% of hypertensives by 2021 and 2030[127]. The study concluded that if hypertension management is conducted proactively by the government, this could result in a 12.7 : 1 annual return on investment by 2021 and an 8.6 : 1 annual return by 2030.

In Greece, Athanasakis et al.[128] conducted an economic evaluation of hypertension control in 2014 using a Markov model for CBA. This study concluded that interventions that promote BP control should be a health policy priority.

In the Netherlands, primary prevention of CVDs in mild hypertension was evaluated using a Markov model. This found that SBP reductions were cost-effective in both a 10-year and lifetime horizon[129].

The above studies provided a good basis and reference for the methodology and international scholarship presented in this thesis. Whether in developed or developing countries, intervention or screening measures at the primary care level were found to be cost-effective or have good value for money. As indicated above, most economic studies adopted a Markov model. For example, the study in the Netherlands[129] built a Markov model that set five states of CVD progression: healthy with hypertension, acute non-fatal CVD, stable non-fatal CVD, CVD death, and non-CVD death. This is similar to the approach adopted by Gu et al.[38] and provides an accurate reference for Markov modelling for hypertension control.

2.6.4 Study gaps in China

In terms of the economic evaluation of disease management in China, the gap is threefold. First, nearly all the studies have focused on CEA or CUA, but neglect CBA. For example, in an evaluation of stroke intervention in China, CBA was not included[130]. In the PhD thesis by Liang Xiao-Hua[131], who was from the Chinese Academy of Medical Sciences and Peking Union Medical College, an economic evaluation of hypertension management in communities was conducted. However, she did not conduct a CBA either[131-132]. Second, although several studies did undertake CBA on hypertension management in primary care settings, the methodology was not performed. For example, a study[133] used the Monte Carlo model for a CBA of a diabetes screening program. However, in the study, only QALYs gained and treatment cost were considered, which didn't make estimation of monetory benefit and was incomplete for the estimation. Another investigation, which was the analysis of curative effect and cost benefit of hypertension patients in a community management model, did not conduct sensitivity analysis[134]. Third, in the process of economic evaluations, the economic impact on individuals in society has not been considered[135].

In 2015, Gu et al. [135] partially addressed the gap discussed above. However, there are at least two points that can be further developed. First, there is still no evidence on the return of investment for the NBPHS program, let alone for the disease management of hypertension. Second, although many reports have emphasized that measures taken at the primary care level would gain a high return for economic growth and social development[9, 136], Gu et al.'s[38] study found that expanded hypertension treatment was only borderline cost-effective in China. From this perspective, this current study provides in-depth evidence for the cost-effectiveness of these measures.

2.7 Brief summary

This chapter has presented a review of studies on hypertension and its health consequences, how to quantify the impact of hypertension as a risk of CVD, the estimation of health outcomes based on risk equations, and economic evaluation methodologies for healthcare interventions. This study aims to estimate the health benefits arising from hypertension control, and the averted morbidity and mortality of diseases. Through a literature review, appropriate methodologies were identified for use in this study.

Comparative analysis and trend analysis are employed for estimation of the role of the NBPHS in management of hypertension from different data sources. Positive results provide a basis for further evaluation in terms of economic return and investment. This is described in Chapter 3.

Regarding risk equations and long-term health outcome modelling, this study developed a Markov model based on Gu et al.'s study (2015), which will be described further in Chapter 4.

As discussed, several healthcare economic evaluations of hypertension interventions have been conducted, such as studies in the Netherlands[129], Greece[128], Bhutan[126], and Vietnam[137]. This study drew on these international investigations by combining health outcome estimation processes with cost and benefit calculations to generate a Markov model framework. A CBA framework was also developed following previous studies[44-45].

The economic and social benefits generated from NBPHS interventions on hypertension in monetary terms were modelled from the following aspects.

(1) Benefits in terms of higher GDP over a longer term, which includes effects of increased labour supply from death or illness averted, productivity increased from fewer workers working while ill, and investment effects associated with a healthier and more vibrant workforce.

(2) Social benefits were estimated in terms of the disease control impact to the

community by estimation of the value of a statistical life year in terms of per capita GDP beyond the economic benefit (Stenberg et al., 2014). To compare the benefits with the costs of the program, the net social benefit, benefit-cost ratio and internal rate of return for such an investment were developed. The main process of economic evaluation is explained further in Chapter 5.

(3) Direct costs saved by the individuals and families, which include medical and associated costs on the illness, carer and transport, are also explained in Chapter 5.

3 Role of the NBPHS on hypertension control

3.1 Introduction

Hypertension control is one of the main targets for reducing CVDs[77, 137], and it is widely acknowledged that community-based interventions of hypertension are effective and cost-effective measures for hypertension control. As part of the NBPHS program, disease management of hypertension was launched in China, but with no intervention-controlled pilot study[15]. It was reported that by the end of 2017, the number of hypertensives managed by the NBPHS had reached 101 million[24]. However, baseline data were not available to evaluate hypertension management. According to government statistical data, the number of hypertensive patients had been increasing gradually from 2009 to 2015[139]. In addition, involvement in the program was based on the willingness of patients who could participate in and drop out of the program at any time. This made it more difficult to calculate the participation rate of the program.

A systematic review of a framework for developing the structure of public health economic models pointed out that it is important to identify the impacts of public health interventions when conducting economic evaluations of public health programs [57].

However, there are few studies that analyze the contribution of regular follow-up, medication, and non-pharmacological therapies in hypertension management[138-140]. Therefore, evaluation of the effectiveness of community-based programs is difficult in terms of linking program attendance to the health outcomes over time.

On the other hand, it is even more difficult to quantify the incremental effectiveness of hypertension control in the NBPHS because of other confounding factors, such as social economic development. The reasons are twofold: (1) both the quality of primary healthcare and people's awareness of hypertension are under continued improvement as society and the economy develops; and (2) many other local or national level programs, which are difficult to detect and observe, may have been implemented at the same time as the NBPHS. To overcome these barriers in an economic evaluation of the NBPHS program, time series trend analysis was employed to predict the hypertension control status of 2015 with data before 2009.

To estimate the effectiveness of hypertension management, relationships of PATC were explored. According to the specifications of hypertension management in the NBPHS program, community health service facilities were obligated to conduct screenings for patients with hypertension, provide treatment and referral, establish management information systems, stratify the risk factors, and implement regular follow-up and management (at least once every three months) [10, 25]. Therefore, theoretically, hypertension management would be improved in terms of awareness, treatment and control. This has been demonstrated in the findings of several studies[15, 66, 85].

To achieve the study aims, it was necessary to find a time series dataset that would reflect the trend of hypertension PATC before and after 2009. Further estimation was made based on the time series prediction model.

There are five sections in this chapter. Section 3.2 presents the full literature review conducted to analyze data related to hypertension PATC from 1990 to the present. In Section 3.3, this data is further analyzed in terms of age-specific characteristics and trends. Section 3.4 focuses on the missing data in the period 1990 to 2009, which was addressed using a Lagrange interpolation polynomial method. A time series prediction model was also established using pre-2009 data. Then a predicted control rate of hypertension was estimated through the model. The difference between the predicted and observed control rate of hypertension in 2015 was seen as representing the effectiveness of the NBPHS. Section 3.5 presents a comparison between the evidence from the literature and the findings discussed in Section 3.4. The final two sections, Sections 3.6 and 3.7, provide a discussion and conclusions.

3.2 Literature review on hypertension PATC from 1990 to the present

3.2.1 Search strategy and selection criteria

Relevant studies on PATC of hypertension in China were searched via the search engine PubMed on 22 November 2018.

Key words included (hypertension OR high blood pressure) AND (prevalence OR epidemiology OR awareness OR treatment OR control) AND (China OR Chinese). The following filters were used: full text; publication date from January 1, 2000 to December 31, 2018. From this initial search, 5, 553 articles were identified. Another three articles were accessed from other sources (personal communication with scholars). In total, 5, 556 articles were reviewed by title and abstract.

3.2.2 Inclusion/exclusion criteria

Articles were included if the following criteria were met: (1) a national representative survey was used, with a multi-stage stratified random (or cluster) sampling method; (2) the age range of the target population was 18 years and above; (3) the survey population structure was weighted according to the national or international population; (4) BP was obtained during field surveys, measured by trained examiners at the time of survey, with an average of two or three measurements employed as the BP values; (5) the article was published in English or Chinese; and (6) hypertension was defined by SBP≥140mmHg or DBP≥90mmHg, and/or administration of anti-hypertensive drugs.

Awareness of hypertension was considered as the self-reporting of any previous diagnosis of hypertension by a healthcare professional among the hypertension population. Treatment of hypertension was considered as self-reported if medication for hypertension had been prescribed within two weeks of the survey. Control of hypertension was defined as hypertensive participants having the following readings: SBP<140mmHg and DBP<90mmHg. Studies in the Hong Kong, Macao Special Administrative Region and Taiwan province were not included.

Surveys undertaken in a population of specific ethnicity, occupation, or age-range were excluded, if that population could not be considered representative of all adults aged 18 and above across the national population. If articles were focused on the same theme and age range, the article with a higher impact factor was selected. Papers that were published as supplementary articles were excluded.

3.2.3 Articles extracted

Once the filtering and exclusion processes had been completed, 117 potential articles remained. These were further filtered by reviewing their abstracts, and 30 articles were selected for data extraction, with 15 more used for further analysis in relation to hypertension management effectiveness (discussed in Section 3.5). The filtering process is illustrated in Figure 3-1 and the selected articles are summarized in Table 3-1 below.

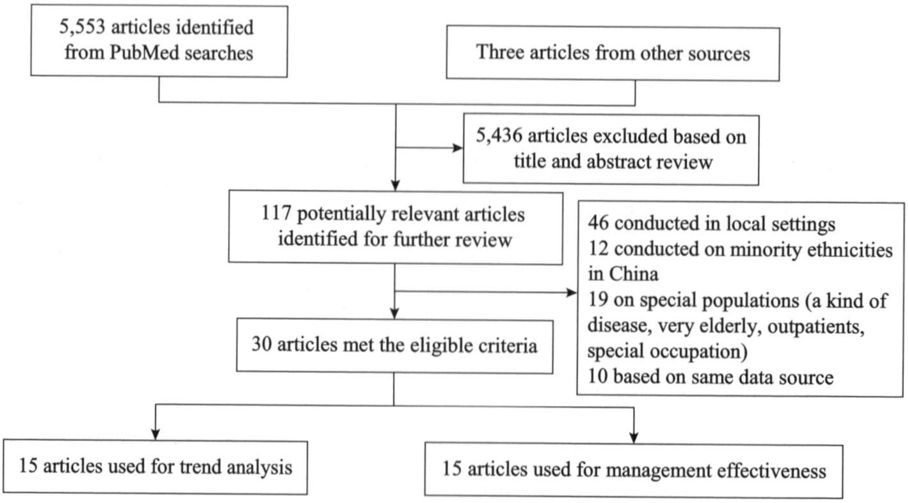

Figure 3-1 Selection of articles for further analysis

Table 3-1 Summary of articles on hypertension prevalence, awareness, treatment, and control in China, 1991-2018

No.	Title of Publication	Year of survey	Survey design	Age range	Analysis methodology	Sample size
1	Trends in prevalence, awareness, treatment and control of hypertension in the middle-aged population of China, 1992-1998[141]	1992-1994 and 1998	China Multi-Centre Study of Cardiovascular Epidemiology: random cluster samples	35-59	Comparative analysis between 1992 and 1998 of PATC	18, 746 (1992-1994) 13, 504 (1998)
2	Hypertension burden and control in China: Analysis of nationwide data 2003-2012[33]	2003-2012	Review	18+	Systematic review	N/A
3	Hypertension in China: Data from the China National Nutrition and Health Survey 2002[142]	2002	CNNHS (China National Nutrition and Health Survey)	18+	Comparative analysis	141, 892
4	Prevalence, awareness, treatment, and control of hypertension in China [143]	2000-2001	InterASIA: 4-stage stratified sampling	35-74	Descriptive analysis (M, SD)	19, 012
5	Trends in prevalence, awareness, treatment, and control of hypertension among Chinese adults 1991-2009 [87]	1991-2009	CHNS	18+	Trend analysis	8, 426-8, 503
6	Hypertension prevalence, awareness, treatment, and control in 115 rural and urban communities involving 47, 000 people from China[144]	2005-2009	PURE (prospective, standardized collaborative study)	35-70	Generalized linear model	153, 996
7	Prevalence of hypertension in China: A cross-sectional study[86]	2007-2008	Cross-sectional survey	20+	Analysis of prevalence of hypertension in China	46, 239

continued

No.	Title of Publication	Year of survey	Survey design	Age range	Analysis methodology	Sample size
8	Hypertension among older adults in low-and middle-income countries: Prevalence, awareness, and control [145]	2007-2010	SAGE	50+	Descriptive analysis (M, F)	13, 348
9	Prevalence, awareness, treatment, and control of hypertension in China: Results from a national survey [65]	2009-2010	Multi-stage, stratified sampling	18+	Analysis of PACT of hypertension in China	50, 171
10	Hypertension and related CVD burden in China [146]	2010	China non-communicable disease surveillance 2010	18+	Literature review (China non-communicable disease surveillance 2010)	N/A
11	The dynamics of hypertension prevalence, awareness, treatment, control and associated factors in Chinese adults: Results from CHNS 1991-2011 [51]	2011	CHNS	18+	CHNS Longitudinal survey	8, 658-12, 474
12	China CVDs report 2015: A summary[77]	2011	CHNS	18+	Literature review	N/A
13	Report on Chinese Residents' Chronic Diseases and Nutrition[147]	2012	Multi-stage, stratified sampling	18+	Descriptive analysis	
14	Status of hypertension in China: Results from the CHS 2012-2015 [33]	2012-2015	China Hypertension Survey	18+	T test and logistic regression	451, 755
15	Burden of hypertension in China: A nationally representative survey of 174, 621 adults[148]	2013-2014	China chronic disease and risk factors surveillance (CCDRFS) survey 2013-2014	18+	With consideration of the complex design, the mode adjusted means and prevalence were estimated and tested in design-based lineal regression and logistic regression	174, 621

Hypertension PATC of adults aged 18 or above or 20 or above from 1991 to 2013 were analyzed. This therefore excluded articles 1, 4, 6, 8 in which the age range did not fit the study population.

The most consistent survey in China is the CHNS, which is a large-scale, national and successive cross-sectional survey. It was designed to identify how the health and nutritional status of the Chinese population has been affected by social and economic factors[149]. According to the guidelines of the NBPHS, adults aged 35 years or above are the main target population for hypertension screening and management. The CHNS dataset not only provides long-term data for further analysis, but also meets the requirement of extracting data related to hypertensives aged 35 years and above at the population level. Two other sources provided national level data that included this age range. These were the study conducted in 2016[144] and the China Hypertension Survey (2012-2015)[33].

Therefore, this study applied both the published data of the CHNS 1991 to 2011 for further analysis and data selected from the full literature review. Data were weighted based on the 2010 Chinese Census.

The full survey data from the CHNS 1991 to 2015 was used for this study. Based on the following criteria, records were excluded: age below 18 years or missing data for age, gender, SBP or DBP.

Finally, 75, 526 records of 24, 410 individuals were retained. From the 2015 CHNS database, there was a total of 11, 525 cases aged 35+ years. Table 3-2 lists hypertension awareness, treatment, and control from 1991 to 2015, which are retrieved from 7 studies as shown in the last column. In each year, the survey was described in terms of survey year, sample size and age range. To analyze the relationship among awareness, treatment and control of hypertension, treatment/awareness and control/treatment (which were both proportions), are generated.

As shown in Table 3-2 above, there was an increasing trend in the PATC of hypertension. From 1991 to 2015, hypertension prevalence increased from 14.13% to 23.20%; awareness increased from 23.19% to 46.90%; treatment increased from

Table 3-2 Relationships among awareness, treatment and control of hypertension

Survey year	Survey	Sample size	Age	Prevalence/%	Awareness/%*	Treatment/%*	Control %*	Treatment/ Awareness**	Control/ Treatment**	Reference or data source
1991	CHNS	8, 436	18+	14.13	23.19	10.88	2.75	0.536	0.250	CHNS *** (1991-2011)
1993	CHNS	7, 906	18+	15.23	18.46	9.45	2.71	0.543	0.257	
1997	CHNS	8, 496	18+	17.51	13.87	8.13	1.70	0.738	0.177	
2000	CHNS	9, 500	18+	17.42	21.28	12.58	3.09	0.697	0.243	
2004	CHNS	8, 843	18+	19.90	23.47	16.18	4.72	0.772	0.277	
2006	CHNS	8, 974	18+	18.58	28.39	19.00	5.10	0.742	0.237	
2009	CHNS	8, 411	18+	21.92	26.46	20.53	6.12	0.874	0.268	
2011	CHNS	12, 490	18+	19.85	36.11	26.52	9.31	0.734	0.351	
2002	CNNHS	141, 892	18+	18.00	25.00	20.00	5.00	0.800	0.250	(Wu et al, 2008)
2003-2012	SR	N/A	20+	26.70	44.60	35.20	11.20	0.789	0.318	(Li et al., 2015)
2009-2010	China National Survey of Chronic Kidney Disease	50, 171	18+	29.60	42.60	34.10	9.30	0.800	0.273	(Wang et al., 2014)
2010	China non-communicable disease surveillance	98, 658	18+	33.70	33.30	23.90	3.90	0.718	0.163	(Xu Y, 2013)

continued

Survey year	Survey	Sample size	Age	Preval-ence/%	Awaren-ess/%*	Treatm-ent/%*	Control %*	Treat-ment/ Aware-ness**	Control/ Treat-ment**	Reference or data source
2013-2014	China Chronic Disease and Risk Factors Surveillance	173, 621	18+	27.80	31.90	26.40	9.15	0.828	0.347	(Li et al., 2017)
2012-2015	China Hypertension Survey	451, 755	18+	23.20	46.90	40.70	15.30	0.868	0.376	(Wang et al., 2018)
2015	CHNS****	13, 980	18+	45.37	19.65	16.12	6.71	0.4331	0.4163	CHNS database, retrieved on May 26, 2019

Notes: *Awareness, treatment and control are presented as percentages of the hypertensive prevalent population.

** Treatment/awareness represents the share of treated patients as the awared and control/treatment represnets the share of patients with hypertension controlled as the treated, which were both expressed in percentages.

***CHNS data were all age standardized on the 2000 or 2010 Chinese Census.

****The HTN prevalence in the age group 18-35 years was extremely high in the CNHS, which seems an exception in the sample population.

As the data set is newly released, it needs further confirmation. In the following section, only the sample aged 35+ years is employed, which is consistent with other studies.

10.88% to 40.70%; and control, although kept at a low level, increased from 2.75% to 15.30%.

Further analysis was made to determine the relationships among awareness, treatment and control. This demonstrated that: (1) treatment/awareness ratios were higher than control/treatment ratios. From 1991 to 2015, the highest control/treatment rate was no more than 0.45, while the lowest treatment/awareness ratio was more than 0.50; (2) after 1997, the treatment/awareness rate was higher than 0.700, which means that if a patient became aware they would be more likely to seek medical advice; and (3) control/treatment ratio kept increasing, which reflects improved adherence on the part of patients, and in part also the role of other factors and players beyond the control of the health system.

From Table 3-2, it should be noted that the data of CHNS 2015 was not reliable. Firstly, in both the CHNS 2009 and CHNS 2011, the adults' hypertension prevalence was about 20%, while the CHNS 2015 showed 45.37%. Also, the awareness and treatment rate of hypertension in the 2015 survey result were both much lower than in the 2009 or 2011 survey results. Secondly, in the meantime in another survey, the CHS 2012-2015, of which the sample size was much larger than the CHNS 2015, the prevalence, awareness, treatment and control results were more consistent with the CHNS surveys during 1991-2011. Therefore, in the following section, data from the CHS 2012-2015 survey was used for the observed status of hypertension in China.

3.3 Age-specific analysis of PATC

Age is an important influencing factor for CVDs[150]. This section analyzes the hypertension PATC trends among different age groups in the past 20 years.

The status of hypertension awareness, treatment and control is shown in Appendix Table A1. From 1991 to 2015, among the hypertensive patients aged 35+ years, awareness increased from 27.10% to 44.91%. Treatment increased from 14.44% to 38.42% and control from 2.87% to 14.72%. In 2015, 85.5% of patients who were aware of their hypertensive condition received anti-hypertensive treatment, with an increase of 32.2% from 1991 to 2015. Among patients who received treatment, the control rate increased from 19.9% in 1991 to 38.3% in 2015. Details are given in Table 3-3.

Table 3-3 Time series dataset for trend analysis of hypertension PATC of adults aged 35+ year in China, 1991-2015

year	Prevalence/%	Awareness/%[a]	Treatment/%[a]	Control/%[a]	Treatment/awareness (proportion)	Treatment/control (proportion)
1991	22.18	27.10	14.44	2.87	0.533	0.199
1993	22.59	26.29	14.00	2.73	0.533	0.195
1997	26.10	18.78	12.12	2.95	0.645	0.243
2000	26.33	30.82	19.81	4.55	0.643	0.230
2004	27.46	33.33	23.95	6.95	0.719	0.290
2006	25.96	37.42	27.91	7.41	0.746	0.265
2007[b]	41.90	41.60	34.40	8.20	0.827	0.238
2009	30.47	37.85	29.54	8.61	0.780	0.291
2011	28.19	50.93	40.05	14.31	0.786	0.357
2015[c]	32.62	44.91	38.42	14.72	0.855	0.383

Notes: a. Awareness, treatment and control are listed as percentages of the hypertensive prevalent population.

b. 2007 data from hypertension prevalence, awareness, treatment, and control rates in 115 rural and urban communities involving 47, 000 people from China[144].

c. Data from the CHS 2012-2015 (Wang et al., 2018).

Figures 3-2 to 3-5 describe hypertension prevalence, awareness, treatment and control trend from 1991 to 2015 for different age groups. The prevalence, awareness, treatment and control of hypertension all showed an increasing trend from 1991 to 2015 in all age groups. It is observed that hypertension awareness, treatment and control are better in the older participants than their young counterparts. The highest prevalence was in the 75+ age group, and the highest awareness, treatment and control were all in the 65-74 age group.

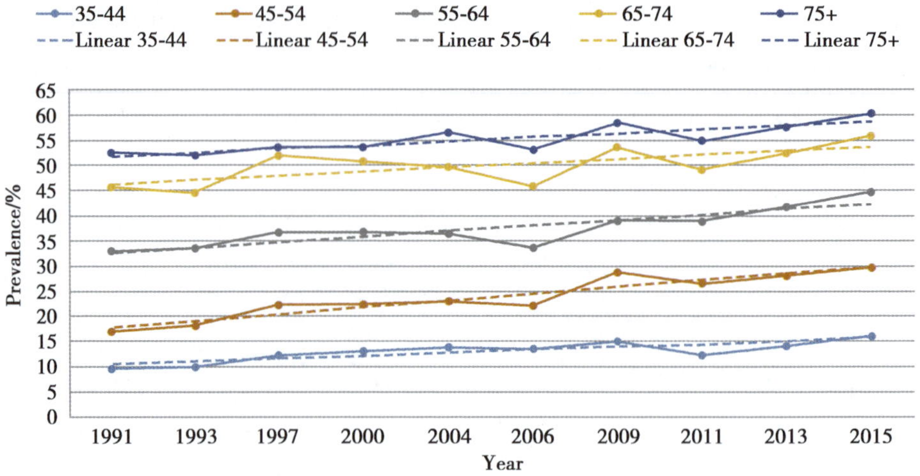

Figure 3-2 Hypertension prevalence among different age groups, 1991-2015

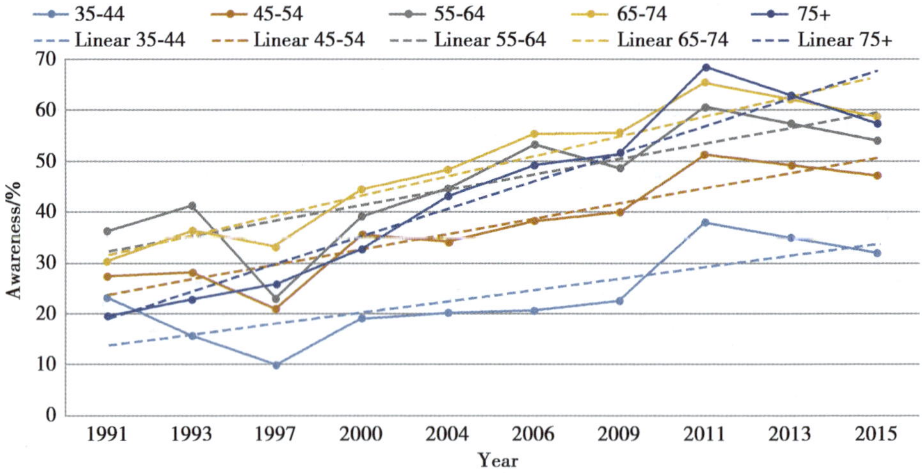

Figure 3-3 Awareness of hypertensives among different age groups, 1991-2015

As illustrated in the figures above: (1) there was a general increasing trend of hypertension PATC from 1991 to 2009 for all age groups; (2) hypertension prevalence increased with age, for adults aged 35 years and above which was higher than 10% and increased sharply, peaking at the oldest age group; and (3) although prevalence peaked in the oldest group, awareness, treatment and control did not necessarily peak in the same way. For most time points analyzed, the highest awareness and treatment rates were seen in the 65-74 age group, and the highest

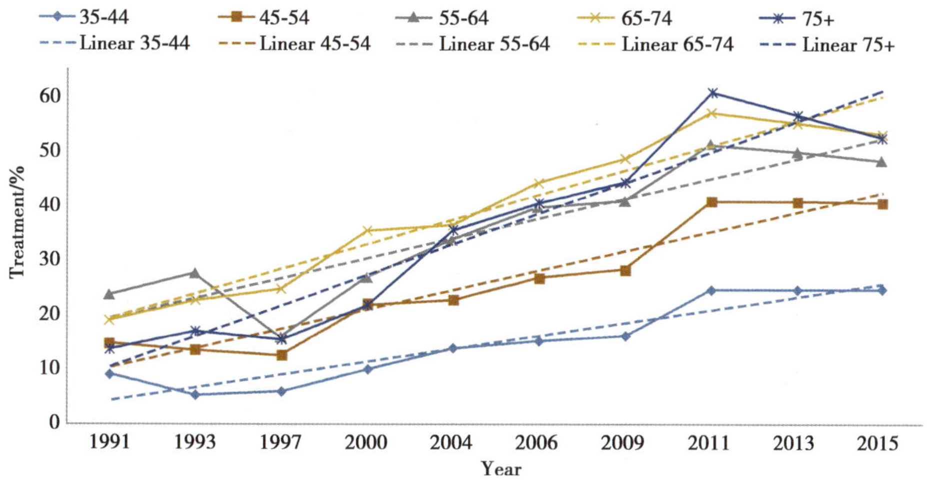

Figure 3-4 Treatment of hypertensives among different age groups, 1991-2015

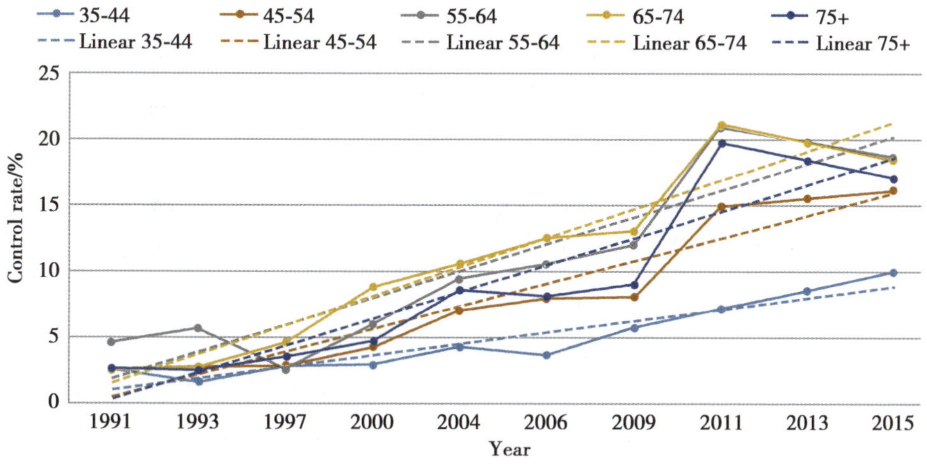

Figure 3-5 Control rate of hypertensives among different age groups, 1991-2015

control rates were seen in the 55-64 age group. An obvious decrease from the 65-74 age group to 75+ age group was observed. As shown in Figure 3.3, although the hypertension rate grew with age while the awareness, treatment, and the control rate decreased with age, the treatment control rate was higher in the younger group than in the elder group. These rates were 40.4%, 40.0%, 38.7%, 34.8% and 32.6%, for age groups 35-44, 45-54, 55-64, 65-74 and 75+, respectively. Details are given in figure 3-6.

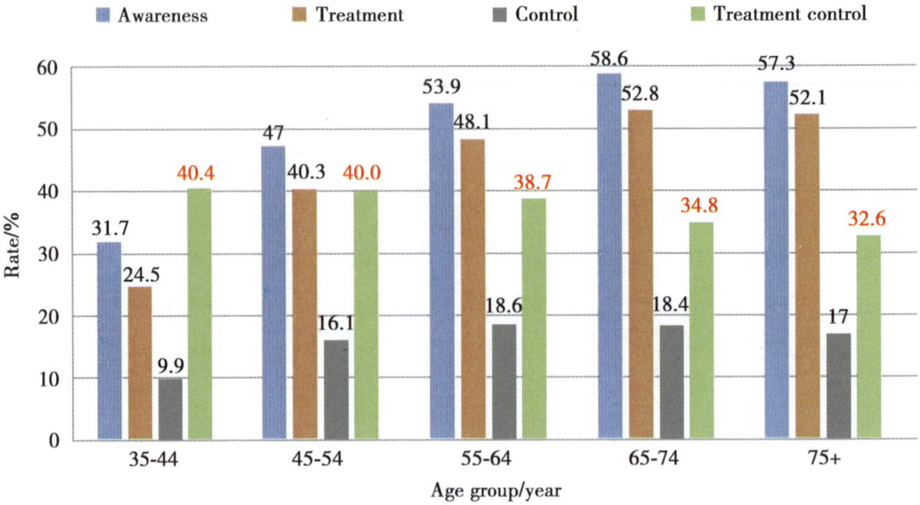

Figure 3-6 Hypertension awareness, treatment, control and treatment control of hypertensives aged 35+ years, surveyed during 2012-2015.

Source: WANG Z, CHEN Z, ZHANG L, et al. Status of Hypertension in China: Results From the China Hypertension Survey, 2012-2015[J]. Circulation, 2018, 137 (22): 2344-2356.

As shown in Table 3-3, from 1991 to 2015, the treatment/awareness ratio kept increasing. In 2015, this ratio was 0.855, which is much higher than the treatment/control ratio. This indicates that if the patient became aware of their hypertension, they would be more likely to seek medical advice, which is the most important step for getting hypertension under control[31, 33]. According to the NBPHS guidelines, the first step in hypertension management is to measure BP during the patient's first visit to a primary healthcare physician. As shown in Table 3-3, the treatment/control ratio was much lower than the awareness/treatment ratio over the 1991 to 2015 period. Therefore, while it is difficult to quantify precisely, it can be inferred from Figure 3-2 to 3-5 that a significant improvement had been reached in terms of awareness through the NBPHS program comparing data of 2015 with that of 2009.

Treatment/awareness is used to reflect the willingness of hypertensives to receive treatment, while treatment/control reflects the effectiveness of treatment among hypertensives[33]. Treatment/awareness after 2009 did not change much compared with that before 2009, which was around 80%. Again, this means that if a person became aware of their hypertension, they would be likely to seek medical advice. The treatment/control rate after 2009 was higher than that before 2009. Some of this improvement could be attributable to the NBPHS program since healthcare became more accessible and more available for hypertensive patients.

As the objective of hypertension management is to achieve properly controlled blood pressure and as the above analysis shows that the impact of awareness and treatment of hypertension can be transformed into hypertension control, the following section conducts further analysis on hypertension control.

3.4 Time series analysis of hypertension control

3.4.1 Data used

Trend analysis was performed using CHNS data from 1991 to 2009[51, 87]. As the data were not continuous or in a time series form with the same intervals, data from other studies were inserted to generate a time series dataset. Hypertension PATC data for adults aged 35 + from 1991 to 2015 are shown in Table 3-3 and Figures 3-2 to 3-5.

The PATC rates before 2010 were age-standardized according to the 2010 Chinese Census data. An age-group analysis was performed, and is presented in the supplementary material (Appendix D).

3.4.2 Statistical analysis

Descriptive analysis on hypertension PATC was conducted to compare trends from scenarios of time and age.

Although the data extracted from the CHNS 1991 to 2011 and from the full literature review is comprehensive, data from 1991 to 2009 in one-year intervals is still not enough for time series analysis. Only 10 years of data were available for the estimation period, which represented a small sample. Therefore, a small sample time series analyzing method was employed based on two Chinese studies[34-35], in which R Language, Lagrange interpolation polynomial was employed to generate values for 1995 based on the data from 1991, 1993, 1997 and 2000, and values for 2002 were generated based on data from 1997, 2000, 2004 and 2006.

Data of control rates for each year from 1991 to 2009 were completed using a Lagrange interpolation polynomial method (the R language program is listed in Appendix B).

Trend analysis was employed on the time series data from 1991 to 2009. With the trend formula generated, a predicted estimate for the year 2015 was generated. Regarding observational control rates of hypertension, estimates from the CHS 2012-2015 were used[35]. By comparing the observed value with the predicted value of the number of patients under hypertension control, the difference was considered to represent the incremental effectiveness of the NBPHS program.

3.4.3 Results

3.4.3.1 Elementary trend analysis of PATC

In a study by Li et al.[149], it was highlighted that in 2000-2001 (n=15, 540), the control rate of hypertensive patients in China was 8.1%, while a similar study in 2005-2009 (n=18, 915) showed that it was 8.2%. This means that the hypertension control rate was at a low level from 2000 to 2009, according to different studies. Figure 3-7 shows the trend of awareness, treatment and control of adults aged 35+ years from 1991 to 2013. An obvious jump can be seen from 2009 to 2011 in hypertension control rate, which provides a basis for further analysis of the role of the NBPHS.

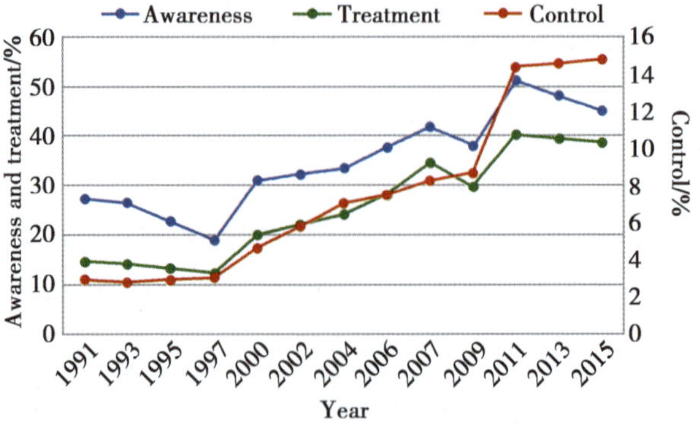

Figure 3-7 Trends of awareness, treatment and control among adults aged 35+, 1991-2015

3.4.3.2 Trend analysis of hypertension control and predictions of 2015

Using a Lagrange interpolation polynomial method, data of hypertension control from 1991 to 2009 were completed, as shown in Table 3-4.

Table 3-4 Completed data of hypertension control rates, 1991-2009

Year	Control rate/%	Year	Control rate/%
1991	2.94	2001	5.26
1992	2.92	2002	5.90
1993	2.85	2003	6.48
1994	2.78	2004	6.95
1995	2.74	2005	7.10
1996	2.78	2006	7.41
1997	2.94	2007	8.20
1998	3.37	2008	8.26
1999	3.95	2009	8.61
2000	4.60		

Given that the trend analysis is based on fewer than 20 data points, a small sample time series analysis was performed, where pre-treatment was performed on small sample data using the Lagrange Interpolation Polynomial method. With SPSS 22.0, time series predicting analysis was performed using an expert-modeler method in which the difference was used to realize time series stationarity to predict the control rate of 2015. According to the expert modeler, a Brown exponential smoothing model was selected for linear trend prediction, as shown in Table 3-5 and Figure 3-8.

The residual auto-correlation function (ACF) showed a random distribution with no outliers, which indicates good model fitness (see Appendix B in supplementary material).

Table 3-5 Model statistics for the time series prediction of hypertension control rate

Model	Number of predictors	Model fit statistics		Ljung-Box Q (18)			Number of outliers
		Stationary *R*-squared	*R*-squared	Statistics	DF	Sig.	
Control-model_1	0	0.162	0.990	3.852	17	1.000	0

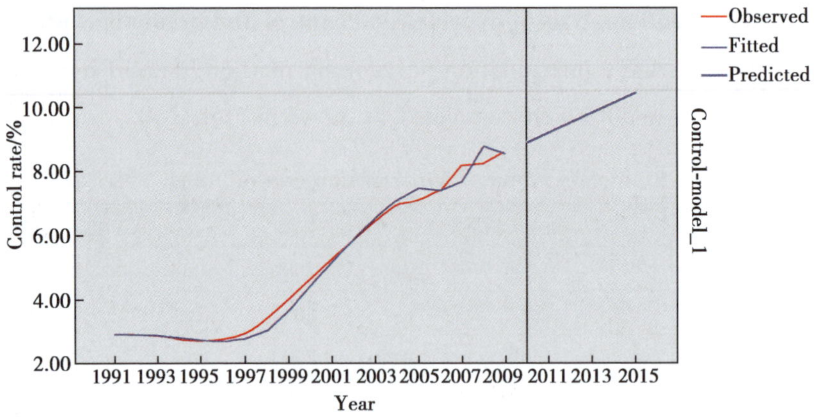

Figure 3-8 Time series trend of hypertension control rate, 1991-2009 and predicted analysis from 2010 to 2015

Table 3-6 is the forecasted control rate of hypertension from 2010 to 2015 based on the model established from 1991 to 2009. Both upper control limit and lower control limit are listed. It is predicted that in 2015, the control rate of hypertension would be 10.46% [95%*CI* (7.33%, 13.59%)] based on the trend from 1991 to 2009.

Table 3-6 Forecasted control rate of hypertension from the prediction model, 2010-2015/%

Model	2010	2011	2012	2013	2014	2015
Forecast	8.92	9.22	9.53	9.84	10.15	10.46
UCL*	9.40	10.13	10.93	11.80	12.73	13.71
LCL**	8.43	8.32	8.13	7.88	7.57	7.20

Notes: *UCL = Upper control limit, **LCL = Lower control limit.

3.4.3.3 Estimation of the role of the NBPHS on hypertension control

This study aimed to use the difference between the predicted control rate and the observed control rate of hypertension to reflect the effectiveness of the NBPHS from 2009 to 2015. The number of adults aged 35+ years was 685, 998, 627, which was estimated based on the age-gender structure of the 2010 Chinese census data.

According to the CHS 2012-2015, the prevalence of hypertension among adults aged 35 or above was 32.62% in 2015[33], while the number of hypertensives aged 35+ in 2015 was 223, 772, 752. The predicted control rate of 2015 was 10.46% [95%*CI*(7.20%, 13.71%)]and the observed control rate was 14.72%. The change of percentage points used as incremental effectiveness was 4.26 [95%*CI*(1.13, 7.39)]. Therefore, it was estimated that from 2009 to 2015, the NBPHS program increased the number of hypertensive patients under control by 9, 532, 719 [95%*CI* (2, 528, 632, 16, 536, 806)].

Age-specific analysis was performed. The predicted control rates and the observed control rate of 2015 for each age group are listed in Appendix Table D3. With the same population data and method, it was estimated that from 2009 to 2015, the NBPHS program increased the number hypertensives under control by 8, 009, 449 (95%*CI*: 1, 581, 856 13, 065, 018), which would be 0 1, 635, 397 1, 564, 164 170, 388 and 617, 939 for males in age groups 35-44, 45-54, 55-64, 65-74 and 74+ respectively, and 0 1, 568, 221 1, 523, 002 169, 167 and 761, 170 for females in each age group, respectively. Although the number of hypertensives under control estimated through age-specific analysis are significantly different from the all-age group analysis, the benefit-cost ratios generated from the two analyses are not significantly different from each other.

In addition, as the raw database of CHS 2012-2015 was not available, the hypertension prevalence and control rate of different genders were not available. Therefore, the prevalence and control rate of the two genders were considered to be the same; and, 75-84 and 85+ age group data were not accessible, so the two age groups were incorporated into people aged 75+, which made the results even less precise. Therefore, an all-age-group analysis was used in the thesis. (Details of the age-specific analysis are shown in Appendix D.)

To verify the estimate from trend analysis and CHS 2012-2015, further evidence was searched in the literature and a range of values of the effectiveness of hypertension control from the NBPHS were obtained from other researchers. Details are in Section 3.5.

3.4.3.4 Sensitivity analysis

To carry out a sensitivity analysis on the trend projection model, the author has done two things: firstly, calculate 95% *CI* around this model, see Table 3-6 (UCL and LCL); and secondly, compared this with another approach, where with data from 1991-2009, a linear regression model for trend analysis model was estimated (Figure 3-9). It was found that the linear regression approach was slightly higher. Therefore, from the above analysis, it can be estimated that the predicted control rate of 2015 would be 10.66%.

The predicted hypertension control rate from the linear regression analysis (10.66%) was 0.2 percentage point higher than the coefficient regression model used in the thesis, which was 10.46%[95%*CI* (7.20%, 13.71%)]. The change was minor and the result from the linear regression model lies in the 95% *CI* of the results from the coefficient regression model. Following that, under the linear regression analysis it was estimated that from 2009 to 2015, the NBPHS program increased the number of hypertensive patients under control by 9, 085, 173, compared with 9, 532, 719 generated from the coefficient regression model. The result still lies in the 95% *CI* (2, 528, 632 16, 536, 806) of the analysis of the thesis.

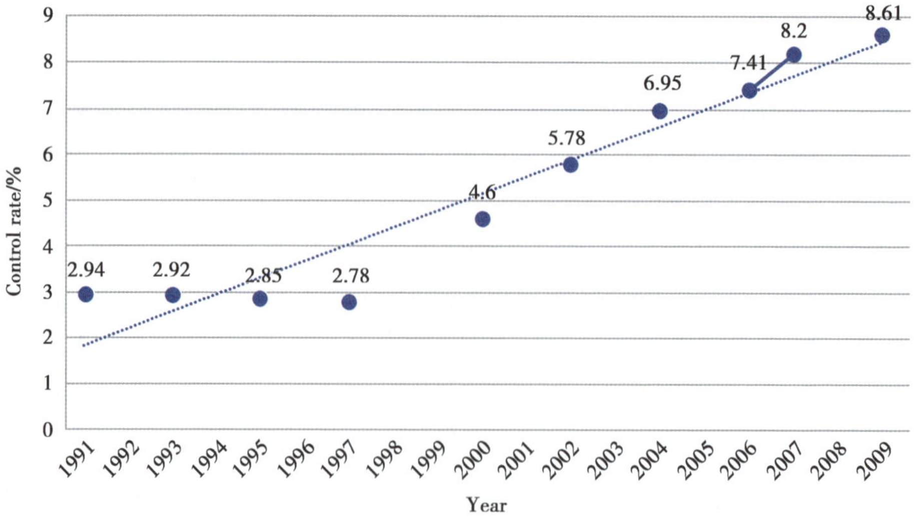

Figure 3-9 Original linear trend analysis on hypertension control rate 1991-2009

Linear trend model: $y = 0.367,2x + 1.483,6$, $R^2 = 0.924,8$

3.5 Evidence from other sources on the role of the NBPHS

3.5.1 Statistical analysis of hypertension management

To quantify the effectiveness of hypertension control, it is essential to know how many hypertensive patients had participated in the NBPHS program. According to the statistical data of the Office of Health Reform of the State Council (OHRSC), the number of patients managed by CHOs from 2010 to 2013 increased from 14.8 million to 85.03 million, as shown in Figure 3-10. By the end of 2017, the number of hypertensive patients managed by the NBPHS program had reached 101, 038, 100, and the annual investment in the NBPHS had reached 55 CNY per capita. By 2018, a total financial commitment of 452.8 billion CNY had been invested into the NBPHS program, of which approximately 248.3 billion CNY came from the central government.

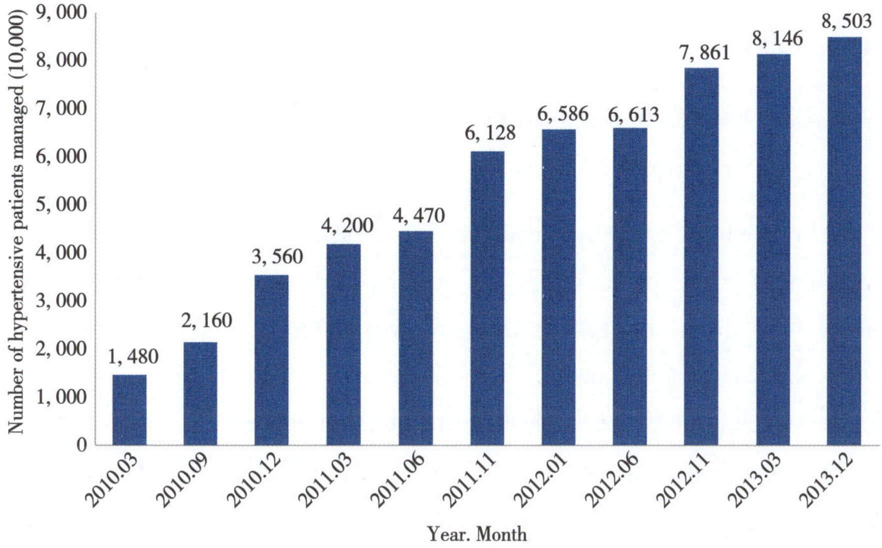

Figure 3-10 Number of hypertensive patients managed under the NBPHS, 2009-2013

Note: The lateral axis is of time, which expresses the year and month in each year, so, 2010.03 is March 2010.

Source: The Office of Health Reform of the State Council of China. Health reform monitoring report 2015, Retrieved April. 15, 2016.

Another estimate was made based on studies evaluating hypertension management at the community level after 1991 and these studies also evaluated the NBPHS. Government statistical data were used to determine the number of hypertensives managed by community health service facilities in China. If this number is multiplied by the control rate of hypertensives under community health service settings, the number of patients controlled can be generated. Based on this, further comparison can be made with estimates from the trend analysis.

As discussed earlier, the prevalence of hypertensives and awareness among hypertensive adults aged 35 or over equaled 32.62% and 44.91% respectively in 2015 [33].It was estimated that the number of hypertensives aged 35+ in 2015 was 223, 772, 752, while 100, 496, 343 hypertensives became aware of hypertension. By the end of 2015, it was reported that about 88.35 million hypertensives were covered by the NBPHS program in China, which means that about 88% of hypertensives with awareness were under a certain level of management within the NBPHS program. Therefore, hypertensives with a level of awareness who were identified in the China Hypertension Survey [33] can be used to represent the hypertensives under management within the NBPHS program in China.

3.5.2 Evidence from other literature on hypertension control within the NBPHS

Many attempts have been made to evaluate the effectiveness of hypertension management programs, in terms of lowering BP and improving hypertension control. To validate the results from trend analysis in this study, a literature review was conducted to analyze the quantitative effectiveness of hypertension management in terms of the number of patients under control.

In comparison to the method of trend analysis that employed hypertension PATC at the general population level, further evidence was based on a community health service setting or a specific evaluation of the NBPHS under the new health reform that began in 2009. Table 3-7 lists four studies with different survey datasets which attempted to analyze the impact of the NBPHS on hypertension management.

Linking data from the literature review with the analysis in Section 3.5.1, which reported that about 88.35 million hypertensives were covered by the NBPHS program in China, four estimates of the effectiveness of hypertension control from the NBPHS, which ranged from 6, 979, 650 to 16, 212, 225, were found as shown in the last row of Table 3-7.

3.5.2.1 An estimate using data before the implementation of the NBPHS

Two studies evaluated the community interventions that preceded the establishment of the NBPHS in 2009. The first was a 2008 follow-up evaluation of a guideline-oriented hypertension management program in Beijing. It focused on patients aged 50+ at high risk of stroke in primary healthcare settings and demonstrated that the rates of awareness, treatment and control of hypertension were 70.0%, 62.1% and 29.6%, respectively[151]. The study concluded that improvement of awareness and treatment in community health service settings would contribute to hypertension control.

A more representative study in China involving 1, 000 community health service centres in urban areas across China, which included a total of 249, 830 identified hypertensive patients, evaluated the association between drug use and BP control in community-based routine practice (see Table 3-7). It was reported that 37% of the patients covered by the Community Health Services Centers were treated. Among the treated patients, 36.5% received monotherapy and 63.5% received combination therapy, of which hypertension control rates were 27.7% and 24.1%, respectively [139]. The general hypertension control rate could reach 27.0% under management of a community health service [33]. According to the studies by the same author group[33] from 2012-2015, the hypertension control rate of the general hypertensive population aged 35+ was 14.72%. The difference between community management hypertensives and the hypertensives at the population level could be estimated as 12.28%. Taking the number of hypertensives covered by the NBPHS by the end of 2013 as the target population, or 85.03 million, the incremental number of hypertensives under control would be 10.44 million (85.03 million*12.28%).

3.5.2.2 An estimate with a before-and after-comparison

For evaluations of the NBPHS hypertension management at the national level in China, only two articles (in English) met the criteria set out in this investigator's

Table 3-7 Control of hypertension under community health management in China

Parameter	Year	Setting	Sample size	Age range (y)	Design	Control (%)	Improvements by NBPHS **	Estimated number of hypertension controlled as effectiveness of the NBPHS***
Hypertension control in community health centres across China	2007-2010	CHS	249, 830	18-79	Purposive sampling	27.0 (*SE*=0.7%)	Improved by 11.7 percentage points	10, 336, 950
Impact of the national essential public health services policy on hypertension control in China	2011-2013	Surveys	4, 958	⩾45	China health and retirement longitudinal study (CHARLS)	Control rate improved by 7.9% (*SE*=2.9%)	Control rate improved by 7.9%	6, 979, 650
Hypertension PACT following China's healthcare reform	2008-2012	Surveys	1, 961 and 1, 836	⩾45	CHARLS	21.7%-36.4%	Improved by 15.3 percentage points	13, 517, 550
Essential public health services' accessibility and its determinants among adults with chronic diseases in China	2013	CHS	1, 367	25-95	Multi-stage stratified random sampling	33.65* (*SE*=1.28%)	Improved by 18.35 percentage points	16, 212, 225

Notes: *The control rate of chronic disease denoted both hypertensive and diabetic patients, which did not display the two diseases separately.

**The CHS 2012-2015 demonstrated that hypertension control of hypertensives aged 18+ was 15.3%, [35]. According to this benchmark, it was estimated that the effectiveness of the NBPHS was the difference between the control of hypertension of hypertensives managed in CHS settings minus that of the general population (15.3%).

***The Estimated number of hypertension controlled as effectiveness of the NBPHS was the Improvements by NBPHS (shown in previous row) multiplied by 88.35 million, which was the number of hypertensives covered by the NBPHS program in China.

search. Both articles used data from the China Health and Retirement Longitudinal Study (CHARLS) using before-after analysis, focusing on Zhejiang and Gansu Provinces. Zhang et al.'s [152] study found that the coverage of the NBPHS program was associated with an increase of 7.9% in the hypertension control rate (*SE* = 2.9%) from 2011 to 2013 in Zhejiang and Gansu Provinces. In Hou et al.'s[66] analysis, the proportion of patients with hypertension under effective control in Gansu and Zhejiang Provinces increased from 21.7% to 36.4% from 2008 to 2012, showing a difference of 14.7 percentage points at the national level. These two studies defined how to evaluate hypertension management under the NBPHS program according to the specifications and guidelines, which focused on hypertension awareness, treatment and control. They also provided more quantitative evaluation evidence on hypertension PATC, using improved methodologies compared with those used in local area studies. However, the target population of CHARLS, which consists of adults aged 45 years and above, is not consistent with that of the NBPHS. Therefore, CHARLS could not be used to fully evaluate the program. Although the above two studies provided evaluation evidence, neither reflected the NBPHS program comprehensively. In the first study [152], the authors defined the patients who received a physical examination paid by the government as hypertension management, while the second study[66] considered hypertension awareness, treatment and control as the contents of hypertension management.

The two analyzes at the national level provided an estimate of hypertension control reflected by a change in percentage points, from 7.9% to 14.7% in the interval of 2011-2013 and 2008-2012. With the targeted hypertensives of 85.03 million, the incremental effectiveness of the NBPHS in terms of the number of people under hypertension control was estimated to be between 6.72 million and 12.50 million.

3.5.2.3 An estimation using a specific evaluation result of the NBPHS

In 2015, Tian et al. further developed the evaluation of the NBPHS program on hypertension and diabetes management. They conducted a cross-sectional study of a national representative hypertensive and diabetic population managed by primary care facilities under the NBPHS, focusing on the accessibility and effectiveness of the NBPHS[15]. This study revealed that patients with hypertension or diabetes were predominantly middle-aged or elderly, with a mean age of 65.26 years. Tian et al. (2015) defined hypertension management under the NBPHS program and effective management as regular follow-ups or check-ups. They concluded that the program provided effective disease management. Of all the participants, 33.65% had their BP or glucose controlled within the normal range for at least three months. Compared with other studies, Tian et al.'s[15] was not conducted using a case-control or longitudinal design. However, it provided comprehensive information on the status of hypertension control. It also provided a comprehensive and specific evaluation of the NBPHS on hypertension and diabetes from the perspective of managed patients.

If the hypertension control rate was 33.65% and the control rate among general hypertensives was 14.72%, the difference would be 18.93 percentage points. With the targeted number of managed hypertensives at 85.03 million, the incremental effectiveness of the NBPHS in terms of hypertension control was estimated to be 16.10 million persons.

Other evaluations were mainly targeted at developed areas in China, which denoted a high control rate in community health service settings. This may not represent the national status. For example, a guideline-oriented primary healthcare hypertension management program in Beijing proved that the hypertension control rate increased from 40.0% to 70.7% in urban areas and increased from 27.9% to 72.9% in rural areas after a 12-month follow-up[153]. This study involved four typical Community Health Service Centres in Beijing, with 140 patients with hypertension recruited in each centre. Studies in developed regions demonstrated that patients covered by the NBPHS program range from 36.1% (in Xuhui, Shanghai) to 83.2% (in Shanghai and Shenzhen) [82]. A study conducted in the Yulin Community Health Service Center of Chengdu proved that after three years of hypertension management [(33 ± 25) months], the hypertension control rate increased from 32% to 85%[154].

The studies discussed in this section provided a range of estimates for the incremental effectiveness of hypertension control. These were based on evaluations of hypertension management in community health service settings and statistical data from the health administrative departments in China. Three estimates were generated from evaluations of hypertension management in community health service settings. By the end of 2015, the incremental number of hypertensive patients with BP under control had reached 10.44 million, 6.72 million to 12.50 million, and 16.10 million. Evidence from other sources showed that by the end of 2015, the influence of the NBPHS on hypertension control ranged from 6.72 million to 16.10 million people.

In Section 3.4, it was estimated that the number of hypertensive patients under control was 9, 532, 719 [95%*CI* (2, 528, 632 16, 536, 806)], which was consistent with other evidence.

3.6 Discussion

This chapter has provided an estimate of the incremental effectiveness of the NBPHS program in terms of hypertension control. Time series analysis showed that the number of hypertensive patients with BP under control increased by 9.53 million from 2009 to 2015, which was attributed to the implementation of the NBPHS. Evidence from other sources was searched to evaluate the incremental effectiveness of the NBPHS in terms of hypertension control. This was based on hypertension management under community health service settings and statistical data from the health administrative departments in China. According to literature analysis of other evidence, the estimated number of those with controlled hypertension ranged from 6.72 million to 16.10 million. The estimate from the trend analysis lies within this range, which strengthened the confidence in the trend analysis.

In-depth analysis showed that awareness is the key influencing factor in hypertension control, encouraging patients to seek medical advice. The NBPHS has played a major role in improving hypertension awareness and, as a consequence, improving hypertension control.

It was discovered that awareness, treatment, and control rates increased with age. However, the treatment control rate was higher in the younger group than in the older group, at 40.4%, 40.0%, 38.7%, 34.8% and 32.6%, for age group 35-44, 45-54, 55-64, 65-74 and 75+, respectively. This suggests that younger patients are not well managed under the current program. A small improvement in awareness, treatment and control of young patients may result in a big increase in hypertension control.

More seriously, age-specific analysis shows that the NBPHS program did not play an effective role in hypertension control for the 35-44 age group (see Appendix D).

Although hypertension control has improved, it has been far from satisfactory[32, 38]. The treatment control rate, which ranged from 0.163 to 0.376, is much lower when compared with international levels[32, 38]. Although the Chinese Guidelines on Hypertension Management in Primary Care Settings[155] align with international hypertension guidelines, hypertensive patients managed under the program may not reduce their BP to a normal level. This may be partly attributable to the insufficient healthcare delivered by primary care facilities[19, 15], based on the limited human resources of primary healthcare in China[19, 66]. International comparisons highlight that there is still a big gap between China and developed countries in terms of hypertension awareness[63].

Some studies revealed that China had marked deficiencies in the availability, cost, and prescription of anti-hypertensive drugs [79]. The low income levels and high health insurance costs may compromise the effectiveness of the NBPHS program for hypertension control[79].

In addition, as China is a large country, accounting for one fifth of the world's population, the urban-rural gap and regional inequality are long-standing national problems [157]. Evidence suggests that education, geographic regions, changes in health status, occupation and other factors were important factors of perceived equality and benefits from the healthcare system generally[158]. In terms of the development of primary care and hypertension management, the same problems exist[32, 159-160]. It was reported that only a small number of patients with hypertension in China were diagnosed, and far less patients among them achieved optimal control [31]. In this sense, the NBPHS still has a long way to go. More health system reform measures should be taken to improve the investment mechanism, human resource management, medication accessibility and availability, and balanced regional development.

This is not the only study to conduct trend analysis of hypertension PATC. On the contrary, many studies have conducted similar analyzes, such as those that employed the CHNS data[51, 87]. However, evidence on the trends before and after the new health reform, which was launched in 2009, has been scarce, so the analysis presented in this chapter is a first and fills some of the identified gaps.

China is a large country with obvious differences within the country and variations in terms of economic development, demographic status, climate, customs, and so forth. It may be argued that it is meaningless to generalize across the entire Chinese population. In response to this concern, it should be stated that the NBPHS program was implemented in 2009 all over China, with national specifications and guided standards related to government investments. In addition, the NBPHS program was a part of the Equalization of Public Health Service in China, which reflects the concept of equalization in its very title. Finally, although this does not represent a tremendous investment per capita on public health, it is the largest basic public health service in the history of China. Therefore, it is necessary to evaluate the NBPHS at the national level, in terms of its contribution to hypertension awareness, treatment and control.

3.7 Limitations

The first limitation in this research is that the time series analysis data came from different sources and were not complete in an interval of one year. This may compromise the achievement of precise prediction. However, the employment of a full literature review and a lagrange interpolation polynomial method improved the confidence, where 95% confidence intervals have been provided for all estimates in this chapter and major results in Chapter 5. Secondly, as explained in the previous section, there is significant variation between regions in China, which makes it difficult to estimate the effectiveness of the NBPHS on hypertension control at the national level. This deficiency could only be solved through the collection of more consistent and complete data sources.

Although the CHNS database provided the most comprehensive and longitudinal information on hypertension PATC in China, it is not the largest representative study in China. Therefore, this study used data from the 2012-2015 Chinese Hypertension Survey[33] for further analysis of the latest information on hypertension control in China. This may have caused data inconsistency.

However, it was evident that data from the CHNS before 2009 were consistent with other studies. For example, the 1991 CHNS showed that the age-standardized hypertension PATC rates among adults aged 18+ were 14.13% (prevalence), 23.19% (awareness), 10.88% (treatment), and 2.75% (control), and those from the 1991 China Hypertension Survey of adults aged 15+ were 13.6%, 26.3%, 12.1%, and 2.8%, respectively. Another example was the similarity between the CHNS 2006 and 2009 and that of a national representative survey between 2005 and 2009, which analyzed hypertension PATC in 115 rural and urban communities involving 47, 000 people from China[144].

After 2009, a significant difference can be seen between the CHNS and other national representative studies. The Chinese hypertension surveys conducted after 2009, indicated that the hypertension control rate reached 13.8% in 2012 and 16.8% roughly in 2015 (Wang et al., 2018). The CHNS 2015 indicated that the control rate of hypertension among adults aged 35+ was 12.17%, while that of the CHNS 2011 was 14.31% and that of the 2015 Chinese Hypertension Survey was 14.72%. Therefore, this study employed the Chinese Hypertension Survey after 2009 as evidence for further analysis.

3.8 Brief summary

The NBPHS program has improved hypertension awareness, treatment and control. It was estimated that from 2009 to 2015, the NBPHS program increased the number of hypertensive patients under control by 9, 532, 719[95%*CI* (2, 528, 632, 16, 536, 806)]. The NBPHS program also played a major role in improving hypertension awareness. This was most obvious among hypertensives aged 55 years or above. However, there is still a way to go in terms of improving hypertension awareness, treatment, and treatment control for primary care facilities, especially for younger hypertensives. Further policy measures should focus on early detection, treatment and control for young hypertensive patients. The main measures inlcude estalish functional basic health care system, strengthening human resources, and making health insurance more efficient and medication more accessible.

4

Health outcome estimation of the NBPHS: A Markov model

4.1 Introduction

Chapter 3 presented a discussion on the effectiveness of the NBPHS in terms of hypertension control and revealed the mechanism through which the NBPHS worked. This provided an estimate of 9, 532, 719 hypertensives having their BP properly controlled from 2009 to 2015 because of the NBPHS. This chapter analyzes the long-term health outcomes of hypertension control. A hypothesized scenario is set in which the NBPHS is not implemented and the 9, 532, 719 hypertensives do not get their BP properly controlled. This is known as the non-NBPHS scenario And he actual (observed) status is the NBPHS scenario. The health consequences of hypertension in the two scenarios (NBPHS and non-NBPHS) are analyzed and compared. The difference represents the health outcomes of the NBPHS program.

As discussed in Chapter 2, CVDs are commonly referenced in the outcome assessment of hypertension intervention. However, if CVDs are considered the main consequence in assessments, it is important to consider other risk factors besides hypertension. This study used the CHNS 2009 data to extract information from a sample of hypertensives on other factors for the two scenarios (i.e., age, gender, BP, blood cholesterol, diabetes, BMI, and smoking). Based on a multi-factor analysis, risk levels in the development of CVDs were ascertained for the two scenarios. To compare the risk levels of the NBPHS scenario and the non-NBPHS scenario, published epidemiological and modelling studies of hypertension were drawn on[40, 107, 114] to generate the model parameters determining disease transitions. For the non-NBPHS scenario, the parameters of the NBPHS scenario were weighted by the relative rates generated.

A risk prediction and long-term health outcome model was developed by Gu et al. in 2015 based on a cost-effectiveness analysis of low-cost medicine for hypertension control[38]. This model was applied and validated in a more recent economic evaluation of intensive hypertension control in China[42]. Based on the above studies, a Markov model was developed to simulate the long-term development of hypertension and estimate related morbidities and mortalities. This is the focus of discussion in this chapter.

There are three further sections in this chapter: Section 4.2 provides a multi-factor analysis of CVD risk in the two scenarios based on the literature review and the CHNS 2009 data; Section 4.3 presents the Markov model and parameter estimations for the two groups; and Section 4.4 outlines the long-term estimations of CHD, stroke and deaths in a predicted 30-year period.

4.2 Analysis of CVD risks among hypertensives

4.2.1 Analysis of risk factors

As discussed in Chapter 2, age, gender, BP, BMI, total cholesterol, smoking and diabetes have been identified as independent variables for ICVDs, mainly focused on CHD and stroke[36, 40, 103]. However, the factors employed in different studies have not been the same. For example, Wu et al.[36] used age, SBP, BMI, total cholesterol, smoking and diabetes to establish a Cox model for the evaluation of ICVDs. Yang et al.[161] developed tools for the prediction of ASCVD in the Chinese population, using age, SBP, total cholesterol, LDL-C, waist circumference, smoking status, diabetes, urban-rural difference, and family history of ASCVD as risk factors. In 2007, the WHO/ISH developed a risk prediction chart for CVD applied to different WHO regions globally, with age, gender, SBP, total cholesterol, smoking status and diabetes mellitus as independent factors[47].

To simulate the relative rates of the two scenarios, a database with information on risk factors had to be employed. The only accessible qualified database was the CHNS 2009. The CHNS was a household-based study aiming to get information on key public health risk factors, demographic, social and economic factors, and health outcomes across ten rounds of surveys from 1989 to 2015. It employed a multi-stage, random cluster process for sampling[149]. Although the CHNS 2015 has been released recently, information about biomarkers, which is necessary for CVD risk analysis, was still not accessible.

In the CHNS conducted in 2009, a total of 9, 552 participants aged 18 years and over were included in the analysis and 1, 025 participants were hypertensives diagnosed by health professionals. The measurements and definitions of hypertension, awareness, treatment and control were explicated elsewhere[51]. Of the hypertensives identified, data from 1, 017 people aged 35 years and above were used for further analysis. The 1, 017 hypertensives were categorized into either the hypertension-controlled group or the hypertension-uncontrolled group (uncontrolled hypertension was defined as SBP/DBP$\geqslant$140/90 mmHg, otherwise controlled).

To conduct risk predictions of CVDs, mean values of age, gender, SBP, DBP, BMI, and total cholesterol were extracted from the CHNS 2009 dataset of the 1, 017 hypertensives. For each age-gender group, the smoking rate and prevalence of diabetes were calculated for the use of risk score equations. Diabetes was defined as a HbA1c value over 6.5% according to the WHO criteria (2011), receiving hypoglycemic treatment, or the answer "Yes" to the question "Has a doctor ever told you that you are diabetic (U24a)". Smoking status was modified based on the response to question U27: "Do you still smoke cigarettes?"

First, descriptive analysis was conducted. G1 and G2 represented the hypertension-controlled group in the NBPHS scenario and the hypertension-uncontrolled group in the non-NBPHS scenario, respectively. They were compared in age-gender specific features for each risk factor. Mean values were compared for age, SPB, DBP, TC, HDL, and low-density lipoprotein cholesterol (LDL-C). A t-test was employed to identify whether differences were statistically significant (P<0.05). Pearson's chi-square analysis was used to identify whether the difference between the two groups, considering the proportion of smoking and diabetes, was statistically significant (P<0.05). Means and proportions of CVD risk factors were calculated for Chinese adults in 10-year age categories. Comparisons were conducted for the difference between the two groups of age-gender specific risk factor distributions. Statistical analyzes were conducted with SPSS 22.0. Figure 4-1 shows the decision tree of the process of the two scenarios established for comparison in this study. Starting from the first cell on the left, the upper two cells stand for the NBPHS scenario and the lower two cells stand for the non-NBPHS scenario.

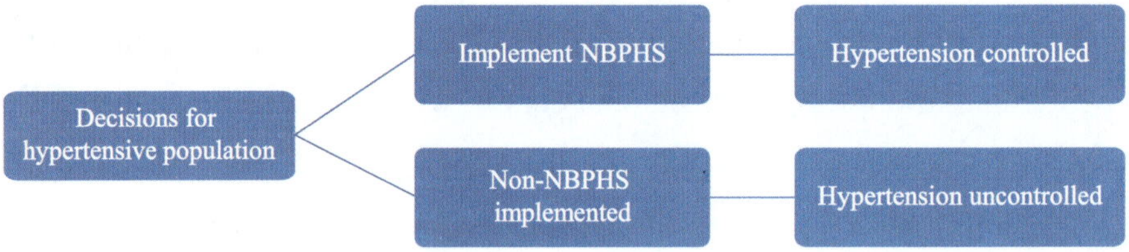

Figure 4-1 Decision tree for NBPHS and non-NBPHS implementation

4.2.2 Results of the risk factor analysis

Among the 1, 017 analyzed participants aged 35+ years who were diagnosed as hypertensives, 44.05% were men and 55.05% women, and 68.53% were hypertension-uncontrolled and 31.47% hypertension-controlled. A significant difference was observed between the hypertension-controlled group and the uncontrolled group in SBP and DBP in all age-gender groups (P<0.05). In the hypertension-controlled group, the mean SBP was around 127mmHg for both males and females; while in the hypertension-uncontrolled group, the mean SBP ranged from 147 to 169mmHg for both genders. There was no significant difference between the two groups for other factors, including mean age, TC, HDL-C, BMI, diabetes rate and smoking rate (*P*>0.05).

Based on the above analysis, out of the eight variables considered to be independent risk factors for CVDs, a difference was only found in BP, which provided a foundation for further analysis of risks among the two groups.

This author has written an article on the above analysis, published in 2018 in the journal *Chinese General Practice*[162]. Details can be seen in this article.

4.3 Method: A Markov model

The CDPM has been the best developed and most widely used model for CVD risk prediction among recent studies[38, 41, 113]. Therefore, this study developed a Markov model for long-term projection based on the CDPM.

To assess the outcomes of NBPHS implementation on hypertension management, the Markov model was used in the two scenarios over a predicted 30-year period. Results were reported for the whole hypertensive population simulated in a closed cohort under NBPHS management, as well as for different age and gender groups.

4.3.1 Markov model development

A Markov model is a state-transition model that is commonly used to evaluate the outcomes of anti-hypertensive treatments[56, 163]. The CDPM was developed based on a Markov model. It was a state-transition, mathematical model for CHD and stroke prevalence, incidence, mortality, and costs in the adult Chinese population, with a cycle length of one year. Researchers have confirmed that the CDPM can be adapted to simulate a closed cohort[38, 40].In this study, the Markov model was used for the hypertensive population in China aged 35+ years following the CDPM [38, 41]. The structure of the Markov model is illustrated in Figure 4-2. In this thesis, CVDs includes stroke and coronary heart disease, and therefore, one state is hidden in Figure 4-2.

The patients of either the hypertension-controlled or the uncontrolled group could shift to one of the six health states: hypertension only; acute heart disease;

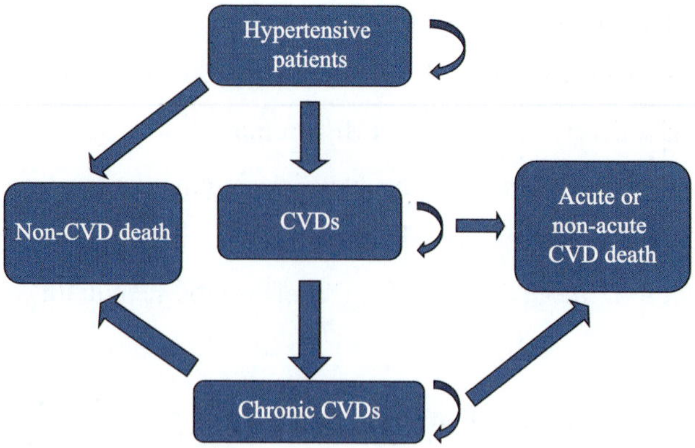

Figure 4-2 Markov model on the progression of CVD in hypertensive patients

acute stroke; chronic CHD; chronic stroke; or death.

The initial stroke or CHD event and its sequelae for 28 days were described in the CDPM model[38, 41].

The cycle of the Markov model was one year. The 28-day case fatality was defined as instant death from acute CHD or stroke. One-year case fatalities of CHD and stroke were calculated based on CHD and stroke mortality, and prior-prevalence of CHD and stroke, aligned with Gu et al.'s study [38].

The non-CVD mortality equaled the all-cause death rate of the population[163] minus CHD mortality and stroke mortality.

Again, the definition of CHD and stroke under the CDPM aligned with Gu et al.'s[38] study. It was assumed that there was no remission to a CVD-free state after a CVD incident. Other health states or diseases were not considered. CHD and stroke were analyzed separately, rather than in the form of CHD, stroke and their combination. A shift between any two health states was defined as a probable transition derived from Gu.et al.'s study[38]. Each state has an annual probability of shifting to a different CVD state. The hypertensive population was stratified by age in 10-year categories and gender.

In this study, the dynamic process of hypertension patients aged 35+ years follows that in the CDPM[38, 41]. Patients remained in the baseline state until a fatal or non-fatal CVD event or death from other non-CVD-related causes occurred. One year was used as the basic simulation cycle. From the stable CVD state, patients could get into a subsequent fatal or non-fatal CVD event or death from non-CVD causes. As shown in Figure 4-3 below, there are six health states: hypertension, CHD, CHD death, stroke, stroke death, and non-CVD death. The state of death is from three causes, which are CHD, stroke and non-CVD causes. Hypertension, CHD and stroke from the last cycle were all fed into the next cycle separately.

TreeAge Pro software 2019 R1.1 (TreeAge Software, Inc., Williamstown, MA, USA) was employed for the calculation of the Markov model. An example of the structure of the model is given in Figure 4-3.

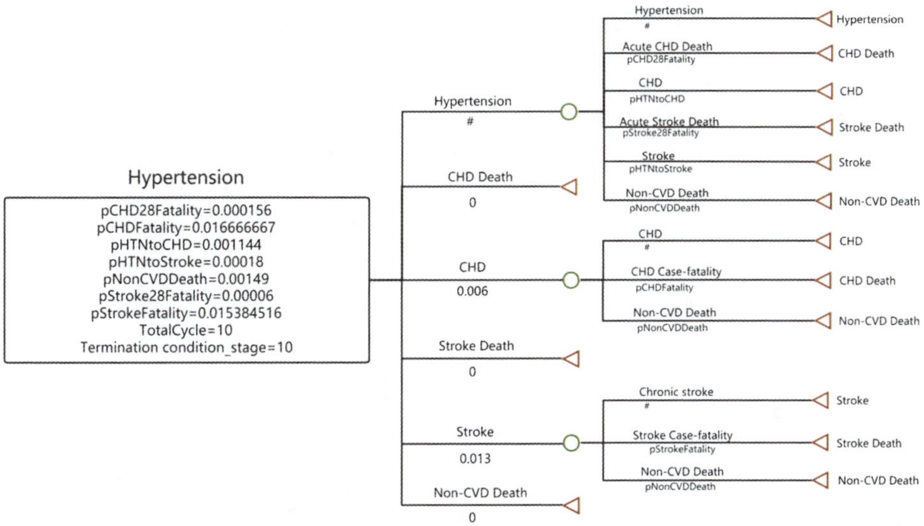

Figure 4-3 Markov model structure, taking the male G1 35-45 age group as an example (1. # equals to 1-sum of values on other branches under the same level; 2. " ○ "means circulation; " △ " means ending.)

4.3.2 Target population

As discussed in Chapter 3, it was estimated that 9, 532, 719 hypertensive patients got their BP under control because of the NBPHS. Because there was no national representative survey available for such a population, this study employed the CHS 2012-2015 to represent the target population in terms of age-gender structure, prevalence and control of hypertension. The CHS was undertaken from October 2012 to December 2015 under a stratified multi-stage random sampling method, involving a nationally representative sample of 451, 755 residents aged over 18 years from 31 provinces in China. The results of the survey were published in 2018[33]. Age-gender structure was weighted according to data from the 2010 Chinese Census. The effectiveness of the NBPHS was quantified by the number of hypertensives under control. The age-gender structure of the controlled hypertensives in the CHS 2012-2015 was considered the same as that of the study population. Another reason for such a simulation is based on the analysis discussed in Chapter 3, which estimated that about 88% of hypertensives aged 35+ years with a level of awareness were under some form of management within the NBPHS program (see Table 4-1).

Table 4-1 Data used for age-standardizing the target population

Age group, years	Population/% [a]	Crude prevalence [b]	Crude control rate [b**]
Men			
35-44	10.2	17.8	9.9
45-54	13.1	30.0	16.1
55-64	14.0	43.5	18.6
65-74	8.9	53.8	18.4
75-84	4.5	56.8	17.0
85+*	0.7	56.8	17.0
Women			
35-44	5.9	10.8	9.9
45-54	11.6	27.8	16.1
55-64	14.2	45.0	18.6
65-74	9.8	58.0	18.4
75-84	5.7	62.7	17.0
85+*	1.3	62.7	17.0

Notes: * Crude prevalence and control rates of people aged 85+ were not specifically described in the China Hypertension Survey and this study considers it the same as that of the 75+ age group.

** The age-sex specific control rates were not described in the China Hypertension Survey and this study considers the control rates of the two sexes were the same.

Source: a. 2010 Chinese Census data, China National Bureau of Statistics.

b. China Hypertension Survey (Wang et al., 2018).

Based on the data extracted from the CHS and the 2010 Chinese Census, further assumptions were made: 1) the 9, 532, 719 hypertensives controlled by the NBPHS had the same age-gender structure as those involved in the CHS 2012-2015 (Wang et al., 2018); 2) in the non-NBPHS scenario, the 9, 532, 719 hypertensives without hypertension control also had the same age-gender structure as those involved in the CHS; and 3) as the hypertension prevalence of the age group aged 85+ years was not available through the CHS 2012-2015[35], the hypertension prevalence and control of this group was assumed to be the same as that of the group aged 75-84.

To calculate the number of hypertensives in each age-gender group: first, the hypertension prevalence and control rate (taken from the CHS 2012-2015) in each age-gender group was weighted by the population in each age-gender group, according to the 2010 Chinese Census; second, the proportion of each age-gender group was multiplied by 9, 532, 719. The results are shown in Table 4-2.

Table 4-2 Weighted structure and number of target hypertensives aged 35+years

Age group, years	Proportion/%	Number of hypertensives
Men		
35-44	6.11	582, 276
45-54	12.71	1, 211, 554
55-64	16.04	1, 529, 342
65-74	10.29	981, 285
75-84	4.64	442, 566
85+	0.79	75, 476
Women		
35-44	3.55	338, 476
45-54	11.29	1, 076, 590
55-64	16.16	1, 540, 445
65-74	11.02	1, 050, 308
75-84	5.96	568, 066
85+	1.43	136, 336
Total	100	9, 532, 719

Data source: Population age-gender structure from the 6th population census and hypertension prevalence of each age-group from 2012-2015 CHS[33].

4.3.3 Parameters for estimating long-term health outcomes

For the hypertension-controlled group and the non-controlled group, middle-term and long-term health outcomes were represented by CVDs avoided and deaths averted, which assumed that the 9, 532, 719 hypertensives were categorized into a closed cohort under the two scenarios.

It was assumed that in the NBPHS scenario (G1), in which the 9, 532, 719 hypertensives got their BP controlled, the model parameters that determine disease shifts were the same as those of the general population extracted from previous studies [38]. In the non-NBPHS scenario (G2), in which the 9, 532, 719 hypertensives did not get their BP controlled, the model parameters that determine disease shifts were weighted by the annual risk ratios of the two groups for each age-gender group.

As discussed earlier, the only risk factor for fatal and non-fatal CVDs was the BP level for the two groups. Parameters for G2 were weighted by the relative risks of G2 to G1 in terms of the SBP level, based on BP and the risk of CVDs in the Chinese population[39]. The SBP levels of the two groups, as evident in the CHNS 2009 data, have been described in Section 1 of this chapter, which also described risk factors of CVDs. The relative risks of CHD and stroke were calculated from the SBP levels[39]. The risk ratio of G1 to G2 was also calculated, as shown in Table 4-3. By comparing the relative rates of G2 and G1, the risk ratios of each age-gender group were generated, also shown in Table 4-3.

Table 4-3 SBP level and relative risks of developing CHD and stroke, G1 and G2

Age group	SBP/mmHg*		Multivariate-adjusted RR as indicated by Gu et al. (2008)					
			CHD			Stroke		
	G1	G2	G1	G2	G2 to G1 ratio	G1	G2	G2 to G1 ratio
Men/yr								
35-44	127	147	1.23	2.03	**1.65**	1.76	3.62	**2.06**
45-54	127	149	1.23	2.03	**1.65**	1.76	3.62	**2.06**
55-64	129	152	1.23	2.03	**1.65**	1.76	3.62	**2.06**
65-74	127	157	1.23	2.03	**1.65**	1.76	3.62	**2.06**
75-84	126	160	1.23	2.84	**2.31**	1.76	5.83	**3.31**
85+	127	157	1.23	2.03	**1.65**	1.76	3.62	**2.06**

continued

Age group	SBP/mmHg*		Multivariate-adjusted RR as indicated by Gu et al. (2008)					
			CHD			Stroke		
	G1	G2	G1	G2	G2 to G1 ratio	G1	G2	G2 to G1 ratio
Women/yr								
35-44	131	155	1.17	1.63	**1.39**	1.98	3.32	**1.68**
45-54	125	152	1.16	1.63	**1.41**	1.59	3.32	**2.09**
55-64	127	156	1.16	1.63	**1.41**	1.59	3.32	**2.09**
65-74	131	156	1.17	1.63	**1.39**	1.98	3.32	**1.68**
75-84	126	164	1.16	2.00	**1.72**	1.59	4.96	**3.12**
85+	138	164	1.17	2.00	**1.71**	1.98	4.96	**2.51**

Note: *The SBP level for each age-gender group was taken from the 2009 CHNS.

The parameters for the Markov model are as follows:

- The age-gender structure of the hypertensive population is as described in Section 4.3.2.
- Prior myocardial infarction (MI), prior stroke, incidence of CHD and stroke, 28-days case fatality and mortality of CHD, and stroke were all adopted from recent epidemiological and modeling studies[38, 105], in which they were well calibrated. It was assumed that prior MI or stroke in the study population was the same as that in the general population.
- Non-CVD mortality was calculated based on 2013 statistics of urban/rural age-gender disease specific mortality[43] and the population structure was based on the 2010 Chinese Census. As the age-gender structure of urban and rural populations was not available, it was assumed that there was no significant difference between those populations. This study adjusted 2013 urban-rural specific mortalities and generated age-gender specific all-cause mortality rates[43]. The non-CVD mortality rates adjusted by age-gender are listed in Appendix Table B3.
- Mortality rates for CHD and stroke were taken from Chan et al.[106] for hypertensives younger than 85 years. Mortality rates were calculated by dividing the number of deaths by the population at risk during a defined time period, usually one year[98]. The CHD mortality and stroke mortality rates for

adults aged 85+ were calculated based on urban and rural age-gender disease specific mortality from the 2014 *Chinese Health Statistic Yearbook*[43] and the age-gender structures were adjusted according to the data from the 2010 Chinese Census.

- The 28-day case fatality rate was used to represent deaths caused by acute CVDs based on Chan et al.'s[106] study in each cycle (one year). The case fatality rate, or the case fatality ratio, is the proportion of deaths of a defined disease as in all individuals diagnosed with the disease over a specific period of time. The case fatality rate was generated by dividing the number of deaths, because of the analyzed disease, over a certain period (one year), by the number of patients with the disease during that time.
- The case fatality rate of CHD or stroke was generated from CHD or stroke mortality and the prevalence of prior MI or prior stroke (used as the general prevalence of CHD or stroke). This was equals to the CHD or stroke mortality minus 28-day case fatality of CHD or stroke.

For details, see Table 4-4 and Appendix Table B4.

All the parameters were in 10-year age categories and the Markov process was run in one-year cycles. Parameters were changed into the next 10-year age groups after running for 10 cycles. Results of hypertension, CHDs, stroke, deaths due to CHD or stroke and non-CVDs death running from the first 10 cycles were fed into the next 10-year age-gender group. Details are provided in Appendix Table B4.

The model started with four states: hypertension only, with prior MI, with prior stroke, and death (0 at the start point). Cumulative incidences of CHD, stroke, instant (28-day) case fatalities, deaths due to chronic CVDs, and deaths due to non-CVD causes in each age-gender group of the target population were estimated under the two scenarios.

In the Markov model, shifts among CVDs, adverse events, and death over the 30-year period were evident. For the age group 75-84, only 10- and 20-year shifts were reported, and for the age group 85+, only 10-year shifts were reported because of the lack of data on life expectancy. In each cycle, the number of CHDs, strokes and deaths were aggregated with the previous cycle over time.

Table 4-4 Parameters and data sources

Parameters	Source
Age-gender specific proportion of hypertensives	The 2010 Chinese Census & Z. Wang et al. (2018)[33]
CHDs	
Prior CHD	(Gu et al., 2015)[38]
Incidence of CHD for G1	(Gu et al., 2015)[38]
Incidence of CHD for G2	Recalculation
28-days case fatality	(Gu et al., 2015)[38]
CHD mortality	(Gu et al., 2015)[38]
CHD case fatality (yearly)	Calculated
Stroke	
Prior stroke	(Gu et al., 2015)[38]
Incidence of stroke for G1	(Gu et al., 2015a)[38]
Incidence of stroke for G2	Recalculation
28-days case fatality	(Gu et al., 2015a)[38]
Stroke mortality	(Gu et al., 2015a)[38]
Stroke case fatality (yearly)	Calculated
Non-CVD mortality	*China Health Statistical Yearbook*, 2014[43]

4.3.4 Sensitivity analysis

Thc CHNS 2009 showed that the difference between G1 and G2 (hypertension control or not) was mainly caused by blood pressure. Although 2015 CHNS didn’t have biomarker data, it did have blood pressure data. And in the CHNS 2015, the measurement of blood pressure and the definition of hypertension was exactly the same as that of CHNS 2009. Therefore, a sensitivity analysis was carried out with the use of 2009 data, and SBP levels of G1 and G2 were analyzed with data from the CHNS 2015, with results shown in Table 4-5-1 and Table 4-5-2. The differences between the CHNS 2009 and 2015 in both the hypertension controlled and uncontrolled groups across all age-groups are quite small, except for 35-45 of women (5.47%) in G1 and 85+ of women in G2 (5.62%). The difference of SBP across all age groups between 2009 and 2015 as a percentage of 2009 was 0.63% for the hypertension controlled group, and 0.60% for hypertension uncontrolled group, as shown in Table 4-5-1 and Table 4-5-2.

Table 4-5-1 SBP of hypertension controlled group of CHNS 2009 and 2015 (G1)

Age group	2009			2015			Difference of SBP between 2009 and 2015 as of 2009 /%
	N	Mean Blood pressure/ mmHg	Standard Deviation	N	Mean Blood pressure/ mmHg	Standard Deviation	
Men/yr							
35-44	10	127.13	5.675	13	129.18	10.14	1.61
45-54	28	127.33	11.195	48	124.62	7.487	−2.13
55-64	35	128.65	10.841	97	127.67	9.02	−0.76
65-74	42	127.44	9.605	117	127.3	8.405	−0.11
75-84	16	126.5	9.022	40	128.25	6.65	1.38
85+	2	127	5.185	2	130.67	6.6	2.89
Women/yr							
35-44	7	131.1	9.863	10	123.93	9.815	−5.47
45-54	43	125.04	9.543	57	126.66	9.751	1.30
55-64	51	126.69	11.169	123	125.52	9.539	−0.92
65-74	63	130.68	8.343	103	126.52	8.472	−3.18
75-84	22	125.52	13.155	41	129.59	7.676	3.24
85+	1	136.67	N/A	4	133.83	4.29	−2.08
Total	320	127.68	10.101	655	126.88	8.743	−0.63

Note: *The SBP level for each age-gender group was taken from the CHNS 2009 and 2015. N/A means not available.

Table 4-5-2 SBP of hypertension controlled group of CHNS 2009 and 2015 (G2)

Age group	2009			2015			Difference in SBP between 2009 and 2015 as of 2009/%
	N	Mean Blood pressure/mmHg	Standard Deviation	N	Mean Blood pressure/mmHg	Standard Deviation	
Men/yr							
35-44	14	147.24	14.556	26	148.53	14.882	0.88
45-54	55	148.63	13.642	106	148.94	15.154	0.21
55-64	74	152.15	18.032	199	152.27	14.904	0.08
65-74	78	156.64	14.886	193	154.94	16.721	-1.09
75-84	38	159.94	19.435	64	154.22	14.54	-3.58
85+	3	156.67	6.11	13	157.79	11.375	0.71
Women/yr							
35-44	11	155.45	28.772	26	150.54	15.361	-3.16
45-54	48	151.88	14.52	111	155.88	16.421	2.63
55-64	97	156.08	14.913	208	153.96	14.788	-1.36
65-74	99	155.8	15.144	234	158.13	17.357	1.50
75-84	56	164.35	23.929	109	157.25	17.1	-4.32
85+	4	163.08	5.865	13	153.92	14.859	-5.62
Total	577	155.43	17.273	1, 302	154.5	16.104	-0.60

Note: *The SBP level for each age-gender group was taken from the CHNS 2009 and 2015. N/A means not available.

4.4 Long-term health outcome estimations

4.4.1 Long-term trends in CVD development and deaths in the two groups

In each projected year, the number of patients developing CHDs, strokes, or dying due to CVDs, and non-CVD deaths in the total were generated in the Markov process.

Figure 4-4 provides a graphic representation of the trends in total deaths over the projected 30-year period for G1 and G2, taking the 35-44 age group of male and female hypertensives as an example. This indicates that at the end of the projection period, the number of deaths due to CVDs in the G2 scenario was higher than in the G1 scenario.

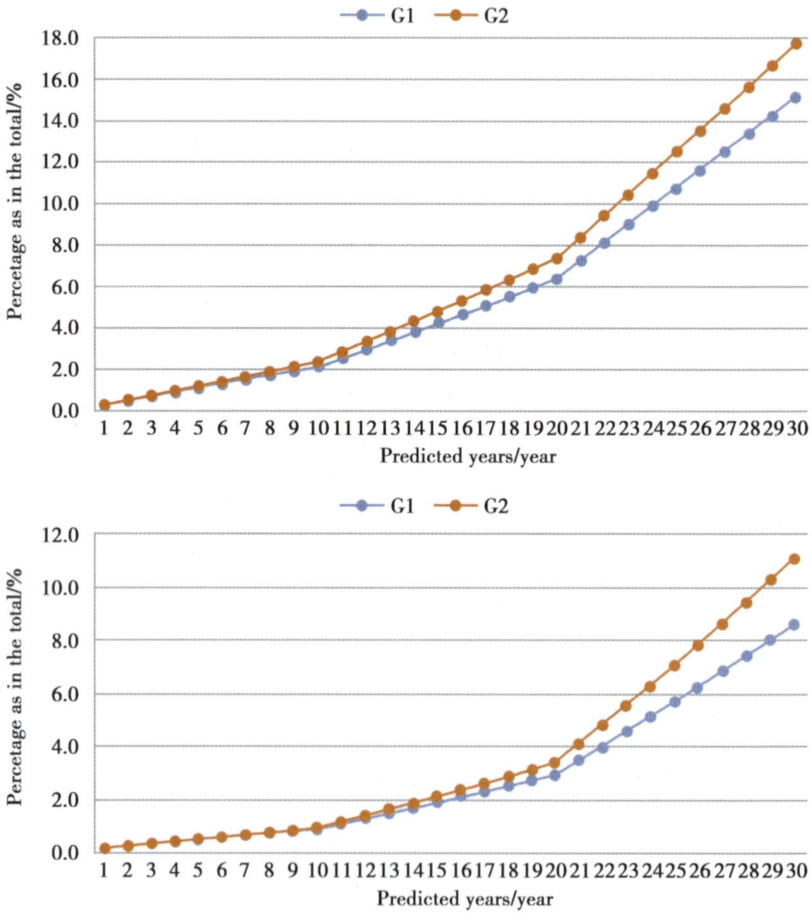

Figure 4-4 Percentages of deaths in G1 (blue) and G2 (orange), for 35-44-year-old males (upper side) and females (below side)

Trends in deaths over the projected 30-year period for all other age-gender groups are presented in Appendix B: Supplementary materials.

4.4.2 Estimates of CVDs and deaths averted

At the end of the 10th projection year in the G1 scenario, compared with G2, 43, 386, 314, 004, and 289, 644 hypertensive patients would have avoided CHD, stroke and death, respectively. At the end of the 20th projection year, 45, 035, 400, 313, and 558, 625 hypertensive patients would have avoided CHD, stroke and death, respectively. At the end of the 30th projection year, 25, 012, 296, 258, and 744, 493 hypertensive patients would have avoided CHD, stroke and death, respectively. Details of these results are provided in Tables 4-6, 4-7, and 4-8. In Table 4-8, there are some negative figures which are generated mainly from older age groups of both genders in the 30-year horizon analysis (age groups of 65-74 and 75-84 years). This is because in the non-NBPHS group, more patients die from CVDs than those in the NBPHS group, which makes less CVDs survivors compared with those, especially for stroke.

4.5 Brief summary

Based on the above analysis, obvious decreases in CVDs and deaths due to CVDs were found in 10-, 20- and 30-year horizon projections due to the implementation of the NBPHS. The G2 scenario (non-NBPHS implementation) had a much higher incidence of CVDs and deaths compared with that of G1. This indicates that the NBPHS was effective in preventing CVDs and averting deaths.

The assumption in the analysis was that there was no significant difference between the hypertension-controlled population under the NBPHS scenario and those in the general population, and between the hypertension uncontrolled population under the non-NBPHS scenario and those in the general population. According to the analysis of the CHNS 2009, BP levels increased with age, which is the same as other findings[35, 147]. It was discovered that the major determinant of CVD risk was BP level in the two simulated groups.

Table 4-6 Running results for a 10-year horizon

Age group	G1			G2			Number of patients avoiding CVD and death		
	CHD	Stroke	Death	CHD	Stroke	Death	CHD	Stroke	Death
Men/yr									
35-44	8, 850	7, 325	11, 961	12, 685	8, 295	13, 241	3, 835	970	1, 279
45-54	20, 764	43, 028	55, 518	27, 332	55, 544	62, 625	6, 568	12, 516	7, 107
55-64	52, 845	171, 455	160, 667	62, 566	235, 985	181, 610	9, 720	64, 529	20, 943
65-74	39, 085	134, 254	250, 126	47, 710	182, 196	281, 718	8, 625	47, 943	31, 591
75-84	10, 657	27, 684	262, 932	13, 782	44, 502	330, 665	3, 124	16, 818	67, 733
85+	196	708	63, 276	214	1, 017	67, 247	18	310	3, 971
Women/yr									
35-44	1, 822	3, 301	2, 901	2, 010	3, 713	3, 061	187	413	160
45-54	15, 382	37, 287	24, 892	16, 788	53, 124	29, 098	1, 406	15, 838	4, 205
55-64	52, 731	151, 827	104, 128	57, 084	231, 981	130, 512	4, 353	80, 154	26, 384
65-74	36, 524	142, 037	188, 712	40, 111	187, 380	215, 570	3, 587	45, 343	26, 858
75-84	16, 363	39, 042	288, 907	18, 303	67, 216	376, 364	1, 941	28, 174	87, 457
85+	529	1, 628	105, 549	550	2, 626	117, 503	21	998	11, 954
Total							43, 386	314, 004	289, 644

Table 4-7 Running results for a 20-year horizon

Age group	G1			G2			Number of patients avoiding CVD and death		
	CHD	Stroke	Death	CHD	Stroke	Death	CHD	Stroke	Death
Male/yr									
35-44	11, 288	11, 640	36, 786	17, 081	18, 271	42, 491	5, 794	6, 632	5, 705
45-54	27, 984	87, 416	165, 285	39, 953	147, 164	191, 465	11, 969	59, 748	26, 180
55-64	49, 619	176, 237	501, 353	63, 760	270, 605	575, 794	14, 141	94, 368	74, 441
65-74	16, 748	49, 410	689, 698	19, 449	76, 986	812, 824	2, 701	27, 576	123, 127
75-84	464	1, 683	413, 651	193	1, 152	434, 930	-271	-531	21, 278
85+	196	708	63, 276	214	1, 017	67, 247	18	310	3, 971
Female/yr									
35-44	2, 675	7, 595	9, 779	3, 278	12, 979	11, 345	603	5, 384	1, 566
45-54	21, 910	86, 113	89, 760	25, 939	153, 118	115, 012	4, 028	67, 005	25, 252
55-64	47, 061	199, 008	362, 939	52, 755	295, 357	438, 796	5, 694	96, 349	75, 857
65-74	22, 513	66, 566	633, 132	23, 385	109, 438	779, 062	873	42, 872	145, 930
75-84	1, 058	3, 309	506, 396	523	2, 912	549, 760	-535	-397	43, 364
85+	529	1, 628	105, 549	550	2, 626	117, 503	21	998	11, 954
Total							45, 035	400, 313	558, 625

Table 4-8 Running results for a 30-year horizon

Age group	G1			G2			Number of patients with avoiding CVD and death		
	CHD	Stroke	Death	CHD	Stroke	Death	CHD	Stroke	Death
Male/yr									
35-44	14, 331	34, 814	87, 775	21, 795	63, 359	102, 978	7, 464	28, 545	15, 203
45-54	33, 031	113, 086	412, 957	45, 871	191, 467	482, 630	12, 840	78, 381	69, 673
55-64	23, 572	67, 940	1, 113, 669	25, 708	107, 119	1, 301, 559	2, 136	39, 179	187, 891
65-74	740	2, 721	935, 116	259	1, 666	970, 908	–481	–1, 055	35, 792
75-84	464	1, 683	413, 651	193	1, 152	434, 930	–271	–531	21, 278
85+	196	708	63, 276	214	1, 017	67, 247	18	310	3, 971
Female/yr									
35-44	5, 111	24, 123	29, 135	6, 516	45, 658	37, 457	1, 405	21, 535	8, 323
45-54	24, 115	128, 254	259, 680	28, 452	200, 737	321, 327	4, 337	72, 483	61, 647
55-64	30, 398	91, 952	970, 678	29, 347	149, 716	1, 189, 612	–1, 051	57, 764	218, 934
65-74	1, 552	4, 928	959, 805	682	3, 973	1, 026, 267	–870	–955	66, 463
75-84	1, 058	3, 309	506, 396	523	2, 912	549, 760	–535	–397	43, 364
85+	529	1, 628	105, 549	550	2, 626	117, 503	21	998	11, 954
Total							25, 012	296, 258	744, 493

This is the first study to analyze hypertension management from this perspective. As discussed in Chapter 3, several studies have attempted to evaluate hypertension management under the NBPHS in terms of improved hypertension control rates and decreased BP levels[15, 65, 154]. However, evidence on the middle-and long-term impacts of hypertension management is scarce. This study has, to an extent, filled this gap.

This study has several strengths. First, a population survey was employed to reflect the real status of risk factors for a hypertensive population. By employing data from the CHNS 2009, the risk factors for hypertension-controlled and uncontrolled populations were compared, including age, gender, BP, total cholesterol, BMI, smoking, and diabetes. To make the analysis more representative, the CHS 2012-2015 was used for the age-gender structure analysis of the hypertensive population. As explained in Chapter 3, estimated based on the CHS 2012-2015[33], the number of hypertensives aged 35+ in 2015 was 223, 772, 752, while 100, 496, 343 hypertensives became aware of their condition. According to statistical data from the health reform report[164], by the end of 2015, about 88.35 million hypertensives were covered by the NBPHS program in China. This means that about 88% of hypertensives with awareness of their condition, were under a certain level of management in the NBPHS program. Therefore, the hypertensives with awareness in the *China Hypertension Survey*[33] can be used to represent the hypertensives under management in the NBPHS program in China. Secondly, by employing a Markov model[38, 113], combined with a risk prediction model[39, 165], a long-term projection was made. This fills a gap in economic evaluation research on hypertension management in China. As hypertension is a "chronic disease", effectiveness should be expressed from a middle-or long-term perspective. This will help policymakers in their long-term decision-making. Thirdly, the analysis provided a clear structure of all simulated states in the projected 30-year period. This provides a basis for all kinds of economic evaluations, including CEA, CUA and CBA, as cost, effectiveness, utility and benefit data can be assigned to each state in each year[117, 166].

People may challenge the assumption that in the non-NBPHS scenario, none of the 9, 532, 719 patients got their BP under control. However, this is a possibility. As discussed in Chapter 3, China still has quite low rates of awareness, treatment, and control in relation to hypertension; and the improvement of awareness, treatment and control has been far from satisfactory. From 1991 to 2015, the control rate of hypertension among adults in China was still lower than 20%, which means that in that 25-year period more than 150 million hypertensives did not have their hypertension properly under control.

It has been suggested that treating all hypertensives in China could prevent about 800, 000 CVD events each year[38]. This study takes this estimation further through longer-term projections and by taking both CVDs and deaths averted into account. Although progress has been achieved, there is still a way to go. The latest data shows that no more than 15% of hypertensives aged 35+ years have their hypertension under control[33]. If all hypertensives had their BP controlled, the number of deaths averted would be many times the current estimates.

This chapter has provided a bridge between Chapter 3 and Chapter 5, linking direct health outcomes with economic outcomes, respectively. The methods used were twofold: a CVD risk estimation model based on Gu et al.'s[38, 39] studies; and a Markov model used for long-term health impact estimation, commonly used in the economic evaluation of healthcare programs[42, 127]. Internationally, economic evaluations of hypertension management in primary care settings have been well conducted, such as studies in Argentina[112], the Netherlands[129], Vietnam[137], and the UK[167]. In China, the evidence in this area is scarce. Again, this study helps fill that gap.

The limitation of this study lies mainly in the data used for analyzing the risk factors of fatal and non-fatal CVDs, which were extracted from the CHNS 2009. If more recent data were available, an up-to-date analysis could be performed.

In conclusion, in a 30-year horizon, the implementation of the NBPHS reduced the incidence of CHD, stroke and deaths by 25, 012 296, 258, and 744, 493, respectively. The Markov model results provided the patient numbers for hypertension, CHD, stroke, and deaths in each simulated year. These were applied to an economic evaluation, discussed in the following chapter.

5

Benefit, cost and return on investment of the NBPHS on hypertension control: An innovative framework

5.1 Introduction

Based on the results discussed in Chapters 3 and 4, this chapter presents an economic evaluation of the investment in hypertension management under the NBPHS, focused on a return on investment based on a benefit-cost analysis.

The return on investment framework on health interventions was developed by the Victoria Institute of Strategic Economic Studies (VISES) of Victoria University (VU) and has been peer-reviewed and validated in a number of different studies. The model was initially developed for maternal and child health[45], and adolescent health[168]. Importantly, it has been used in the evaluation of interventions for NCDs, namely CVDs [44] and mental health [169]. These studies covered a number of countries and all included China in the analysis. More recently, the framework has been used in individual countries, such as India and Burundi[170].

All these studies included health outcome models and economic models. The health outcomes were modelled using the One Health Tool (OHT). This is a Markov-based model, which uses an integrated approach to evaluate costs and health benefits[45-46, 165]. For this study, a Markov model was developed, as presented in Chapter 4. The economic model developed by VISES at Victoria University was then adapted[44-45, 169], using demographic and labour force data for China from the UN and the ILO, based on Chinese published data.

An important concern in economic evaluation is to determine the perspective of analysis, which can be individual, societal, enterprise or insurance[171-173]. The NBPHS was implemented at the national level and aimed to provide quality-equalized and quantity-equalized services to all people across China, to benefit individuals, families, organizations and even the whole society. Therefore, this study adopted a social perspective, in line with similar international studies[137]. When considering the NBPHS as an incremental investment in supporting the hypertensive population, the benefits of the program should include the cost saved by reducing CHD and stroke, improved health of the labour force and consequent increases in productivity, and social benefits, which can be converted into monetary terms[173].

5.2 Conceptual framework

As discussed in Chapter 2, there are four types of economic evaluations of healthcare programs (CMA, CUA, CEA and CBA). CBA is considered the broadest form of analysis, because it could ascertain whether the beneficial outcomes of a program justify the cost[120]. Benefits are defined by assigning monetary values to the outcomes of healthcare programs[120].

The conceptual framework of this study is summarized in Figure 5-1. It mainly consists of two parts. The first part (pink background) involves the specification of the direct and indirect improvements in health outcomes generated, and the time frame of those improvements, which were discussed in Chapter 4. The second part (blue background) of the framework represents the calculation of the economic and social benefits derived from improved health outcomes.

Within the framework, the economic costs are defined as the cost of hypertension management in the NBPHS. However, as discussed in Chapter 1, with

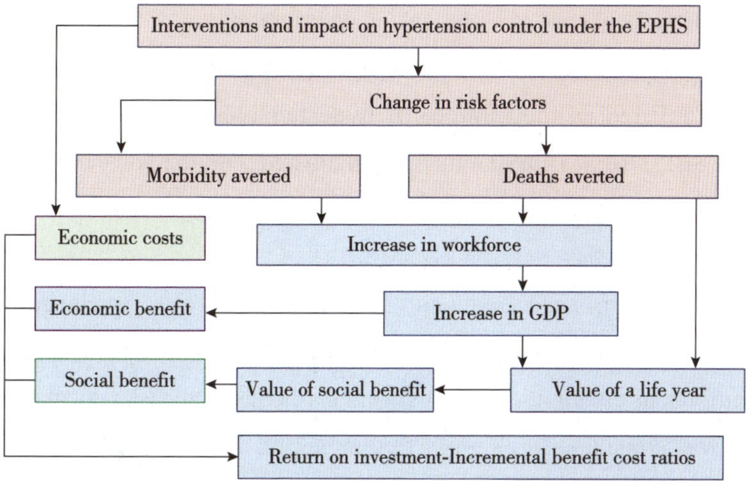

Figure 5-1 The VISES framework for return on investment of health interventions

the implementation of the NBPHS, patients would become more aware of the need for treatment and receive better treatment. This might result in greater consumption of healthcare services from the patient side, thus increasing the cost of treatment. On the other hand, as discussed in Chapter 4, control of hypertension would result in a decrease in CHD and stroke, which would save healthcare expenditure. To estimate the long-term benefit, healthcare expenditure, which was considered part of the cost of the intervention, was calculated in both hypertension-controlled and uncontrolled scenarios. To do this, the cost of illness (CoI) framework developed by the WHO was employed[30] with data from the China National Health Development Research Center's household survey conducted over 17 provinces in China[52].

5.2.1 Interventions, costs and benefits

5.2.1.1 Interventions and costs

It has been clearly defined that the intervention referred to in this study is the hypertension management component of the NBPHS in China across a specific time frame (2009 to 2015). Hypertension management includes the screening of adults aged 35+ upon their first visit to a GP in community health service facilities, regular follow-ups with monitoring and evaluation, advice on hypertension control, and referral to hospitals in case of hypertension deterioration.

The direct health outcome of this initiative would be hypertension control, which was defined as the number of hypertensives with BP being properly controlled (SBP/DBP≤140/90 mmHg)[26] compared with the non-NBPHS scenario. The number was estimated to be 9, 532, 719 from 2009 to 2015, as detailed in Chapter 3.

As for long-term health outcomes, a Markov model was developed following the CDPM employed by Gu et al.[38] in terms of CVDs and deaths (see Chapter 4). The differences in the number of deaths and cardiovascular events between the two scenarios was considered to signify the impact of the NBPHS health promotion investment.

5.2.1.2 Modelling the benefits of improved health outcomes

Premature death of members of the labour force would have an impact on future contributions to GDP. People who continued to live with disease would suffer from disability caused by that disease and may discontinue working as part of the labour force or may continue working with somewhat impaired productivity. Consequently, a reduction in the incidence of CVD would likely result in greater workforce participation and increased productivity. Better health in older age groups would also potentially lead to increased participation by older workers, a phenomenon evident in many developed countries [44]. Estimating these impacts on the labour force and productivity, which can be transformed into GDP, was therefore an important task of the model. To do this, this study followed an innovative study which used the VISES economic model for benefit estimation[44], while taking into account the *China guidelines for pharmacoeconomic evaluations*[171].

The defined period for the model projection was set as 2016 to 2045 and benefits were generated from both mortality and morbidity averted. The economic impacts of avoided mortality were calculated based on the labour force participation of each age, gender, and year category. The contribution to economic outcomes of the NBPHS program was calculated by multiplying the number of people in each age-gender group by a productivity rate that varied according to age and year. Each subsequent year of the age-specific participation rate was applied to that cohort to calculate the labour force for that cohort in that year. Average death rates by age were also calculated. The labour force in any year was obtained by adding together all the cohorts up to that year. The participation rates used were for those currently in that age group.

Labour force participation rates by gender and age, and the population and death rates were accessed from the ILOSTAT database[174]. Data for GDP was sourced from the World Bank Development Indicators[175]. Death rates were obtained from the UN *World Population Prospects* forecasts[46].

In each age-gender group, the average ages of the hypertensiveswere calculated based on the CHNS 2009 in 12 age-gender categories (male/female, 35-, 45-, 55-, 65-, 75- and 85+). The persons in this study represented the sum of all persons of working age, employed or unemployed. According to the ILO (2017), for the age group aged 65+ years, the labour force participation rates of males and females were 27.6% and 15.2%, respectively in 2016. Therefore, in the economic benefit estimation of this study, the maximum age of those in the labour force was assumed to be 70 years. GDP per person in the labour force was calculated by dividing total GDP by the total labour force.

Considering social benefits, it was assumed that the social and economic components of the value of a life year saved were distinguished. This approach has been used frequently in previous studies[44-45, 169]. Similarly, the maximum age for social benefit estimation was 80 years, in line with the parameters used in these studies.

5.2.1.3 Benefits estimation from morbidity averted

In this study, morbiditics only included CHD and stroke. Estimates of benefits from morbidity averted CHD and stroke were provided based on severity and their distribution. The chronic states of CHD and stroke was considered as morbidity, and the acute state was incorporated in mortality. As described in the latest Global Burden of Disease (GBD) study on morbidity[176], there are four levels of severity of angina pectoris: asymptomatic, mild, moderate, and severe. Mild angina is described as having chest pains during strenuous physical activity, moderate angina refers to chest pains during moderate physical activity, and severe angina occurs during minimal physical activity. The last of these levels was considered to be severe enough to prevent the person from working and was treated as equivalent to death for the purposes of analysis. The other two severity levels were considered equal to complete health and were not included in the benefit estimation for morbidity averted. A similar approach was taken in analyzing stroke morbidity. Chronic stroke has five severity levels: mild, moderate, moderate plus cognition problems, severe, and severe plus cognition problems[176]. The latter three severity levels all resulted in some difficulties in mobility (e.g. using the hands and dressing, being confined to bed or a wheelchair), or cognitive abilities (e.g. speaking, thinking and remembering things), and dependence levels (e.g. needing to be fed, toileted, and/or dressed). The mild and moderate levels were excluded, and were considered equal to complete health.

Based on severity distributions[48], the number of patients with CHD or stroke in each year with the above severity levels were generated for each age-gender group in the two scenarios. The benefit estimation was determined to be the difference in these numbers between the non-NBPHS scenario and the NBPHS scenario. Details are provided in Table 5-1.

Table 5-1 Severity levels and distribution used for CHD and stroke in the analysis

CHD			Stroke		
Severity level	Distribution (proportion)	Disability weight	Severity level	Distribution (proportion)	Disability weight
Asymptomatic angina	30.40	0	Mild	18.60	0
Mild angina	24.00	0.033	Moderate	42.80	0.02
Moderate angina	12.60	0.080	Moderate plus cognition problems	22.70	0.07
Severe angina	33.00	0.167	Severe	11.70	0.32
			Severe plus cognition problems	1.60	0.55

5.2.1.4 Net present value (NPV)

Net present value (NPV) was employed to estimate both the economic and social benefits of the program designed for hypertension control. NPV is the difference between the present value of cash inflows and that of cash outflows over a period. NPV is mainly employed in capital budgeting and investment planning to analyze the outcome of an investment[54]. It is calculated as follows.

$$NPV=\sum_{ti=1}^{n}\frac{R_t}{(1+i)^t}$$

where:

R_t = net cash inflow-outflows during a single period;

ti = discount rate or return that could be earned in alternative investments;

t = number of timer periods, which is a year in this study.

A return on investment framework was used to compare the benefit generated from the intervention with the cost of the NBPHS on hypertension management under a certain discount rate over the projected period. Parameters for estimations are listed in Table 5-2.

Table 5-2 Parameters input for health outcomes and cost benefit analysis

Category	Unit	Value	Source and publication year
Incremental cost			
Lower estimate	Billion CNY	24.66	Expert consultation
Middle estimate		35.97	Jq et al.(2015); Zhao et al. (2015)
Upper estimate		44.38	Xiao et al. (2014)
Incremental effectiveness in hypertension control (number of patients)		9, 532, 719	Trend analysis discussed in Chapter 3
GDP per capita 2017	CNY	58, 681	World Bank (2017)
Discount rate	%	0, 2, 3, 5	Liu et al. (2011)
Productivity growth rate from 2013 to 2017	/	/	World Bank (2017)
Population and death rate	/	/	UN Department of Economic and Social Affairs, Population Division (2017)

Remarks: N/A means not applicable.

5.2.2 Target population structure and assumptions

The target population was the 9, 532, 719 hypertensives in the NBPHS scenario and the hypothesized non-NBPHS scenario in 2016. It was assumed that the two scenarios had the same age-gender structure and distribution as the national hypertensive population[33]. This model projected the population by age and gender for China in a 30-year period from 2015 to 2045, based on the population data of China from the UN statistics. The labour force comprises all persons of working age who furnish the supply of labour for the production of goods and services during a specified time-reference period. It refers to the sum of all persons of working age who are employed and those who are unemployed. The series is part of the ILO estimates and is harmonized to account for differences in national data and scope of coverage, collection and tabulation methodologies, as well as for other country-specific factors. Data for 1990-2015 are estimates, while 2016-2030 data are projections. The dataset was updated as of July 2017 (UN Department of Economic and Social Affairs, Population Division, 2017). Number of annual deaths of the male and female population by five-year age group, region, sub-region and country for the years 2015-2050 (thousands of annual deaths) were from the UN as well.

It was also considered likely that the increasing incidence of chronic disease in an economy or several economies would have dynamic effects on growth[135]. However, such an effect was very difficult to estimate and therefore the migration and dynamic growth effects were not included.

5.2.3 Sensitivity analysis

To address uncertainty around mean incremental costs and benefits, a univariate sensitivity analysis was performed, with only one variable analyzed every time while controlling for other variables at their mean or base-case value. Whenever possible, the analysis was conducted using the upper and lower bounds of previous estimates, including costs and health outcomes. Moreover, the following range of discount rates of costs and socio-economic benefits were applied: 0, 2%, 3%

and 5%.

5.2.4 Analysis of cost of illness (CoI)

As explained earlier, there was the potential for healthcare expenditure to increase under the NBPHS scenario because of the cost of medications used for hypertension control. To address this concern, this study analyzed the direct CoI.

Based on data availability, the direct CoI saved was calculated in reference to reduced CHDs and stroke, using the CoI methodology recommended by the WHO[177]. Direct CoI is calculated in person-years multiplied by average direct cost of each patient in each illness, taking the probability of seeking medical care into account. Calculation was based on the survey conducted by the China National Health Development Research Center (CNHDRC) in the 2014 household health service interview survey.

CHD includes angina pectoris, myocardial infarction and other IHD, and stroke includes cerebrovascular disease as in the survey design of the CNHDRC. The direct CoI was estimated annually and composed of direct medical expenditure and direct non-medical expenditure, which were sub-categorized into inpatient related expenditure and outpatient expenditure. This was calculated based on each disease, with the probability of seeking healthcare taken into account in each population with the disease analyzed (i.e., hypertension, CHD and stroke in this study)[85]. The non-inpatient healthcare expenditure was calculated from two weeks of expenditure multiplied by 26 (as there are 52 weeks in a year), while the inpatient related expenditure was calculated from annual expenditure as designed by the data source survey.

The CoIs of CHD and stroke in the hypertension-controlled group are considered the same as that in the hypertension-uncontrolled group. The annual CoI was generated by adding the two expenditure figures together. The formula used is as follows:

Direct medical expenditure = (hypertensive population × outpatient visit rate of a fortnight × average outpatient expenditure per person time × 26 + hypertensive population × self-treatment rate of a fortnight × average self-treatment expenditure per person time × 26 + hypertensive population × admission rate of inpatient care × average inpatient expenditure of each admission)

Direct non-medical expenditure = (hypertensive population × outpatient visit rate of a fortnight × average outpatient related cost per person time × 26 + hypertensive population × admission rate of inpatient care × average non-medical expenditure of each admission)

Definitions of each term used in the above formulas are provided in Table 5-3.

Table 5-3 Definitions of terms used in the CoI calculation

Terms used	Definitions and calculating methods
Outpatient visit rate of a fortnight	The number of patients who received outpatient care during the past fortnight before the survey as a share of the total number of hypertensives.
Average outpatient expenditure per person time	Generated by dividing the total expenditure of outpatient medical care of hypertensives by the number of hypertensives.
Self-treatment rate of a fortnight	The number of patients who conducted self-treatment during the past fortnight before the survey as a share of the total number of hypertensives. This mainly denotes expenditure on drug purchasing from a pharmacy, nutritional treatment by family members, and so forth.
Average self-treatment expenditure per person time	Generated by dividing the total expenditure of self-treatment of hypertensives by the number of hypertensives.
Average outpatient related cost per person time	The total outpatient related cost divided by the number of patients who received outpatient care during the past fortnight. This denotes expenditure on transportation, nutrition, taking care of patients, and so forth.
Admission rate of inpatient care	The number of patients who received inpatient care during the past year before the survey as a share of the total number of hypertensives.
Average inpatient expenditure of each admission	Calculated by dividing the total expenditure of inpatients by the number of patients for each disease.
Average non-medical expenditure of each admission	Calculated by dividing the total inpatient related non-medical care cost divided by the number of patients who received inpatient care during the past year. This denotes expenditure on transportation, nutrition, taking care of the patients, and so forth.

The above methodology was developed by the WHO (2009), and has been widely used and validated. In 2014, this researcher co-authored an article using the same methodology with a similar dataset[52], which included an analysis of the CoI of hypertension, CHD and stroke, providing a good basis for this current study. The article analyzed the prevalence of NCDs and the economic burden on patients in eight typical cities in China. The survey, employed in this thesis, included 9, 677 hypertensives and patients who sought healthcare in the past year and who were further analyzed, including 9, 166 hypertensives, 1, 047 patients with CHD, and 736 patients with stroke[52].

5.3 Results of intervention costs, benefits and return on investment

5.3.1 Investment into hypertension management under the NBPHS

The NBPHS program, as discussed in Chapter 2, was established to provide free basic public health services, including hypertension management, to the entire population of China[15]. Initially, funding for the program was provided by the government on the basis of 15 CNY per capita each year (2009 to 2010). This was increased to 25 CNY in 2011, 30 CNY in 2013, 35 CNY in 2014 and 40 CNY in 2015[178]. According to the 2010 Chinese Census, the population of China was 1, 332, 810, 869. Therefore, it was estimated that over 246.57 billion CNY (around 36.64 billion USD at an exchange rate of 6.73 CNY per USD) was invested in this program.

The 2009 to 2015 investment from the NBPHS on hypertension control was considered to be the cost identified in the economic evaluation framework in this study. Although the total investment of the NBPHS was easy to estimate, the investment on different categories varied. The results varied from study to study, considering how much had been invested into hypertension management during the estimated period. In 2014, for example, a study by the World Bank estimated that about 18% of the investment was spent on the hypertension management of the patients, representing around 44.38 billion CNY in total (or 6.59 billion USD)[12]. A study on the fund allocation measurement of basic public health service in communities[179], which was based on workload, estimated that 20.4% of the NBPHS fund was allocated to chronic disease management, including both hypertension and diabetes. However, this study did not indicate how much had been allocated to hypertension alone [179]. Another study in Shenzhen, conducted by the same research team as the study above[180], provided further details of cost on hypertension and diabetes. This indicated that the cost of hypertension was 2.51 times that of diabetes. As the study from the World Bank[12] denoted that proportions of the total budget for the management of patients with hypertension only and diabetes only were 18% and 7%, respectively, it can be inferred that the cost of hypertension was 2.57 times that of diabetes. The studies conducted by Zhao et al.[179] and that by Xiao et al.[12] revealed the same results on the ratio of hypertension to diabetes, although their estimations on the cost of hypertension as proportions of the NBPHS fund were different. Taking the 2015 studies[12] as the criteria for funds allocated to hypertension management, these indicated that hypertension and diabetes management took a 20.4% share of the total funding and the cost of hypertension was 2.51 times that of diabetes. The proportion of the total budget of the NBPHS for hypertension management was 14.59%. Multiplying the total funding by 14.59%, we get to know that 35.97 billion CNY (5.34 billion USD) was invested in hypertension management from 2009 to 2015.

However, in February 2019, a focus group discussion was conducted with Chinese experts, coming to an agreement that only about 10%-12% of the NBPHS fund was used for the management of hypertension in China. Therefore, another lower estimate of 10% was employed in this study for estimation, which was equivalent to 24.66 billion CNY.

To sum up, three estimates were employed for further analysis based on the literature and expert panel discussion: 24.66 billion CNY, 35.97 billion CNY and 44.38 billion CNY.

5.3.2 Mortality and morbidity averted

To conduct the benefit estimation, deaths and morbidity averted were assigned a monetary value. The difference between deaths in the non-NBPHS group and those in the NBPHS group can be considered as deaths averted because of the implementation of the program. In the NBPHS scenario, the deaths in the 10–, 20–, and 30-year scenarios were 1, 519, 570 3, 577, 605, and 5, 857, 687, respectively; while the counterparts in the non-NBPHS scenario were 1, 809, 214 4, 136, 230, and 6, 602, 179, respectively. It was estimated that the number of deaths averted was 289, 644, 558, 625, and 744, 493 at a 10–, 20– and 30-year prediction horizon, respectively (see Table 5-4 below). The number of deaths in each predicted year was also listed in the Markov results, where the year and ages of the dead were also displayed. Details of these deaths are provided in Appendix Tables C3-1 and C3-2.

Table 5-4 Deaths in the two groups and deaths averted in projected years

Prediction cycle	NBPHS scenario	Non-NBPHS scenario	Death averted (lives saved)
10-year horizon	1, 519, 570	1, 809, 214	289, 644
20-year horizon	3, 577, 605	4, 136, 230	558, 625
30-year horizon	5, 857, 687	6, 602, 179	744, 493

In terms of morbidity averted, this study took CHD and stroke into account. The difference between morbidities in the non-NBPHS group and those in the NBPHS group can be considered as morbidity averted because of the implementation of the program. The numbers of hypertensives with CHD at the 10–, 20– and 30-year horizons were 65, 093 83, 165, and 69, 293, respectively, while those of stroke were 386, 888 590, 021, and 562, 666, respectively (see Table 5-5).

Table 5-5 Numbers of hypertensives with CHD and stroke in the two groups projected

Prediction cycle	CHD	Stroke
	Number of hypertensives	
10-year horizon	65, 093	386, 888
20-year horizon	83, 165	590, 021
30-year horizon	69, 293	562, 666

The number of people with CHD or stroke in the predicted year was also listed in the Markov results, where the year and ages were also displayed, and weighted by GDP or productivity to generate economic and social benefits. Details are provided in Appendix Tables C4.1-C4.4.

The economic benefit arising from the deaths and morbidity averted was calculated using a return on investment model developed by VISES. This model uses average productivity per worker to estimate the economic output produced. The growth path for this productivity is assumed to increase at a rate based on historical trends in China but approaches that of high income countries over time. The social benefit can be generated by multiplying the number of patients in each age and gender group in each year by 0.5 of GDP per capita in the specified year.

5.3.3 Return on investment and benefit-cost ratio

Using a standard model of economic evaluation, total economic and social benefits were calculated by aggregating all the above data in each year. GDP increases due to death and morbidity averted were calculated at the discount rates of 0, 2%, 3% and 5%. The projected economic benefits in NPVs would be 330, 523 (95%*CI*: 87, 674, 573, 372), 210, 745 95%*CI*: (55, 902, 365, 588), 169, 857 (95%*CI*: 45, 056, 294, 658) and 112, 310 (95%*CI*: 29, 791, 194, 829) million CNY under the above 4 discount rates, respectively. With social benefit included, the total benefit would be 605, 047 (95%*CI*: 160, 494, 1, 049, 600), 347, 956 (95%*CI*: 92, 298, 603, 614), 267, 297 (95%*CI*: 70, 903, 463, 691), and 161, 698 (95%*CI*: 42, 892, 280, 504) million CNY. Benefit-cost ratios and internal rate of return were calculated with different estimates of the cost of hypertension management under the NBPHS. Given that hypertension management accounts for 14.59% of the NBPHS funding: the benefit-cost ratios would be 8.9 (95%*CI*: 2.36, 15.44), 6.6 (95%*CI*: 1.75, 11.45), 6.0 (95%*CI*: 1.59, 10.41), and 4.9 (95%*CI*: 1.30, 8.50), at the discount rates of 0, 2%, 3% and 5%; and if the social benefit is included, the benefit-cost ratios would be 25.1 (95%*CI*: 6.66, 43.54), 17.6 (95%*CI*: 4.67, 30.53), 15.4 (95%*CI*: 4.08, 26.72), and 11.9 (95%*CI*: 3.16, 20.64), at the discount rates of 0, 2%, 3% and 5%. The internal rate of return would be 14.6% (95%*CI*: 3.87%, 25.33%) if considering only the economic benefit, and 20.7% (95%*CI*: 6.45%, 42.15%) if social benefit is included. Details are provided in Tables 5-6 and 5-7.

Table 5-6 Cost and return on investment at different discount rates (million CNY)

Discount rate	Return on investment (95%*CI*)		Cost (95%*CI*)		
	GDP-deaths averted, NPV	Social benefit, NPV	10% of the NBPHS funding	14.59% of the NBPHS funding	18% of the NBPHS funding
0%	3, 305.23 (876.74, 5, 733.72)	6, 050.47 (1, 604.94, 10, 496.00)	255.26	395.40	443.83
2%	2, 107.45 (559.02, 3, 655.88)	3, 479.56 (922.98, 6, 036.14)	217.27	336.54	377.20
3%	1, 698.57 (450.56, 2, 946.58)	2, 672.97 (709.03, 4, 636.91)	194.99	302.04	338.01
5%	1, 123.10 (297.91, 194, 829)	1, 616.98 (42, 892, 280, 504)	158.37	245.32	273.88

Table 5-7 Benefit-cost ratios at different discount rates and internal rate of return

Cost	Benefit-cost ratios under different discount rates				Internal rate of return(95%*CI*)/%
	0 (95%*CI*)	2% (95%*CI*)	3% (95%*CI*)	5% (95%*CI*)	
18% of the NBPHS funding as cost					
GDP-deaths averted eocnomic benefit/cost	7.2 (1.91, 12.49)	5.4 (1.43, 9.37)	4.8 (1.27, 8.33)	3.9 (1.03, 6.77)	12.9 (3.42, 22.38)
GDP-deaths averted eocnomic benefit plus social benefit/cost	20.4 (5.41, 35.39)	14.3 (3.79, 24.81)	12.5 (3.32, 21.68)	9.6 (2.55, 16.65)	18.8 (4.99, 32.61)
14.59% of the NBPHS funding as cost					
GDP-deaths averted eocnomic benefit/cost	8.9 (2.36, 15.44)	6.6 (1.75, 11.45)	6.0 (1.59, 10.41)	4.9 (1.30, 8.50)	14.6 (3.87, 25.33)
GDP-deaths averted eocnomic benefit plus social benefit/cost	25.1 (6.66, 43.54)	17.6 (4.67, 30.53)	15.4 (4.08, 26.72)	11.9 (3.16, 20.64)	20.7 (5.49, 35.91)
10% of the NBPHS funding as cost					
GDP-deaths averted eocnomic benefit/cost	12.9 (3.42, 22.38)	9.7 (2.57, 16.83)	8.7 (2.31, 15.09)	7.1 (1.88, 12.32)	17.9 (4.75, 31.05)
GDP-deaths averted eocnomic benefit plus social benefit/cost	36.7 (9.73, 63.67)	25.7 (6.82, 44.58)	22.4 (5.94, 38.86)	17.3 (4.59, 30.01)	24.3 (6.45, 42.15)

Age-specific analyses were performed, which showed that the benefit-cost ratios and internal rate of return would be less than the all-age-group analysis. With age-specific analysis based on the CHS 2012-2015 data, at a discount rate of 3% and given that 14.59% of the NBPHS funding was spent on hypertension management, the BCR would be 5.9. With social benefit included, the BCR would be 15.1. The internal rate of return would be 14.7% and 20.4%. Details are in Appendix D.

5.3.4 CoI analysis

The CoI of hypertension, CHD and stroke were calculated using the CoI framework. Among the 9, 166 hypertensives, 1, 047 patients with CHD, and 736 patients with stroke, the number of patients under two-week healthcare and inpatient care were extracted. The results were used for weighting expenditure in the hypertensive population. Details are provided in Table 5-8.

Table 5-8 Expenditure of hypertensives who sought healthcare in the year prior to the CNHDRC survey 2014

Situation of hypertensive patients	Number of patients	Two-week healthcare expenditure (CNY)	Annual inpatient care expenditure (CNY)
Hypertension controlled	7, 054	392, 167	1, 856, 960
Hypertension uncontrolled	2, 112	87, 945	680, 683
CHD	1, 047	118, 981	4, 457, 273
Stroke	736	113, 839	6, 338, 632

Based on total direct CoI of hypertension, CHD and stroke, and the number of patients for each disease in the hypertension-controlled and uncontrolled groups, the annual CoI of the three diseases was generated. The CoI of hypertension in the hypertension-controlled group was more than that of the hypertension-uncontrolled group. It is hypothesized that the CoI of CHD and stroke in the two groups are the same. Based on the CNHDRC survey 2014, it was estimated that annual direct CoI of patinets with hypertension with blood pressure controlled and uncontrolled, CHD and stroke were 1, 708.72 CNY, 1, 404.95 CNY, 7, 211.82 CNY and 12, 633.76 CNY, respectively.

Through the Markov model, the probabilities of each illness (hypertension only, hypertension with CHD, and hypertension with stroke) were projected for the 30-year period from 2016. Aggregated person-years were generated from the above results, as shown in Table 5-9. This denotes that in each age-gender group, there were many more CHD and stroke patients in the non-NBPHS scenario than in the NBPHS scenario.

Table 5-9 Aggregated person-years for each illness at the end of the 30-year predicted period

Group	NBPHS (hypertension-controlled)			Non-NBPHS (hypertension-uncontrolled)		
	Hypertension	CHD	Stroke	Hypertension	CHD	Stroke
Male						
35-44	15, 774, 791	385, 036	494, 318	15, 236, 919	563, 014	763, 971
45-54	28, 925, 971	1, 042, 323	2, 618, 662	26, 704, 540	1, 402, 874	4, 050, 810
55-64	26, 811, 417	2, 324, 601	6, 108, 210	22, 235, 813	2, 855, 632	8, 843, 384
65-74	11, 093, 710	1, 542, 623	3, 806, 906	8, 217, 278	1, 862, 944	5, 172, 743
75-84	2, 829, 335	526, 010	975, 734	1, 633, 406	674, 884	1, 385, 107
85+	267, 002	34, 976	69, 733	220, 257	41, 678	85, 155
Female						
35-44	9, 528, 274	89, 048	294, 487	9, 265, 155	106, 115	497, 553
45-54	27, 035, 525	712, 319	2, 560, 542	25, 036, 257	810, 456	4, 103, 754
55-64	30, 016, 795	2, 139, 024	6, 489, 494	25, 131, 870	2, 354, 465	9, 785, 280
65-74	14, 108, 563	1, 623, 837	4, 397, 236	10, 797, 864	1, 771, 355	6, 136, 027
75-84	4, 322, 289	775, 930	1, 325, 807	2, 677, 173	875, 451	2, 001, 330
85+	569, 880	71, 819	127, 464	442, 573	85, 147	174, 885

Note: The prediction duration of the age group 75-84 and 85+ is 20 years and 10 years, respectively, based on parameter availability and average life expectancy in the Chinese population.

Total direct CoI in the projected 30 years of the two groups was calculated through weighting the total person-years by CoI of hypertension, CHD and stroke. The results showed that the total direct cost of hypertension, CHD and stroke for the hypertension-controlled group in the projected 10, 20, and 30 years was

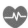

262, 141.37 521, 912.78 and 738, 025.82 million CNY, respectively, and for the hypertension-uncontrolled group was 272, 198.41 576, 172.47 and 847, 288.39 million CNY, respectively, without consideration of the discount rate. There was a difference of 111, 416.33 million CNY between the cost of hypertension in the uncontrolled group and the controlled group. Given that the investment for hypertension was 35.97 billion CNY (14.90% of the total NBPHS investment), the CoI saved from hypertension was calculated as 3.10 times the investment. As CoI was only used as a reference for analysis, whose results were not used in the main analysis, 95% CI were not calculated. Details are provided in Table 5-10.

Table 5-10 CoI of the two groups over the projected years (million CNY)

Prediction cycle	NBPHS scenario	Non-NBPHS scenario	CoI averted
10-year horizon	262, 141.37	272, 198.41	10, 057.04
20-year horizon	521, 912.78	576, 172.47	56, 412.80
30-year horizon	738, 025.82	847, 288.39	111, 416.33

5.4 Discussion

The potential health and economic benefits of hypertension management are very high. It was calculated that such an intervention as the NBPHS had the potential to avert 744, 000 deaths in China over a 30-year period. In addition to the health benefits, investment in implementing these interventions would generate broader benefits to the economy. At the discount rate of 0, 2%, 3% and 5%, the projected economic benefits in NPVs would be 330, 523 210, 745, 169, 857 and 112, 310 million CNY, respectively, and with social benefit included, the total benefit would be 605, 047 347, 956 267, 297, and 161, 698 million CNY, respectively. Benefit-cost ratios and internal rate of return were calculated with different estimates of the cost of hypertension management under the NBPHS. Given that hypertension management accounts for 14.59% of the NBPHS funding: the benefit-cost ratio would be 6.0 at a discount rate of 3%, and if the social benefit is included, the benefit-cost ratio would be 15.4 at the same discount rate. The internal rate of return is 14.6% if considering only the economic benefit and

20.7% if social benefit is included. These results are higher than those in a recent study conducted on investing in NCDs, which suggested an average ratio of 5.6 for economic returns and 10.9 if social returns are included[44]. This means that hypertension management delivered by a primary care system under the NBPHS represents a very high return on investment.

To address the concern that such an investment may increase the cost of hypertensive treatment, the total direct cost of hypertension, CHD and stroke were analyzed. The results show that 111, 416.33 million CNY would be saved in the projected period, with no discount rate considered. Given that the investment for hypertension is 35.97 billion CNY (14.90% of the total NBPHS investment), the CoI saved from hypertension management is 3.10 times of the investment.

The results also show that the social benefit is greater than the economic benefit. The main reason is that the health outcomes generated from the younger groups are less efficient than those from the older groups, as discussed in Chapter 3. As indicated by the economic evaluation model, the labour force participation and productivity rates of young people are much higher than for their older counterparts. If further measures can be taken on young hypertensives, more young lives will be protected and much greater economic benefits will be generated.

This chapter has discussed the development of an integrated economic evaluation framework for hypertension based on previous studies. Using epidemiological parameters that have been well validated and calibrated[38-39], a health outcome model based on a Markov process was developed in terms of CVD mortality and morbidity. Following the studies of VISES[44-45, 168-169], a social and economic benefit estimation framework was developed and applied in this study. In this sense, this study contributes to the knowledge of economic evaluation on hypertension management through primary care in China.

The model was based on previous studies that conducted benefit analyzes with similar frameworks on mental health[169], CVDs[44], maternal and child health and adolescents[45, 168]. This study developed a framework for hypertension interventions in the Chinese primary healthcare settings, which may be used for rolling out other healthcare programs in China or in other developing countries.

This study conducted a conservative analysis. It may have underestimated the benefits from the following three aspects:

(1) In the Markov model, CHD and stroke as consequences of hypertension are considered here, which may underestimate the benefit. It is known that kidney diseases can also result from hypertension[82]. However, because the epidemiological parameters were not accessible, kidney diseases were not considered.

(2) The cut-off age for economic benefit estimation was set at the age of 70, which was based on the labour force participation rate and previous frameworks[44-45]. However, a recent study from the World Bank argued that people do not become economically inactive just because they reach a certain age. Older people can be part of the labour force as household participants, volunteers, and in mobilizing other community activities[181]. With the growth in the number and proportion of older people globally, more and more measures are needed to explore and release the productivity of the elderly[182]. Therefore, the estimation of labor force is also conservative.

(3) The social value of a life year is considered to be 0.5 GDP per capita, which is also quite conservative. Previous reviews have provided a broad range for the value of a life year, which is 2-4 times GDP per capita[45]. Following the published studies on NCDs, by distinguishing between the social and economic components, the social benefit of each life year was assigned a value of 0.5 GDP per capita to people aged 70-80 years[44]. However, as China is aging rapidly, healthy life expectancy will be prolonged[170], with a lot more people living healthy lives beyond the age of 80 years. This means more social benefit will be generated.

Limitations: This estimate of the costs and benefits of increased investment in hypertension management is elementary, and estimates would change with different assumptions. However, both the economic and individual health benefits were predicted to be more than five times the costs by 2045. Therefore, the economic and social returns on investment studied here would be very high, and this would be unlikely to change with reasonable variations in assumptions.

5.5 Brief summary

This study has indicated that the potential health and the economic benefits of hypertension management under the NBPHS are very high. The benefit-cost ratio would be 6.0, given that the cost of hypertension management accounts for 14.59% of the NBPHS investment; and with social benefit included, the benefit-cost ratio would be 15.3, at a discount rate of 3%. An economic evaluation framework for hypertension management has been developed and can be applied to other chronic diseases in primary healthcare settings in or out of China. If further investment is made on younger hypertensives, much more will be gained in terms of labour force participation and productivity improvements.

6

Discussion and conclusion of the book

6.1 General description

In this thesis, the impact of the NBPHS on hypertensives from 2009 to 2015 in China has been estimated, in terms of hypertension control, morbidity and mortality averted, and economic and social benefits generated.

6.1.1 Hypertension control from the NBPHS

According to the 2009 *Opinion on deepening health system reform in China*[183], the NBPHS represented the largest investment in hypertension management from 2009 to 2015[8, 12, 136]. Considering the NBPHS as an incremental investment into a primary care system on hypertension control, this study sought to quantify the number of hypertensives who were able to get their blood pressure under control because of the program. To this end, a small-sample time series model of hypertension control rates from 1991 to 2009 was established to analyze the trend of hypertension control before 2009.

To access national representative data before 2009, a full literature review was conducted, and the CHNS data were used as the main source, supplemented by data from the reviewed publications. Control rate data for each year from 1991 to

2009 were completed using a Lagrange interpolation polynomial method (discussed in Chapter 3). Using a time series prediction model based on the data from 1991 to 2009, the predicted control rate for 2015 was calculated as 10.46%[95%*CI* (7.33%, 13.59%)]. Using data from the CHS 2012-2015 as observed information, the incremental effectiveness from the trend analysis was 4.26% compared with the observed control rate (14.72%) of hypertension in 2015. Based on population data extracted from the 2010 Chinese Census, it was estimated that 9, 532, 719 hypertensives had their BP properly controlled (under 140/90mmHg).

In addition, age-specific trend analyzes of hypertension awareness, treatment and control were undertaken based on data from 1991 to 2015. It was found that the highest awareness and treatment rates were in the 65-74 age group, and the highest control rates were observed among the 55-64 age group. This indicated that people aged over 55 years were under the best hypertension management and younger patients were in an unsatisfactory management status. Further analysis demonstrated that poor awareness was responsible for unsatisfactory management among the young hypertensives.

Although there were some uncertainties, this analysis provided a method of estimation of the effectiveness of a large interventional program for hypertension in China. The unsatisfactory management status of young hypertensives provides a guide to policy priorities in the next stages of the NBPHS.

6.1.2 Estimation of the long-term health outcomes from the NBPHS

Based on the incremental number of hypertension patients under control, two scenarios were established for evaluating long-term health outcomes. In the NBPHS scenario, 9, 532, 719 hypertension patients had their BP properly controlled, while in the non-NBPHS scenario, 9, 532, 719 hypertension patients did not have their BP properly controlled.

Multi-factor risk analysis of developing CVDs was undertaken with a sample of hypertensives from the 2009 CHNS to simulate the two scenario groups[51, 87]. It was discovered that the most significant risk factor for CVDs was blood pressure level, where blood pressure, diabetes, blood cholesterol, smoking, and BMI were considered.

To make long-term projections, a Markov model was established following the CDPM, which had been well developed and calibrated. For the NBPHS scenario, the model parameters determining the disease transitions were extracted from a recent published study [38]; as for the non-NBPHS scenario, the parameters were weighted by risk ratios of the two scenarios for each age-gender group according to BP and risk of CVD in China[38, 113].

The expected numbers of deaths under the NBPHS scenario with hypertension management were calculated by age and gender and used to compare with the hypothesized scenario (the non-NBPHS). The non-NBPHS scenario had a much higher incidence of CVDs and deaths compared with that of the NBPHS scenario. At the end of the 30th projection year, 25, 012 296, 258, and 744, 493 hypertensive patients would be protected from CHD, stroke and death, respectively. In addition, the Markov model provided estimates of the number of hypertensives, CHD, stroke, CVD-related deaths, and non-CVD deaths each year during the projected period.

6.1.3 Costs, benefits and return on investment analysis of the NBPHS

From 2009 to 2015, over 246.57 billion CNY (around 36.64 billion USD, at an exchange rate of 6.73 CNY per USD) was invested in the NBPHS. It was estimated that about 10% to 18% (three estimates were employed for further calculation, which were 10%, 14.59% and 18%)[12, 179, 180, 184] of the fund was used for the management of hypertension. These estimates–24.66 billion, 35.97 billion and 44.38 billion CNY, which were 0%, 14.59% and 18% of the fund, respectively-were used for a range of further analyzes on the cost of the NBPHS on hypertension management from 2009 to 2015.

A benefit-cost metric was employed for economic evaluation in this study from a societal perspective. Based on the VISES innovative framework of economic evaluation on health interventions[44-45], economic and social benefits were estimated based on labour force participation and GDP increases resulting from deaths prevented and morbidity averted. The economic benefits were estimated based on increased workforce participation of the working age population. The estimation was made on hypertensives aged 18 to 70 years. Social benefit was considered equal to 0.5 GDP per capita, where estimation was made on hypertensives with a maximum age of 80 years.

At the discount rates of 0, 2%, 3% and 5%, the projected economic benefits in NPVs would be 330, 523 210, 745 169, 857 and 112, 310 million CNY, respectively, and with social benefit included, the total benefit would be 605, 047 347, 956 267, 297, and 161, 698 million CNY, respectively. Benefit-cost ratios and internal rate of return were calculated with different estimates of the cost of hypertension management under the NBPHS. Given that hypertension management accounts for 14.59% of the NBPHS funding, the benefit-cost ratio would be 6.0, at a discount rate of 3%; and if the social benefit is included, the benefit-cost ratio would be 15.4 at the same discount rate. The internal rate of return would be 14.6% if only considering economic benefit and 20.7% if social benefit is included. This is higher than the result of a recent study conducted on investing in NCDs, which demonstrated that the average ratio would be 5.6 for economic returns and 10.9 if social returns are included[44]. Conpared with the above study, hypertension management delivered by the primary care system under the NBPHS represents a very high return on investment.

To check whether such an investment may increase the cost of treatment of hypertensives, the total direct cost of hypertension, CHD and stroke based on previous studies[48, 85] and available datasets[52] was analyzed. The results show that 92, 841.07 million CNY will be saved in the projected period with no discount rate considered. Given that the investment for hypertension is 35.97 billion CNY (14.90% of the total NBPHS investment), the CoI saved from hypertension would be 2.58 times of the investment.

6.2 Contribution to knowledge and policy implications

The economic evaluation framework of hypertension management under the NBPHS presented in this study highlights some important findings that have implications for policy-makers in China.

6.2.1 A good return on investment for hypertension management under the NBPHS

This study provided an overall effectiveness estimation of the NBPHS focused on hypertension control at the national level. It demonstrated that interventions through the NBPHS on hypertensives can result in improvement in awareness, treatment and control, substantial reductions in mortality and morbidity, and an increase in benefits.

Compared with the non-NBPHS scenario, it was estimated that with the implementation of the NBPHS, from 2009 to 2015, 9, 532, 719 hypertension patients had their BP properly controlled. Based on this, it is estimated that 744, 493 deaths would be prevented in the period 2016 to 2045 in China. It was estimated that a one-CNY input could generate a 6.0 to 15.2 CNY output when comparing the investment with economic and social benefits, using NPV with a discount rate of 3.0%. Another study, from which economic metrics were also drawn for this study, reported that the benefit-cost ratio of the maternal and child health program in China was 3.8[45]. This program was implemented in 2005-2006, aimed at elevating the number of births through hospital delivery and reducing maternal mortality. The Stenberg et al.[45] study further confirms the research conclusions of other studies, including the findings of the CHS 2012-2015[33], which concluded that the improvement in hypertension levels may be partially attributed to healthcare reform and community-based standardized BP management programs launched by the government.

The high benefit-cost ratio in this evaluation of the NBPHS indicates that for chronic disease interventions, it was a good decision to invest in the primary care system in China. It is significant that the management of chronic disease could combat the CVD challenge. These findings might also encourage further financial investment from the government.

6.2.2 A way to go to achieve policy goals

The latest statistical data showed that by the end of 2017, the number of hypertensives under the control of NBPHS primary care facilities had reached 101.04 million. The CHS 2012-2015 revealed that the number of hypertensives aged 35+ in 2015 was 246, 479, 307. This means that about 41% of all hypertensives aged 35+ and 88% of hypertensives with some level of awareness were under the management of the NBPHS program. However, more than half of hypertensives, unaware of the onset of hypertension and its related conditions, were still not covered by the program.

A number of studies have been conducted on the PATC of hypertension at regional and national levels. For example, Li et al[32]. conducted a systematic review of hypertension burden and control in 31 provinces (autonomous regions, municipalities directly under the central government) in China through an analysis of nationwide data from 2003 to 2012. They reported that 48 studies before 2012 provided prevalence data, while 30 studies provided awareness, treatment and control data. Li et al.[32] also found that among hypertensive patients aged 20 to 79 years, the awareness, treatment and control rates were 44.6%, 35.2% and 11.2%, respectively.

The most recent and largest-sample study, with results published in *The Lancet* in October 2017, reported that the awareness, treatment and control rates of hypertensive adults aged 35-75, were 36.0%, 22.9% and 5.7%, respectively[79]. Although a convenience sampling strategy was employed, which may compromise the representativeness of the sample, the results reflected the unsatisfactory status of hypertension management in China. Results from the CHS 2012-2015 indicated that hypertension PATC rates among adults aged 18 years or above, were 23.2%, 46.9%, 40.7% and 15.3%, respectively[33]. Although the awareness, treatment and control rates improved after 2009, there were still gaps compared with international levels[31-32]. Global comparisons also indicated that the effectiveness of hypertension management in China was far from satisfactory. Although the hypertension management care package was designed to improve awareness, treatment and control rates, these rates were still at a relatively low level nationally[33, 79, 148, 185]. This presents some policy implications, which are explained as follows.

First of all, further investment should be made into hypertension management in the primary care system through the NBPHS. Such a conclusion is drawn from the evidence of the benefit-cost analysis. In addition, a previous study by the author and supervisor concluded that the management of hypertension played a role in hypertension control that was independent of medication compliance[16].

Secondly, it is necessary to take measures to strengthen the primary healthcare system in China, such as in the capacity building of human resources and information systems[186]. Although all enablers are important, several factors should be further prioritized, and root causes of unsatisfactory hypertension management need further clarification. The root cause can be summarized as a "weak primary care system" , and factors include insufficient investment, lack of high quality workers, and the low capacity of healthcare delivery[12, 66, 75].

Lack of high quality workers in the primary care system has been discussed frequently[12, 66]. According to the author's experience, the root causes of the lack of high quality workforce are twofold. The first is that the policy design for the implementation of the NBPHS was irrational. The NBPHS was implemented in primary care settings in 2009 in a nation-wide manner. Among all the service items, some were implemented even before 2009, such as vaccination and infectious disease reports, and some were additional, such as the management of hypertension and diabetes, and the health management of aged people. However, the number of health staff in primary care facilities, known as "bianzhi" , was determined based on services before 2009. "Bianzhi" was the number of staff determined for public institutions according to their function in China[187]. For example, the staffing standard policy for community health service facilities was released in 2006. This defined the healthcare delivery function and gave CHS facilities a staffing standard of 7-8 health staff members for every 10, 000 citizens[21, 187]. In rural areas, the staffing standard was revised in 2011 to one health staff member per 1, 000 citizens and required a recheck of staffing standards every five years[22, 187]. Although in rural areas the staffing standard was adequate for China as it was released after 2009, it was far more difficult to enroll health professionals[12]. It is also more difficult to incentivize staff in primary facilities as the salary is lower than in other health facilities in China, plus a sound performance-oriented management system has not yet been established[188]. Therefore, it is difficult to attract new medical and public health graduates, and retain qualified professionals in these facilities[12].

For chronic disease management, a sound information system is also needed to collect accurate data for performance evaluations. However, if one is put in place, the primary care facilities in China do not have the technological capabilities to manage evaluations. In an article published in *Chinese Health Economics* in 2017[189], the importance of improving information systems for primary healthcare practice in China is explained, using the UK Quality and Outcome Framework as an international example.

Some researchers have argued that drug accessibility and availability has also influenced the unsatisfactory disease management status of hypertension, indicating that although low-cost generic anti-hypertensive medications are available, the current treatment approaches are still ineffective[139, 151].

Two recent studies analyzed trends in hypertension awareness, treatment and control in 12 high-income countries[190] and the state of hypertension care in 44 low- and middle-income countries[63]. These studies revealed that high-income countries had a much better performance on hypertension management than low-income countries, and the analysis of hypertension management performance of low-income countries concluded that higher GDP per capita is an important contributor to hypertension control. However, among the low-and middle-income countries, some had good performance on hypertension control, such as countries in Latin America and the Caribbean[62]. China is among the low-and middle-income countries. It is worthwhile for China to learn from similar countries to improve performance on hypertension management.

Another concern is that China has obvious regional differences. Several studies have evaluated the NBPHS program on hypertension control in China across different regions, such as Beijing[18], Shanghai and Shenzhen[191], and Gansu and Zhejiang[65]. These studies revealed that the impact of the NBPHS varied from region to region. For in-depth analysis, the author conducted a regional analysis at the national level using the household interview survey data (discussed in Chapter 5)[52]. In the analysis, regression analysis is used to estimate the impact of management provided under the NBPHS on hypertension control, adjusting for the effects of other determinants. From this analysis, a high interaction between hypertension management and geographical region was detected. Further analysis demonstrated that the primary healthcare information management system is the main factor accounting for the difference across regions, which has been highlighted above.

6.2.3 Hypertension management of younger patients should be strengthened

This study also found, in line with previous studies (Hou et al., 2016; Li et al., 2017), that older hypertensives were managing their hypertension better than their younger counterparts, for whom the status of disease management was poor[65, 148].

This study linked all studies on prevalence, awareness, treatment and control together through trend analysis and provided evidence by analyzing the relationship between prevalence, awareness, treatment and control, especially in age-gender specific characteristics. The positive focus on the aged was also the result of the design of the project[8]. One of the reasons for this was that among the NBPHS items, several others were focused on older people's health management, including health record files, and health education programs. These records provided overlapping effectiveness data on hypertension control. However, in-depth analysis revealed that the treatment control rate of younger patients was a little better than that of the aged patients. For example, the treatment control rates of the 35-44, 45-54, 55-64, 65-74 and 75+ age group were 40.4%, 40.0%, 38.7%, 34.8% and 32.6%, respectively. This denoted that among the young hypertensives, poor awareness was responsible for unsatisfactory management.

As discussed in Chapter 5, the social benefit generated is more than the economic benefit. One of the reasons for this is that the health outcomes generated from younger groups are less efficient than those of the aged group. As indicated in the economic evaluation model, the labour force participation and productivity rates of young people are much higher than those of their older counterparts, and for the aged group, the benefit is mainly generated from a social perspective. If further measures can be taken on young hypertensives, more young lives will be protected from premature death and more economic benefits will be generated.

6.2.4 Evidence-based policy making can be strengthened

This study provides a framework of policy tools for a return on investment framework in evaluating healthcare programs at both national and regional levels. Such an approach can be applied to other areas and systems. The Chinese government established an investment mechanism in the NBPHS, which steadily increased by 5 CNY per capita each year. It is now necessary to ascertain whether such an increase was enough for further policy measures. In addition, a dynamic adjustment mechanism should be established in the NBPHS service package for service items in the program, such as hypertension management. To these ends, the effectiveness analysis framework and economic evaluation framework of this study can be applied from financial or social perspectives.

6.3 Strengths and limitations

6.3.1 An integrated evaluation of health outcomes is established

First, this research increased our knowledge of the feasibility and desirability of applying a comprehensive framework to evaluating chronic disease management programs in community health organizations (CHOs) in China. The dynamic process of hypertension management evaluation can be simulated based on the data of prevalence, awareness, treatment and disease control, including complications of CVDs.

The small-sample time series model established in this study has provided a perspective from which to analyze the impact of the NBPHS on hypertension control. This excluded the impact of socio-economic confounding. To identify the impact of interventions, most of the time, case-control or intervention-control design was needed[167, 192]. This study made it possible to evaluate a healthcare program in a data-limited environment.

By developing an epidemiological framework and a Markov model, a longer-term projection model for health outcomes of CVDs was established. By employing the CHNS 2009, the analysis considered other factors of CVD risks, including biomarker information. Through relationship analysis of the CHS 2012-2015[139] data and hypertension management statistical data from the National Health Commission, this study analyzed hypertensives according to age-gender structures. This strengthened the representativeness of the study. To the knowledge of the author, this is the first study to evaluate the NBPHS program in China at the national level in an integrated manner.

6.3.2 An innovative model of economic evaluation is developed

Economic evaluations of hypertension management and interventions have been developed in many countries. In Vietnam, a screening program for managing identified hypertension to prevent CVDs was evaluated from an economic perspective with a cost-effectiveness framework[136]. In Greece, the economic benefits of hypertension control was quantified, concluding that cardiovascular events prevention by controlling blood pressure could avert morbidity, thereby leading to great cost savings[128]. However, such evidence was much less developed in China. It also overcame the contingent deficiency of benefit estimation in traditional economic evaluation frameworks[121].

An integrated economic evaluation framework on hypertension was developed based on previous studies. In China, Gu et al.[38, 39] provided calibrated epidemiological parameters for the estimations of health outcomes in terms of CVD mortality and morbidity. Based on the VISES economic approach[44-45], a social and economic benefit estimation framework was developed and applied to this research. As reviewed in Chapter 2, the most recent and integrated studies for economic evaluation on hypertension were both from medical treatment perspectives[38, 42]. In this sense, this study added knowledge to economic evaluation on disease management of hypertension in primary care settings in China.

The benefits of the hypertension management program as identified in this research include, not only the cost of disease interventions avoided and human capital gained, but also an individual's impact in society, in terms of social value, which equals to 0.5 GDP per capita for each life year[44-45].

6.3.3 Strengths of the study

Although many models and estimations were undertaken in this study with a level of hypothesizing, accuracy was improved by adopting a multi-factor analysis model for CVD risk estimation with the latest epidemiological data[38-39] and employing national representative data. This allowed for the generation of scenario modelling, based on evidence-based global epidemiological protocols. This analysis aligns with previous and ongoing modelling efforts[38, 46, 121], and made full use of the data currently available in China, as highlighted in the methods section. Moreover, the analysis made a start to identify and estimate the economic benefits from averted morbidity, instead of only reduced mortality for NCDs in China. This is applicable to other interventions, such as diabetes, mental health problems and even cancers.

A series of data were extracted and used to improve the accuracy of the analysis. A full literature review was used to extract data on hypertension PATC from 1991 to 2018, providing a good basis for time series analysis. The CHNS 2009 database, which provided bio-marker data of hypertensives in China, was employed to analyze CVD risks in hypertension-controlled and uncontrolled scenarios. Well-calibrated parameters of CVD risks from a recent study by Gu et al. [193], who were among the pioneers leading CVD studies in China, were employed for long-term health outcome estimation under a Markov model. The CHS 2012-2015 and the 2010 Chinese Census were used to improve the representativeness of the analysis in terms of age-gender structure.

6.3.4 Limitations

6.3.4.1 Data availability

In this study, a clear pathway for estimation of direct and long-term health outcomes, and economic impact was established. Although data from different sources were accessed, there was still a limitation in terms of the precision of calculations. Like most economic modelling, a hypothesis was applied when no data was accessible. Although systemic review was employed for extracting data from the past 30 years, the CHNS data was used as the main source. Experts at a meeting conducted in February 2019 pointed out that the data may not be as representative as that of the China Hypertension Survey, considering survey point selection and sample size.

Another limitation in terms of data is that for multi-factor CVD risk analysis, this study adopted the 2009 data as a compromise. Although the CHNS 2015 was released before the submission of the thesis, it did not provide the 2015 bio-marker data. If 2015 data could be accessed, the accuracy of the analysis would be further improved. A further limitation, as discussed in Chapter 4, is that the parameters of CVD risk estimation for people aged 75+ year were not available.

6.3.4.2 Hypothesis in the modelling may underestimate the benefits

In the Markov modelling process, CVD was put in a Markov chain, 28-day-fatal CVD was only considered to happen once in the whole process of estimation, which may underestimate the benefits generated. In addition, to estimate the health consequences of hypertension, only CVDs were considered. Other health consequences, such as kidney disease[194], were not considered. This may be another cause for underestimation of benefits.

In addition, there is still a debate in social benefit estimation about how much should be assigned on a life year as social benefit. In this study, the value of 0.5 GDP per capita is conservative and may have underestimated the benefits generated[45].

6.4 Conclusions and policy recommendations

First, the results generated are significant for further studies and policy making. This research calculated the amount of money to be saved from the interventions by the NBPHS, providing evidence for the investment in chronic diseases at the primary care level in monetary terms. This research built on Stenberg et al.'s study[45], which showed very high returns for such interventions (4.8 for economic benefit and 8.7 for total benefits at a discount rate of 3% for the period to 2035) in women and children's health. In comparison, the NBPHS program had a higher return to investment ratio, creating an enormous impact in this field in terms of research, policy making and implementation.

This study enriches the scarce economic evaluation evidence on hypertension management in China. Sensitivity analysis was performed by varying estimates of cost and discount rates. This is applicable to other items of the NBPHS program, and of its value to other health interventions, such as cancer screening and early interventions in China.

Second, this study indicated the great benefits of hypertension interventions in primary healthcare settings in China and the necessity for further investment in the management of hypertension. This research has provided the Ministry of Health with a framework from this perspective, as well as an indication of how much more is needed to better implement the program. The findings of this research enhance our understanding of the reasons for prioritizing such investments to reduce the burden of NCDs in China.

Policy recommendations to the government are summarized in three points.

(1) To further implement the NBPHS program in terms of increased investment and strengthening the primary healthcare system through its human resources systems.

(2) To strengthen information management systems and improve the performance evaluation of primary healthcare facilities[189]. Information technologies should be applied to chronic disease management to improve their performance and work efficiencies[136].

(3) Young hypertensives and people at high risk should be prioritized in the next stage of the NBPHS. Most young patients are part of the workforce and assume that they are in good health.

There has been a call for developing functional community healthcare facilities in China that mainly provide healthcare services to employees of companies or work units. So far, however, these facilities have had poor results[195-196]. Other young patients are part of the migrant population, which denotes that healthcare services should be strengthened for this population group[160].

6.5 How further progress can be made

When considering the benefit estimation framework, societal gains will be generated not only in the health sector, but also in economic growth and social empowerment. Some of these benefits were difficult to calculate. To enhance the understanding of the potential societal gains of investment in NCDs, subsequent analysis is recommended to explore the impact of reducing NCDs regionally based on previous work.

Regarding further study in China, the following investigations would be beneficial: (1) case studies on specific regions can be undertaken based on the framework established at the national level; (2) a cohort study on chronic diseases in primary care settings could be conducted, providing accurate information on blood pressure, diabetes, smoking status and other risk factors for CVDs; and (3) the economic analysis approaches used in this study could be applied to other items of the NBPHS, such as diabetes management, serious mental disease management, and other health programs in China.

References

[1] GERALD B, GU X Y. Health sector reform: lessons from China[J]. Soc Sci Med, 1997, 45 (3): 351-360.

[2] TANG S, MENG Q, CHEN L, et al. Tackling the challenges to health equity in China[J]. Lancet, 2008, 372 (9648): 1493-1501.

[3] YANG G, KONG L, ZHAO W, et al. Emergence of chronic non-communicable diseases in China[J]. Lancet, 2008, 372 (9650): 1697-1705.

[4] Division of Global Health Protection, Global Health, Centers for Disease Control and Prevention. Global Noncommunicable Diseases Fact Sheet [EB/OL]. (2023-2-3) [2023-8-11] https://www.cdc.gov/globalhealth/healthprotection/resources/fact-sheets/global-ncd-fact-sheet.html.

[5] YANG G, WANG Y, ZENG Y, et al. Rapid health transition in China, 1990-2010: findings from the Global Burden of Disease Study 2010[J]. Lancet, 2013, 381 (9882): 1987-2015.

[6] The National Centre for Cardiovascular Diseases, China (2013). *Report on cardiovascular diseases in China* (2013 ed.) [M]. Beijing: Encyclopedia of China Publishing House.

[7] Ministry of Health of China. *Opinions on implementing the 9 national basic public health services*. Beijing[EB/OL]. (2018-6-6) [2019-7-1].https://www.gov.cn/jrzg/2009-07/10/content_1362010.htm.

[8] YIP W C, HSIAO W C, CHEN W, et al. Early appraisal of China's huge and complex healthcare reforms[J]. Lancet, 2012, 379 (9818): 833-842.

[9] World Bank. Toward a healthy and harmonious life in China: Stemming the rising tide of non-communicable diseases. 2011, Retrieved from http://wwwwds.worldbank.org/external/default/WDSContentServer/WDSP/IB/2011/07/25/000333037_20110725011735/Rendered/PDF/634260WP00Box30official0use0only090.pdf

[10] The National Health and Family Planning Commission of China. *The notice to well*

undertake the national basic public health service 2013. Beijing[EB/OL]. (2013-6-14) [2018-6-6].www.natcm.gov.cn/yizhengsi/gongzuodongtai/2018-03-24/2794.html

[11] The National Health Commission of China. (2018). *Notice of implementing the national basic public health service programme 2018 of China*. Beijing[EB/OL]. (2018-6-20) [2019-6-6]. www.nhc.qov.cn/cms-search/xxak/getManuscriptXxqk.htm?id=acf4058c09d046b09addad8abd395e20

[12] XIAO N, LONG Q, TANG X, et al. A community-based approach to non-communicable chronic disease management within a context of advancing universal health coverage in China: progress and challenges[J]. BMC Public Health, 2014, 14 Suppl 2 (Suppl 2): S2.

[13] Centre for Project Supervision and Management, National Health and Family Planning Commission (2013). *Annual report on essential public health services performance evaluation*. Preprinted[EB/OL].(2014-6-1) [2016-7-1].

[14] Community Health Association of China. (2015). *Report of periodical evaluation on the national essential public health programs*[EB/OL]. (2016-4-2) [2016-7-1].

[15] TIAN M, WANG H, TONG X, et al. Essential Public Health Services' Accessibility and its Determinants among Adults with Chronic Diseases in China[J]. PLoS One, 2015, 10 (4): e0125262.

[16] YIN D, WONG S T, CHEN W, et al. A model to estimate the cost of the National Essential Public Health Services Package in Beijing, China[J]. BMC Health Serv Res, 2015, 15: 222.

[17] WANG H, GUSMANO M K, CAO Q. An evaluation of the policy on community health organizations in China: will the priority of new healthcare reform in China be a success?[J]. Health Policy, 2011, 99 (1): 37-43.

[18] World Bank Group, World Health Organization, Ministry of Finance, et al (2016). Deepening health reform in China. Growth analysis health measurement project [EB/OL]. (2016-07-22) [2018-6-6] https://openknowledge.worldbank.org/handle/10986/24720.

[19] HUNG L M, SHI L, WANG H, et al. Chinese primary care providers and motivating factors on performance[J]. Fam Pract, 2013, 30 (5): 576-586.

[20] General Office of the State Council. Outline of the National Medical and Health Service System Plan[EB/OL]. [2019-6-27] https://www.gov.cn/zhengce/content/2015-03/30/content_9560.htm?trs=1

[21] State Commission Office of Public Sectors Reform, Ministry of Health, Ministry if Finance, Ministry of Civil Affairs, China. (2006). *The guide opinion of staffing standard of community health service facilities in urban areas in China*. Beijing[EB/OL]. (2006-8-18) [2018-6-6]. www.nhc.qov.cn/cms-search/xxak/getManuscriptXxqk.htm?id=acf4058c09d046b09addad8abd395e20.

[22] State Commission Office of Public Sectors Reform, China. *The guide opinion of the staffing standard of the township hospitals in China*. Beijing[EB/OL]. (2011-5-10) [2016-7-1]. https://www.doc88.com/p-9337129116206.html.

[23] LI X, LU J, HU S, et al. The primary health-care system in China[J]. Lancet, 2017, 390 (10112): 2584-2594.

[24] The National Health Commission of China. (2018). *Report on the progress of the essential public health services in China*. Beijing[EB/OL]. (2018-12-10) [2019-3-30]

[25] Hypertension management writing group of 2018 (2019). 2018 Chinese guidelines for the management of hypertension. *Chinese Journal of Cardiovascular Medicine*, *24* (1), 24-56.

[26] WANG J G. Chinese Hypertension Guidelines[J]. Pulse (Basel), 2015, 3 (1): 14-20.

[27] FU W, ZHAO S, ZHANG Y, et al. Research in health policy making in China: out-of-pocket payments in Healthy China 2030[J]. BMJ, 2018, 360: k234.

[28] Ministry of Finance, National Development and Reform Commission, Ministry of Civil Affairs, Security, Ministry of Human Resources and Social Security & Ministry of Health. (2009). *The opinion of improving policies of government investment into health*. Beijing[EB/OL]. (2009-7-1) [2018-6-6]. https://www.gov.cn/ztzl/ygzt/content 1661057.htm

[29] Ministry of Finance & Ministry of Health of China. The notice of issuing management regulation of funding of the national basic public health services of China[EB/OL]. (2010) [2019-6-27] https://wenku.baidu.com/view/bbe7bf0390c69ec3d5bb7565.html?_wkts_=1691731301117&bdQuery=%E8%B4%A2%E6%94%BF%E9%83%A8+%E5%8D%AB%E7%94%9F%E9%83%A8+%E5%9B%BD%E5%AE%B6%E5%9F%BA%E6%9C%AC%E5%85%AC%E5%85%B1%E5%8D%AB%E7%94%9F%E6%9C%8D%E5%8A%A1%E9%A1%B9%E7%9B%AE%E8%B5%84%E9%87%91%E7%AE%A1%E7%90%86+2010

[30] Department of Health Systems Financing. Geneva: World Health Organization. *WHO guide to identifying the economic consequences of disease and injury*[EB/OL]. (2020-12-15) [2023-8-11]. https://www.who.int/home/search?indexCatalogue=genericsearchindex1&searchQuery=WHO%20guide%20to%20identifying%20the%20economic%20consequences%20of%20disease%20and%20injury&wordsMode=AnyWord.

[31] BUNDY J D, HE J. Hypertension and Related Cardiovascular Disease Burden in China[J]. Ann Glob Health, 2016, 82 (2): 227-233.

[32] LI D, LV J, LIU F, et al. Hypertension burden and control in mainland China: Analysis of nationwide data 2003-2012[J]. Int J Cardiol, 2015, 184: 637-644.

[33] WANG Z, CHEN Z, ZHANG L, et al. Status of Hypertension in China: Results From the China Hypertension Survey, 2012-2015[J]. Circulation, 2018, 137 (22): 2344-2356.

[34] Duan, Yiping. (2015). Application of small sample time series analysis in process of Encounter Phase. *Ordnance Industry Automation*, 2015-09, 34 (9), 92-96.

[35] REN J, ZHU J, SHAO Y. (2005). A Study of Data Processing of Small-Style book Time Seties[J]. Journal of Force Engineering University (Natural Science Edition), 6 (3), 71-73.

[36] WU Y, LIU X, LI X, et al. Estimation of 10-year risk of fatal and nonfatal ischemic cardiovascular diseases in Chinese adults[J]. Circulation, 2006, 114 (21): 2217-2225.

[37] ZHANG X F, ATTIA J, D'ESTE C, et al. A risk score predicted coronary heart disease and stroke in a Chinese cohort[J]. J Clin Epidemiol, 2005, 58 (9): 951-958.

[38] GU D, HE J, COXSON P G, et al. The Cost-Effectiveness of Low-Cost Essential Antihypertensive Medicines for Hypertension Control in China: A Modelling Study[J]. PLoS Med, 2015, 12 (8): e1001860.

[39] GU D, KELLY T N, WU X, et al. Blood pressure and risk of cardiovascular disease in Chinese men and women[J]. Am J Hypertens, 2008, 21 (3): 265-272.

[40] Baan CA, Bos, G, Jacobs-van der Bruggen MAM. Modeling chronic diseases: the diabetes module. (2005) [2018-7-1]. https://rivm.openrepository.com/rivm/bitstream/10029/256901/3/260801001.pdf.

[41] MORAN A, GU D, ZHAO D, et al. Future cardiovascular disease in china: markov model and risk factor scenario projections from the coronary heart disease policy model-china[J]. Circ Cardiovasc Qual Outcomes, 2010, 3 (3): 243-252.

[42] XIE X, HE T, KANG J, et al. Cost-effectiveness analysis of intensive hypertension control in China[J]. Prev Med, 2018, 111: 110-114.

[43] The National Health and Family Planning Commission of China. (2014b). *China health statistical yearbook 2014*. Peking Union Medical College Publishing House, Beijing.

[44] BERTRAM M Y, SWEENY K, LAUER J A, et al. Investing in non-communicable diseases: an estimation of the return on investment for prevention and treatment services[J]. Lancet, 2018, 391 (10134): 2071-2078.

[45] STENBERG K, AXELSON H, SHEEHAN P, et al. Advancing social and economic development by investing in women's and children's health: a new Global Investment Framework[J]. Lancet, 2014, 383 (9925): 1333-1354.

[46] United Nations, Department of Economic and Social Affairs, Population Division (2017). World Population Prospects: The 2017 Revision, DVD Edition.

[47] Organization W H.Package of essential noncommunicable (PEN) disease interventions for primary health care in low-resource settings.[J].Geneva: World Health Organization, 2010.

[48] BURSTEIN R, FLEMING T, HAAGSMA J, et al. Estimating distributions of health state severity for the global burden of disease study[J]. Popul Health Metr, 2015, 13: 31.

[49] HODGSON T A, MEINERS M R. Cost-of-illness methodology: a guide to current practices and procedures[J]. Milbank Mem Fund Q Health Soc, 1982, 60 (3): 429-462.

[50] POPKIN B M, DU S, ZHAI F, et al. Cohort Profile: The China Health and Nutrition Survey—monitoring and understanding socio-economic and health change in China, 1989-2011[J]. Int J Epidemiol, 2010, 39 (6): 1435-1440.

[51] GUO J, ZHU Y C, CHEN Y P, et al. The dynamics of hypertension prevalence, awareness, treatment, control and associated factors in Chinese adults: results from CHNS 1991-2011[J]. J Hypertens, 2015, 33 (8): 1688-1696.

[52] Qin J, ZhangY, Fridman M, Sweeny K, Zhang L, Lin C, et al. (2021) The role of the Basic Public Health Service program in the control of hypertension in China: Results from across-sectional health service interview survey. PLoS ONE 16 (6): e0217185. https://doi.org/10.1371/journal.pone.0217185

[53] Claxton K, Sculpher M, Culyer A, et al.Discounting and cost-effectiveness in NICE-stepping back to sort out a confusion[J].Health Economics, 2010, 15(1):1-4.DOI:10.1002/hec.1081.

[54] Jason F. (2023) Net present value (NPV) [EB/OL]. (2023-05-24) [2023-08-11]. https://www.investopedia.com/terms/n/npv.asp

[55] Centre for Health Statistics and Information of China. 2008 English abstract of *analysis report of national health services survey of China*[EB/OL]. (2010-09-21)[2018-07], http://www.nhc.gov.cn/mohwsbwstjxxzx/s8211/201009/49166.shtml.

[56] PERMAN G, ROSSI E, WAISMAN G D, et al. Cost-effectiveness of a hypertension management programme in an elderly population: a Markov model[J]. Cost Eff Resour Alloc, 2011, 9 (1): 4.

[57] Georgetown University Health Policy Institute. Disease Management Programs: Improving health while reducing costs?[EB/OL] (2004) [2018-07-01]. https://hpi.georgetown.edu/management/

[58] SQUIRES H, CHILCOTT J, AKEHURST R, et al. A Framework for Developing the Structure of Public Health Economic Models[J]. Value Health, 2016, 19 (5): 588-601.

[59] TSIACHRISTAS A, CRAMM J M, NIEBOER A, et al. Broader economic evaluation of disease management programs using multi-criteria decision analysis[J]. Int J Technol Assess Health Care, 2013, 29 (3): 301-308.

[60] SCULPHER M J, PANG F S, MANCA A, et al. Generalisability in economic evaluation studies in healthcare: a review and case studies[J]. Health Technol Assess, 2004, 8 (49): iii-iv, 1-192.

[61] World Health Organization. Noncommunicable diseases: hypertension[EB/OL]. (2015-06-29) [2018-12-01]. https://www.who.int/features/qa/82/en/

[62] GELDSETZER P, MANNE-GOEHLER J, MARCUS M E, et al. The state of hypertension care in 44 low-income and middle-income countries: a cross-sectional study of nationally representative individual-level data from 1.1 million adults[J]. Lancet, 2019, 394 (10199): 652-662.

[63] JOFFRES M, FALASCHETTI E, GILLESPIE C, et al. Hypertension prevalence, awareness, treatment and control in national surveys from England, the USA and Canada, and correlation with stroke and ischaemic heart disease mortality: a cross-sectional study[J]. BMJ Open, 2013, 3 (8): e003423.

[64] Unger T, Borghi C, Charchar F, et al. 2020 International Society of Hypertension global hypertension practice guidelines[J]. Journal of Hypertension 38(6):982-1004.

[65] WANG J, ZHANG L, WANG F, et al. Prevalence, awareness, treatment, and control of hypertension in China: results from a national survey[J]. Am J Hypertens, 2014, 27 (11): 1355-1361.

[66] HOU Z, MENG Q, ZHANG Y. Hypertension Prevalence, Awareness, Treatment, and Control Following China's Healthcare Reform[J]. Am J Hypertens, 2016, 29 (4): 428-431.

[67] GAKIDOU E, AFSHIN A, ABAJOBIR A A, et al. (2017). Global, regional, and national comparative risk assessment of 84 behavioural, environmental and occupational, and metabolic risks or clusters of risks, 1990-2016: a systematic analysis for the Global Burden of Disease Study 2016[J]. The Lancet, 2017, 390 (10100): 1345-1422.

[68] W, J, PUGH. (1996). HEALTH AND NUMBERS-BASIC BIOSTATISTICAL METHODS[J].Statistics in Medicine, 1996.DOI: 10.1002/ (SICI) 1097-0258 (19960730) 15：14<1603: : AID-SIM344>3.

[69] SAMET J, WIPFLI H, PLATZ E, et al. "Morbidity rate." In a Dictionary of Epidemiology (5th ed.) [M]. Oxford: Oxford University Press, 189.

[70] JENG J S, LEE T K, CHANG Y C, et al. Subtypes and case-fatality rates of stroke: a hospital-based stroke registry in Taiwan (SCAN-Ⅳ)[J]. J Neurol Sci, 1998, 156 (2): 220-226.

[71] HARRINGTON R A. Case fatality rate[EB/OL]. (2017) [2018-9-12]. https://www.britannica.com/science/case-fatality-rate

[72] STARE J, MAUCORT-BOULCH D. Odds ratio, hazard ratio and relative risk[J]. Metodoloski Zvezki, 2016, 13 (1): 59-67.

[73] KOTCHEN T A, HAJJAR I. Trends in Prevalence, Awareness, in the United States, 1988-2000[J]. JAMA, 2003, 290 (2): 199-206.

[74] LU J, LU Y, WANG X, et al. (2017). Prevalence, awareness, treatment, and control of hypertension in China: data from 1.7 million adults in a population-based screening

study (China PEACE Million Persons Project)[J]. Lancet, 2017, 390 (10112): 2549-2558. http://dx.doi.org/10.1016/S0140-6736(17)32478-9

[75] BAI Y, ZHAO Y, WANG G, et al. Cost-effectiveness of a hypertension control intervention in three community health centers in China[J]. J Prim Care Community Health, 2013, 4 (3): 195-201.

[76] GOODING H C, MCGINTY S, RICHMOND T K, et al. Hypertension awareness and control among young adults in the national longitudinal study of adolescent health[J]. J Gen Intern Med, 2014, 29 (8): 1098-1104.

[77] CHEN W W, GAO R L, LIU L S, et al. China cardiovascular diseases report 2015: a summary[J]. J Geriatr Cardiol, 2017, 14 (1): 1-10.

[78] WANG J, NING X, YANG L, et al. Trends of hypertension prevalence, awareness, treatment and control in rural areas of northern China during 1991-2011[J]. J Hum Hypertens, 2014, 28 (1): 25-31.

[79] SU M, ZHANG Q, BAI X, et al. Availability, cost, and prescription patterns of antihypertensive medications in primary health care in China: a nationwide cross-sectional survey[J]. Lancet, 2017, 390 (10112): 2559-2568.

[80] BAJOREK B V, LEMAY K S, MAGIN P J, et al. Management of hypertension in an Australian community pharmacy setting-patients' beliefs and perspectives[J]. Int J Pharm Pract, 2017, 25 (4): 263-273.

[81] JAMES P A, OPARIL S, CARTER B L, et al. 2014 evidence-based guideline for the management of high blood pressure in adults: report from the panel members appointed to the Eighth Joint National Committee (JNC 8)[J]. JAMA, 2014, 311 (5): 507-520.

[82] GU J, ZHANG X J, WANG T H, et al. Hypertension knowledge, awareness, and self-management behaviors affect hypertension control: a community-based study in Xuhui District, Shanghai, China[J]. Cardiology, 2014, 127 (2): 96-104.

[83] XU J, PAN R, PONG R W, et al. Different Models of Hospital-Community Health Centre Collaboration in Selected Cities in China: A Cross-Sectional Comparative Study[J]. Int J Integr Care, 2016, 16 (1): 8.

[84] TU Q, XIAO L D, ULLAH S, et al. Hypertension management for community-dwelling older people with diabetes in Nanchang, China: study protocol for a cluster randomized controlled trial[J]. Trials, 2018, 19 (1): 385.

[85] Qin, J., Zhang, Y., Zhang, L., Rui, D, Mao, L, Wang, L., & Wu, N. (2014). Prevalence of non-communicable disease and economic burden of patients in 8 typical cities in China. Chinese Journal of Public Health, 30(1), 5-7. https://doi.org/10.11847/zgggws2014-30-01-02

[86] GAO Y, CHEN G, TIAN H, et al. Prevalence of hypertension in china: a cross-sectional study[J]. PLoS One, 2013, 8 (6): e65938.

[87] XI B, LIANG Y, REILLY K H, et al. Trends in prevalence, awareness, treatment, and control of hypertension among Chinese adults 1991-2009[J]. Int J Cardiol, 2012, 158 (2): 326-329.

[88] Peter T.Preventing the cardiovascular complications of hypertension[J].European Heart Journal Supplements, 2004(suppl_H):h37-h42.DOI:10.1093/eurheartj/6.suppl_h.h37.

[89] HAMILTON M, THOMPSON E M, WISNIEWSKI T K. THE ROLE OF BLOOD-PRESSURE CONTROL IN PREVENTING COMPLICATIONS OF HYPERTENSION[J]. Lancet, 1964, 1 (7327): 235-238.

[90] LEWINGTON S, CLARKE R, QIZILBASH N, et al. Age-specific relevance of usual blood pressure to vascular mortality: a meta-analysis of individual data for one million adults in 61 prospective studies[J]. Lancet, 2002, 360 (9349): 1903-1913.

[91] LEWINGTON S, LACEY B, CLARKE R, et al. The Burden of Hypertension and Associated Risk for Cardiovascular Mortality in China[J]. JAMA Intern Med, 2016, 176 (4): 524-532.

[92] TURNBULL F, NEAL B, NINOMIYA T, et al. Effects of different regimens to lower blood pressure on major cardiovascular events in older and younger adults: meta-analysis of randomised trials[J]. BMJ, 2008, 336 (7653): 1121-1123.

[93] Tadege GM (2017) Survival Analysis of Time to Cardiovascular Disease Complication of Hypertensive Patients at Felege Hiwot Referal Hospital in Bahir-Dar, Ethiopia: A Retrospective Cohort Study. J Biom Biostat 8: 369. doi: 10.4172/2155-6180.1000369

[94] Mamun A A, Williams G M, Peeters A, et al. (2020). Risk factors and compression of cardiovascular morbidity: a life history analysis of the 46-year follow-ups of the Framingham Heart Study[C]//World Congress on Heart Disease.Medimond, International Proceedings Division, 2006. DOI:http://espace.library.uq.edu.au/view/UQ:177652.

[95] D'AGOSTINO R B, LEE M L, BELANGER A J, et al. Relation of pooled logistic regression to time dependent Cox regression analysis: the Framingham Heart Study[J]. Stat Med, 1990, 9 (12): 1501-1515.

[96] BENJAMIN E J, LEVY D, VAZIRI S M, et al. Independent risk factors for atrial fibrillation in a population-based cohort. The Framingham Heart Study[J]. JAMA, 1994, 271 (11): 840-844.

[97] SINGER D E, NATHAN D M, ANDERSON K M, et al. Association of HbA1c with prevalent cardiovascular disease in the original cohort of the Framingham Heart Study[J]. Diabetes, 1992, 41 (2): 202-208.

[98] HARRIS T, COOK E F, GARRISON R, et al. Body mass index and mortality among nonsmoking older persons. The Framingham Heart Study[J]. JAMA, 1988, 259 (10):

1520-1524.

[99] PREIS S R, HWANG S J, COADY S, et al. Trends in all-cause and cardiovascular disease mortality among women and men with and without diabetes mellitus in the Framingham Heart Study, 1950 to 2005[J]. Circulation, 2009, 119 (13): 1728-1735.

[100] VISRODIA K, SINGH S, KRISHNAMOORTHI R, et al. Systematic review with meta-analysis: prevalent vs. incident oesophageal adenocarcinoma and high-grade dysplasia in Barrett's oesophagus[J]. Aliment Pharmacol Ther, 2016, 44 (8): 775-784.

[101] D'AGOSTINO RB Sr, VASAN R S, PENCINA M J, et al. General cardiovascular risk profile for use in primary care: the Framingham Heart Study [J]. Circulation, 2008, 117 (6): 743-753.

[102] KUULASMAA K, TUNSTALL-PEDOE H, DOBSON A, et al. Estimation of contribution of changes in classic risk factors to trends in coronary-event rates across the WHO MONICA Project populations[J]. Lancet, 2000, 355 (9205): 675-687.

[103] YANG X, LI J, HU D, et al. Predicting the 10-Year Risks of Atherosclerotic Cardiovascular Disease in Chinese Population: The China-PAR Project (Prediction for ASCVD Risk in China) [J]. Circulation, 2016, 134 (19): 1430-1440.

[104] LAW M R, WALD N J, MORRIS J K, et al. Value of low dose combination treatment with blood pressure lowering drugs: analysis of 354 randomised trials[J]. BMJ, 2003, 326 (7404): 1427.

[105] UNAL B, CAPEWELL S, CRITCHLEY J A. Coronary heart disease policy models: a systematic review[J]. BMC Public Health, 2006, 6: 213.

[106] CHAN F, ADAMO S, COXSON P, et al. Projected impact of urbanization on cardiovascular disease in China[J]. Int J Public Health, 2012, 57 (5): 849-854.

[107] CHENG J, ZHAO D, ZENG Z, et al. The impact of demographic and risk factor changes on coronary heart disease deaths in Beijing, 1999-2010[J]. BMC Public Health, 2009, 9: 30.

[108] Zhang, X. (2015). *Economic evaluation on dyslipidemia of aged people in China based on MARKOV Model*. Master Thesis[D]. Beijing: Peking University Health Science Centre, Beijing, China.

[109] BARTON P, BRYAN S, ROBINSON S. Modelling in the economic evaluation of health care: selecting the appropriate approach[J]. J Health Serv Res Policy, 2004, 9 (2): 110-118.

[110] WEINSTEIN M C, COXSON P G, WILLIAMS L W, et al. Forecasting coronary heart disease incidence, mortality, and cost: the Coronary Heart Disease Policy Model[J]. Am J Public Health, 1987, 77 (11): 1417-1426.

[111] LIGHTWOOD J M, COXSON P G, BIBBINS-DOMINGO K, et al. Coronary heart disease

attributable to passive smoking: CHD Policy Model[J]. Am J Prev Med, 2009, 36 (1): 13-20.

[112] KONFINO J, MEKONNEN T A, COXSON P G, et al. Projected impact of a sodium consumption reduction initiative in Argentina: an analysis from the CVD policy model—Argentina[J]. PLoS One, 2013, 8 (9): e73824.

[113] MORAN A, ZHAO D, GU D, et al. The future impact of population growth and aging on coronary heart disease in China: projections from the Coronary Heart Disease Policy Model-China[J]. BMC Public Health, 2008, 8: 394.

[114] CHAN F, Adamo S, Coxson P, et al. Projected impact of urbanization on cardiovascular disease in china[J]. Int J Public Health, 2012, 57: 849-854.

[115] Gagniuc, Paul A. (2017). Markov Chains (From Theory to Implementation and Experimentation) || Absorbing Markov Chains[M].John Wiley & Sons, Inc. 2017.

[116] SONNENBERG F A, BECK J R. Markov models in medical decision making: a practical guide[J]. Med Decis Making, 1993, 13 (4): 322-338.

[117] HOANG V P, SHANAHAN M, SHUKLA N, et al. A systematic review of modelling approaches in economic evaluations of health interventions for drug and alcohol problems[J]. BMC Health Serv Res, 2016, 16: 127.

[118] World Health Organization. International Statistical Classification of Diseases and Related Health Problems (ICD)[EB/OL].(2019-5) [2022-12-02]. https://www.who.int/classifications/icd/en/

[119] MYERS R P, LEUNG Y, SHAHEEN A A, et al. Validation of ICD-9-CM/ICD-10 coding algorithms for the identification of patients with acetaminophen overdose and hepatotoxicity using administrative data[J]. BMC Health Serv Res, 2007, 7: 159.

[120] DRUMMOND M F, SCULPHER M J, TORRANCE G W, et al. Methods for the economic evaluation of health care programmes[M].3rd ed. Oxford: Oxford University Press, 2005.

[121] DRUMMOND M F, SCULPHER M J, CLAXTON K, et al. Methods for the economic evaluation of health care programmes[M].4th ed. Oxford: Oxford University Press, 2015.

[122] ZHANG D, WANG G, JOO H. A Systematic Review of Economic Evidence on Community Hypertension Interventions[J]. Am J Prev Med, 2017, 53 (6S2): S121-S130.

[123] HUANG Y, REN J. Cost-benefit analysis of a community-based stroke prevention program in Bao Shan District, Shanghai, China[J]. (2010).International Journal of Collaborative Research on Internal Medicine & Public Health, 2010, 2 (9): 307-316.

[124] HUANG Y, WANG S, CAI X, et al. Prehypertension and incidence of cardiovascular disease: a meta-analysis[J]. BMC Med, 2013, 11: 177.

[125] MURPHY K, TOPEL R. The value of health and longevity[J]. J Polit Econ, 2006, 114:

871-904.

[126] DUKPA W, TEERAWATTANANON Y, RATTANAVIPAPONG W, et al. Is diabetes and hypertension screening worthwhile in resource-limited settings? An economic evaluation based on a pilot of a Package of Essential Non-communicable disease interventions in Bhutan[J]. Health Policy Plan, 2015, 30 (8): 1032-1043.

[127] NUGENT R, BROWER E, CRAVIOTO A, et al. A cost-benefit analysis of a National Hypertension Treatment Program in Bangladesh[J]. Prev Med, 2017, 105S: S56-S61.

[128] ATHANASAKIS K, KYRIOPOULOS I I, BOUBOUCHAIROPOULOU N, et al. Quantifying the economic benefits of prevention in a healthcare setting with severe financial constraints: the case of hypertension control[J]. Clin Exp Hypertens, 2015, 37 (5): 375-380.

[129] STEVANOVIć J, O'PRINSEN A C, VERHEGGEN B G, et al. Economic evaluation of primary prevention of cardiovascular diseases in mild hypertension: a scenario analysis for the Netherlands[J]. Clin Ther, 2014, 36 (3): 368-384.e5.

[130] Tian, H., Guo, Z., Song, G., & Wei, Q. (2000). Cost-effectiveness Analysis on Tianjin Non-communicable Diseases Prevention and Control Project Conducted from 1991-1996. Chin J Prev Contr Non-Commun Dis. 5: 196-197;221

[131] Liang, X. (2011). A health economic evaluation for hypertension management in communities and a meta-analysis of the effect of mobile phone intervention for diabetes on glycemic control. *Doctor Thesis*.Peking Union Medical College, Beijing, China.

[132] LIANG X, CHEN J, LIU Y, et al. The effect of hypertension and diabetes management in Southwest China: a before-and after-intervention study[J]. PLoS One, 2014, 9 (3): e91801.

[133] Li, R., Wang, Z., Yu, S., & et al. (2003). Application of Monte Carlo Model in Cost-Benefit Analysis of Diabetes Screening. *Chinese Journal of Public Health Management*, (19), 240-242.

[134] Tang, S. (2011). Analysis on curative effect and cost effectiveness of hypertension patients in the community intervention management model. *Medicine and Society*, *24*, 66-68.

[135] MUKHOPADHYAY K, THOMASSIN P J. Economic impact of adopting a healthy diet in Canada[J]. J Public Health (Oxf), 2012, 20 (6): 639-652.

[136] World Bank, World Health Organization. (2019). *Deepening health reform in China: Building High-Quality and Value-Based Service Delivery*.Washington, DC: 2019 International Bank for Reconstruction and Development/The World Bank and World Health Organization.

[137] NGUYEN T P, WRIGHT E P, NGUYEN T T, et al. Cost-Effectiveness Analysis of Screening for and Managing Identified Hypertension for Cardiovascular Disease Prevention

in Vietnam[J]. PLoS One, 2016, 11 (5): e0155699.

[138] HE J, MUNTNER P, CHEN J, et al. Factors associated with hypertension control in the general population of the United States[J]. Arch Intern Med, 2002, 162 (9): 1051-1058.

[139] WANG Z, WANG X, CHEN Z, et al. Hypertension control in community health centers across China: analysis of antihypertensive drug treatment patterns[J]. Am J Hypertens, 2014, 27 (2): 252-259.

[140] WONG M C, WANG H H, WONG S Y, et al. Performance comparison among the major healthcare financing systems in six cities of the Pearl River Delta region, mainland China[J]. PLoS One, 2012, 7 (9): e46309.

[141] WANG Z, WU Y, ZHAO L, et al. Trends in prevalence, awareness, treatment and control of hypertension in the middle-aged population of China, 1992-1998[J]. Hypertens Res, 2004, 27 (10): 703-709.

[142] WU Y, HUXLEY R, LI L, et al. Prevalence, awareness, treatment, and control of hypertension in China: data from the China National Nutrition and Health Survey 2002[J]. Circulation, 2008, 118 (25): 2679-2686.

[143] GU D, REYNOLDS K, WU X, et al. Prevalence, awareness, treatment, and control of hypertension in china[J]. Hypertension, 2002, 40 (6): 920-927.

[144] LI W, GU H, TEO K K, et al. Hypertension prevalence, awareness, treatment, and control in 115 rural and urban communities involving 47, 000 people from China[J]. J Hypertens, 2016, 34 (1): 39-46.

[145] LLOYD-SHERLOCK P, BEARD J, MINICUCI N, et al. Hypertension among older adults in low-and middle-income countries: prevalence, awareness and control[J]. Int J Epidemiol, 2014, 43 (1): 116-128.

[146] Wang L, Li ZH. Epidemiological Survey of Non-communicable Diseases 2010. Chinese Community Doctors, Comprehensive Edition, 2011, 27(32):323-323.

[147] Disease Prevention and Control Bureau of the Ministry of Health of China. (2015). *Report on Chinese Residents' Chronic Diseases and Nutrition*. Beijing: China people's health publishing house, 2015.

[148] LI Y, YANG L, WANG L, et al. Burden of hypertension in China: A nationally representative survey of 174, 621 adults[J]. Int J Cardiol, 2017, 227: 516-523.

[149] LI H, LIU F, XI B. Control of hypertension in China: challenging[J]. Int J Cardiol, 2014, 174 (3): 797.

[150] WANG J, ZHANG L. Response to "hypertension control prevalence estimates should account for age" [J]. Am J Hypertens, 2014, 27 (11): 1427.

[151] LI H, LIU F, XI B. Control of hypertension in China: challenging[J]. Int J Cardiol, 2014,

174 (3): 797.

[152] JIANG B, LIU H, RU X, et al. Hypertension detection, management, control and associated factors among residents accessing community health services in Beijing[J]. Sci Rep, 2014, 4: 4845.

[153] WANG X, LI W, LI X, et al. Effects and cost-effectiveness of a guideline-oriented primary healthcare hypertension management program in Beijing, China: results from a 1-year controlled trial[J]. Hypertens Res, 2013, 36 (4): 313-321.

[154] Zhao F, Zheng J Z, Chen B, et al. Analyses on the effect of community-based intervention on hypertension[J]. Chin J Epidemiol, 2023, 24 (10): 897-900.

[155] Revising Committee of Chinese Guidelines on Hypertension Management in Primary Care Settings.. 2014 Chinese Guidelines on Hypertension Management in Primary Care Settings [J].Chin J Health Manage, 2015, 9(1): 10-30.

[156] HESKETH T, ZHOU X. Hypertension in China: the gap between policy and practice[J]. Lancet, 2017, 390 (10112): 2529-2530.

[157] WU J X, HE L Y. Urban-rural gap and poverty traps in China: a prefecture level analysis. Applied Economics, 2018, 50 (30), 3300-3314.

[158] ZHAI S, WANG P, DONG Q, et al. A study on the equality and benefit of China's national health care system[J]. Int J Equity Health, 2017, 16 (1): 155.

[159] TANG, X, YANG, J, LI, W, et al. (2013). Urban and rural differences of blood pressure and hypertension control in Chinese communities: pure china study[J]. J Am Coll Cardiol, 61 (10 suppl. 1): E1350.

[160] ZHU Y. China's floating population and their settlement intention in the cities: beyond the Hukou reform. Habitat International, 2007, 31 (1): 65-76.

[161] Yang, X., Li, J., Hu, D., et al. (2016). Predicting the 10-year risks of atherosclerotic cardiovascular disease in Chinese population: The China-PAR Project (Prediction for ASCVD Risk in China). Circulation, 134(19), 1430-1440. https://doi.org/10.1161/CIRCULATIONAHA.116.022367

[162] Zhang, Y., Liu, F., Pu, L., Qin, J., & Sweeny, K. (2018). Effectiveness prediction of community-based hypertension management in China: An analysis based on risk prediction models. *Chinese General Practice*, 21(17), 2082-2087.

[163] SESSO H D, CHEN R S, L'ITALIEN G J, et al. Blood pressure lowering and life expectancy based on a Markov model of cardiovascular events[J]. Hypertension, 2003, 42 (5): 885-890.

[164] Li Bin. Report of the State Council on the Progress of Deepening the Reform of the Medical and Health System in the 18th Meeting of the Standing Committee of the 12th

National People's Congress on 22, Dec. 2015[J]. 2016(1):4.DOI: CNKI: SUN: CWGB. 0. 2016-01-039.

[165] WU C Y, HU H Y, CHOU Y J, et al. High Blood Pressure and All-Cause and Cardiovascular Disease Mortalities in Community-Dwelling Older Adults[J]. Medicine (Baltimore), 2015, 94 (47): e2160.

[166] STANDFIELD L, COMANS T, SCUFFHAM P. Markov modeling and discrete event simulation in health care: a systematic comparison[J]. Int J Technol Assess Health Care, 2014, 30 (2): 165-172.

[167] PENALOZA-RAMOS M C, JOWETT S, MANT J, et al. Cost-effectiveness of self-management of blood pressure in hypertensive patients over 70 years with suboptimal control and established cardiovascular disease or additional cardiovascular risk diseases (TASMINSR) [J]. Eur J Prev Cardiol, 2016, 23 (9): 902-912.

[168] SHEEHAN P, SWEENY K, RASMUSSEN B, et al. Building the foundations for sustainable development: a case for global investment in the capabilities of adolescents[J]. Lancet, 2017, 390 (10104): 1792-1806.

[169] CHISHOLM D, SWEENY K, SHEEHAN P, et al. Scaling-up treatment of depression and anxiety: a global return on investment analysis[J]. Lancet Psychiatry, 2016, 3 (5): 415-424.

[170] SWEENY K, FRIEDMAN H S, SHEEHAN P, et al. A Health System-Based Investment Case for Adolescent Health[J]. J Adolesc Health, 2019, 65 (1S): S8-S15.

[171] Liu, G., Hu, S., & Wu, J. (2011). China guidelines for pharmacoeconomic evaluations[J]. *China Journal of Pharmaceutical Economics*, 3, 6-48.

[172] LUHNEN M, PREDIGER B, NEUGEBAUER E, et al. Systematic reviews of health economic evaluations: a protocol for a systematic review of characteristics and methods applied[J]. Syst Rev, 2017, 6 (1): 238.

[173] DEHMER S P, BAKER-GOERING M M, MACIOSEK M V, et al. Modeled Health and Economic Impact of Team-Based Care for Hypertension[J]. Am J Prev Med, 2016, 50 (5 Suppl 1): S34-S44.

[174] International Lablor Organization. ILOSTATS Data[EB/OL]. (2019) [2020-7-1]. https://ilostat.ilo.org/data/

[175] World Bank. World Development Indicators[EB/OL]. (2019) [2020-7-1]. https://datacatalog.worldbank.org/dataset/world-development-indicators

[176] JAMES S L, ABATE D, ABATE K H, et al. Global, regional, and national incidence, prevalence, and years lived with disability for 354 Diseases and Injuries for 195 countries and territories, 1990-2017: a systematic analysis for the Global Burden of Disease Study 2017[J]. The Lancet, 2018, 392 (10159): 1789-1858.

[177] JO C. Cost-of-illness studies: concepts, scopes, and methods[J]. Clin Mol Hepatol, 2014, 20 (4): 327-337.

[178] Department of Primary Care, National Health and Family Planning Commission (2015). Policy explanation of how to implement basic public health service program in China. Preprinted. [2016-7-1]. http://www.nhc.gov.cn/jws/s3577/201709/9cb26d17f691491bb3bb0f139bbf3ff1.shtml

[179] Zhao, Z., Chen, X., & Zhou, Y. (2015). Measurement of fund allocation proportion of basic public health service in community based on workload. *Chinese General Practice*, 18 (10), 1124-1128.

[180] Jinquan, C., Lu, Z., Zhao, Z., & et al. (2015). An overview of Cost Study of Basic Public Health Service in Community. *Chinese General Practice*, 18 (10), 1115-1119.

[181] Flochel T, Ikeda Y, Moroz H, et al.Macroeconomic Implications of Aging in East Asia Pacific[J].World Bank Other Operational Studies, 2015.

[182] MURRUGARRA, E. (2011). Employability and productivity among older workers: A policy framework and evidence from Latin America. *SP Discussion Paper*, (1113), 1-64 [EB/OL]. [2016-7-1]. http://documents.shihang.org/curated/zh/582931468276366754/pdf/632300NWP0111300public00BOX361509B.pdf

[183] Communist Party of China Central Committee. (2009). Opinions of the Communist Party of China Central Committee and the State Council on Deepening the Health Care System Reform (No. 5) [EB/OL]. [2016-7-1]. https://www.gov.cn/jrzg/2009-04/06/content 1278721.htm

[184] How, W., Zhao, Z., Xia, T., & et al. (2016). The budget prediction of basic public health service in the community. *Chinese Journal of General Practice*, 14 (6), 879-882.

[185] SHEN Y, WANG X, WANG Z, et al. Prevalence, awareness, treatment, and control of hypertension among Chinese working population: results of a workplace-based study[J]. J Am Soc Hypertens, 2018, 12 (4): 311-322.e2.

[186] HUANG K, SONG Y T, HE Y H, et al. Health system strengthening and hypertension management in China[J]. Glob Health Res Policy, 2016, 1: 13.

[187] Xu, G. (2010). Staffing standard in public institution: Orientation, mechanism and coping strategies. *Journal of Renmin University of China*, (5), 143-150.

[188] Qin, J., Zhang, L., Lin, C., Zhang, X., & Zhang, Y. (2016). Scale and allocation of human resources in primary health care system in china after new health reform. *Chinese General Practice*, 19 (4), 378-381. https://doi.org/10.3969/j.issn.1007-9572.2016.04.003

[189] Zhang, Y., Qin, J., Zhang, L., & Lin, C. (2017). Incentive system analysis of family doctor Contracted services in China based on QOF of England. *China Health Economics*, 36 (12),

116-119. DOI: 10.7664/CHE20171232

[190] ZHOU B, DANAEI G, STEVENS G A, et al. Long-term and recent trends in hypertension awareness, treatment, and control in 12 high-income countries: an analysis of 123 nationally representative surveys. The Lancet, 2019, 6736 (19): 1-13.

[191] LI H, WEI X, WONG M C, et al. A comparison of the quality of hypertension management in primary care between Shanghai and Shenzhen: a cohort study of 3, 196 patients[J]. Medicine (Baltimore), 2015, 94 (5): e455.

[192] HUSEREAU D, DRUMMOND M, PETROU S, et al. Consolidated Health Economic Evaluation Reporting Standards (CHEERS) statement[J]. Eur J Health Econ, 2013, 14 (3): 367-372.

[193] The Centre of National Cardovascular Disease of China. (2017). *Guideline for Hypertension Prevention and Control in Primary Care Facilities under the National Essential Public Health Service Program*. Beijing.

[194] PEñALOZA-RAMOS M C, JOWETT S, SUTTON A J, et al. The Importance of Model Structure in the Cost-Effectiveness Analysis of Primary Care Interventions for the Management of Hypertension[J]. Value Health, 2018, 21 (3): 351-363.

[195] Liu, X., Du, J., Guo, A., Han, Z., Liu, J., Bo, X., & Liu, G. (2013). Investigation on occupational population's demand, utilizations and influencing factors of community health service in Desheng Community, Beijing. *Chinese General Practice*, 16 (11C). https://doi.org/10.3969/j.issn.1007-9572.2013.11.097

[196] Wang, F., Li, Y., Ding, X., Liu, L., Zhou, W., & Hu, T. (2012). Status of functional community health services and problem analysis. *China Health Service Management*, (12), 894-896. https://doi.org/1004-4663 (2012) 12-894-03

Appendices

Appendix A Supplementary material for Chapter 3

Table A1 Hypertension PATC of different age groups in China, 1991-2015

Group	1991	1993	1997	2000	2004	2006	2009	2011	2015
Prevalence									
18-24	2.44	4.21	4.70	3.65	4.50	3.71	3.80	2.37	4.00
25-34	3.74	5.92	6.59	6.35	6.94	5.80	7.84	5.95	6.10
35-44	9.50	9.87	12.14	12.93	13.67	13.41	14.82	12.11	15.90
45-54	16.95	18.06	22.12	22.33	22.92	22.16	28.66	26.48	29.60
55-64	32.84	33.43	36.61	36.71	36.36	33.55	38.88	38.76	44.60
65-74	45.56	44.53	51.97	50.74	49.64	45.83	53.56	49.20	55.70
75+	52.44	51.97	53.53	53.58	56.39	53.05	58.35	54.74	60.20
Awareness									
18-24	8.82	7.84	6.12	3.03	0	11.11	0	7.14	5.70
25-34	22.97	7.92	7.87	11.40	9.47	11.94	9.72	9.64	14.70
35-44	23.04	15.46	9.78	18.95	20.08	20.43	22.36	37.81	31.70
45-54	27.18	28.00	20.85	35.37	34.02	38.02	39.78	51.07	47.00
55-64	36.08	41.12	22.86	38.97	44.47	53.02	48.50	60.41	53.90
65-74	30.08	36.25	32.97	44.39	48.25	55.18	55.52	65.32	58.60
75+	19.49	22.69	25.69	32.56	42.91	49.04	51.38	68.15	57.30

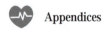

continued

Group	1991	1993	1997	2000	2004	2006	2009	2011	2015
Treatment									
18-24	0	3.92	2.04	0	0	0	0	0	3.40
25-34	9.46	2.97	3.15	4.39	3.16	4.48	6.94	2.41	8.40
35-44	8.90	5.15	5.78	9.82	13.64	15.05	15.85	24.38	24.50
45-54	14.56	13.33	12.39	21.89	22.54	26.59	28.10	40.64	40.30
55-64	23.58	27.51	15.83	26.77	33.58	39.50	40.63	51.12	48.10
65-74	18.70	22.50	24.59	35.20	36.29	43.97	48.34	56.75	52.80
75+	13.56	16.81	15.28	21.51	35.22	40.23	44.00	60.42	52.10
Control									
18-24	0	3.92	0	0	0	0	0	0	0.60
25-34	4.05	1.98	0	1.75	1.05	1.49	2.78	0	3.30
35-44	2.62	1.55	2.67	2.81	4.17	3.58	5.69	7.07	9.90
45-54	2.43	2.67	2.82	4.21	6.97	7.91	8.03	14.84	16.10
55-64	4.55	5.62	2.51	6.00	9.38	10.50	12.02	20.91	18.60
65-74	2.44	2.50	4.59	8.74	10.52	12.47	12.96	21.04	18.40
75+	2.54	2.52	3.47	4.65	8.50	8.05	8.92	19.67	17.00

Note: The rate of awareness, treatment and control were of the prevalent hypertensives.

Source: 1991-2011 data from the CHNS, and 2015 data from Wang et al. (2018).

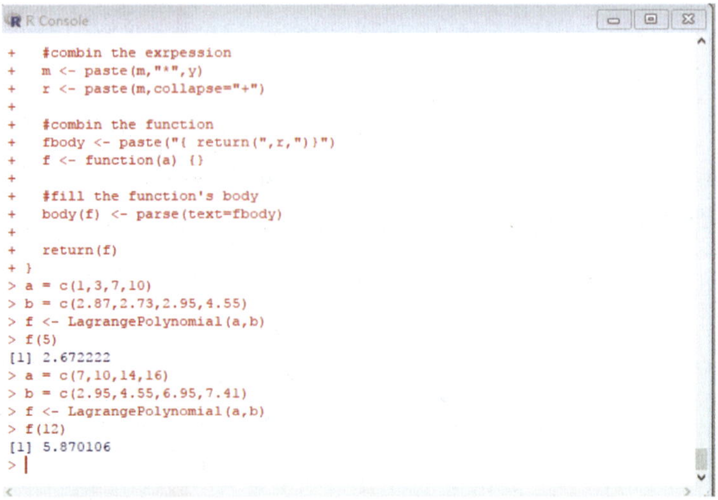
R Console
```
+   #combin the exrpession
+   m <- paste(m,"*",y)
+   r <- paste(m,collapse="+")
+
+   #combin the function
+   fbody <- paste("{ return(",r,")}")
+   f <- function(a) {}
+
+   #fill the function's body
+   body(f) <- parse(text=fbody)
+
+   return(f)
+ }
> a = c(1,3,7,10)
> b = c(2.87,2.73,2.95,4.55)
> f <- LagrangePolynomial(a,b)
> f(5)
[1] 2.672222
> a = c(7,10,14,16)
> b = c(2.95,4.55,6.95,7.41)
> f <- LagrangePolynomial(a,b)
> f(12)
[1] 5.870106
>
```

Figure A1 Screen shot of R Console to realize Lagrange interpolation polynomial

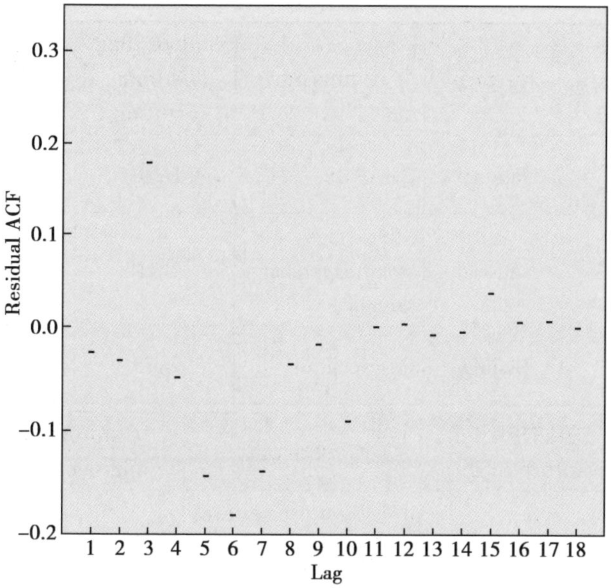

Figure A2 Residual ACF of the time series model for hypertension control, 1991-2009

Table A2 Summary of articles on hypertension prevalence, awareness, treatment, and control in China, 1991-2018

Authors	Study period/ Year	Region	Sampling	Study setting (U=urban; R=rural)	Age range/yr	Sample size
Jiang et al., 2014	2008	Beijing	Cluster	U	⩾50	9, 397
Liang et al., 2014	2009	Chongqing	Cluster	U	⩾18	6, 681
Wang et al., 2014	2007-2010	National	Stratified cluster	U	18-79	249, 830
Li et al., 2015	2010-2011	Shanghai & Shenzhen	Multi-stage random sampling	U	⩾18	3, 196
Gu et al., 2014	2011	Xuhui, Shanghai	Cluster	U	⩾35	3, 328
Zhang et al., 2014	2011	Yulin CHSC (Chengdu)	Cluster	U	⩾35	3, 191
Hou et al., 2016	2008, 2012	National Zhejiang & Gansu	CHARLS	U&R	⩾45	1, 961 1, 836

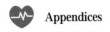

continued

Authors	Study period/Year	Region	Sampling	Study setting (U=urban; R=rural)	Age range/yr	Sample size
Zhang et al., 2018	2011, 2013	National	CHARLS	U&R	≥45	4, 958
Tian et al., 2015	2013	National	Multi-stage stratified random sampling	U&R	≥35	2, 173
Wang et al., 2013	2013	Beijing	Case-control	U&R	≥18	436

Authors	SBP/DBP lowered/mmHg	Control rate	Control rate improved (%)	Duration of follow-up
Jiang et al., 2014	N/A	45.8% with regular therapy	N/A	N/A
Liang et al., 2014	3.5 (3.2-3.7)/ 2.9 (2.7-3.2)	N/A	N/A	1 year
Wang et al., 2014	N/A	25.5%	37%. monotherapy 27.7% combination 24.1%	N/A
Li et al., 2015	N/A	83.2% 76.3%	N/A	2 years
Gu et al., 2014		36.1		
Zhang et al., 2014	(147 ± 17) *vs.* (133 ± 8), (83 ± 11) *vs.* (75 ± 6)	32% *vs.* 85%	53%	(33 ± 25) Months
Hou et al., 2016	N/A	21.7% 36.4%	14.7	N/A
Zhang et al., 2018	N/A	27.3% 35.5%	7.9%	N/A
Tian et al., 2015	N/A	33.65%	N/A	N/A
Wang et al., 2013	N/A	42.1% *vs.* 34.3% urban/ 30.7% *vs.* 10.0% rural 70.7% *vs.* 40.0% urban and 72.9% *vs.* 27.9% in rural	7.8%-urban 20.7%-rural 30.7%-urban 45%-rural	3 months 1 year

Note: U = urban area and R = rural area.

Appendix B Supplementary material for Chapter 4

Table B1 Characteristics and age-group specific risk factors, comparison of hypertensive population grouping by hypertension control or not, male

Age group	Group	N	Age/yr (mean±SD)	SBP/ mmHg (mean±SD)	DBP/ mmHg (mean±SD)	TC/($mmol \cdot L^{-1}$) (mean±SD)	HDL-C/ ($mmol \cdot L^{-1}$) (mean±SD)	BMI/($kg \cdot m^{-2}$) (mean±SD)	Diabetes/n (%)	Smoking/n (%)
35~44	G1	10	41.86 ± 1.66	127 ± 6	83 ± 4	4.97 ± 0.71	1.24 ± 0.32	24.9 ± 1.85	2/10 (20.0)	8/10
	G2	22	41.09 ± 2.48	147 ± 15	101 ± 10	5.18 ± 1.10	1.16 ± 0.44	27.3 ± 3.12	4 (18.2)	11 (50.0)
t (Chi-squared) value			0.895	4.13	5.49	0.55	−0.55	2.11	0.015	2.57
P value			0.378	<0.01	<0.01	0.59	0.59	0.04	0.903	0.14
Age group	**Group**	**N**	**Age (mean±SD)**	**SBP/ mmHg (mean±SD)**	**DBP/ mmHg (mean±SD)**	**TC/($mmol \cdot L^{-1}$) (mean±SD)**	**HDL-C/ ($mmol \cdot L^{-1}$) (mean±SD)**	**BMI/($kg \cdot m^{-2}$) (mean±SD)**	**Diabetes/n (%)**	**Smoking/n (%)**
45~54	G1	28	49.24 ± 3.41	127 ± 11	84 ± 6	4.84 ± 0.96	1.14 (1.02-1.40)*	25.7 ± 3.82	6 (21.4)	18 (64.3)
	G2	66	50.29 ± 2.97	149 ± 14	100 ± 11	5.21 ± 0.98	1.25(1.06-1.51)*	26.1 ± 3.25	13 (19.7)	37 (56.1)
t (Chi-squared) value			−1.501	7.12	7.23	1.68	−1.62* (Z value)	0.54	0.037	0.55
P value			0.137	<0.01	<0.01	0.10	0.11* (P value)	0.59	0.848	0.50

continued

Age group	Group	N	Age (mean±SD)	SBP/ mmHg (mean±SD)	DBP/ mmHg (mean±SD)	TC/(mmol · L^{-1}) (mean±SD)	HDL-C/ (mmol · L^{-1}) (mean±SD)	BMI/(kg · m^{-2}) (mean±SD)	Diabetes/n (%)	Smoking/n (%)
55~64	G1	35	60.03 ± 3.01	129 ± 11	83 ± 6	5.12 ± 0.91	1.24 ± 0.31	25.0 ± 2.66	9 (25.7)	15 (42.9)
	G2	91	60.24 ± 2.92	152 ± 18	97 ± 13	4.97 ± 0.85	1.27 ± 0.37	24.7 ± 3.11	17 (18.7)	44 (48.4)
t (Chi-squared) value			−0.369	7.12	6.40	−0.88	0.54	−0.46	0.763	0.31
P value			0.713	<0.01	<0.01	0.38	0.59	0.65	0.382	0.69
Age group	Group	N	Age (mean±SD)	SBP/ mmHg (mean±SD)	DBP/ mmHg (mean±SD)	TC/(mmol · L^{-1}) (mean±SD)	HDL-C/ (mmol · L^{-1}) (mean±SD)	BMI/(kg · m^{-2}) (mean±SD)	Diabetes/n (%)	Smoking/n (%)
65~74	G1	42	69.23 ± 3.03	127 ± 10	80 ± 7	4.61 ± 0.85	1.28 ± 0.34	23.4 ± 3.55	6 (14.3)	20 (47.6)
	G2	91	69.13 ± 2.78	157 ± 15	91 ± 11	5.10 ± 0.94	1.31 ± 0.38	23.4 ± 3.76	20 (22.0)	32 (35.2)
t (Chi-squared) value			0.196	11.48	5.87	2.35	0.43	3.25	1.081	1.87
P value			0.845	<0.01	<0.01	0.02	0.67	0.00	0.298	0.19
Age group	Group	N	Age (mean±SD)	SBP/ mmHg (mean±SD)	DBP/ mmHg (mean±SD)	TC/(mmol · L^{-1}) (mean±SD)	HDL-C/ (mmol · L^{-1}) (mean±SD)	BMI/(kg · m^{-2}) (mean±SD)	Diabetes/n (%)	Smoking/n (%)
75~84	G1	16	78.57 ± 2.63	126 ± 9	77 ± 9	4.61 ± 0.89	1.30 ± 0.34	23.3 ± 3.47	3 (18.8)	6 (37.5)
	G2	42	78.89 ± 2.49	160 ± 19	92 ± 11	5.00 ± 0.79	1.31 ± 0.39	23.4 ± 3.77	10 (23.8)	12 (28.6)
t (Chi-squared) value			−0.429	6.56	4.80	1.63	0.08	0.09	0.171	0.43
P value			0.669	<0.01	<0.01	0.11	0.94	0.93	0.680	0.54

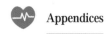

continued

Age group	Group	N	Age (mean±SD)	SBP/ mmHg (mean±SD)	DBP/ mmHg (mean±SD)	TC/(mmol · L^{-1}) (mean±SD)	HDL-C/ (mmol · L^{-1}) (mean±SD)	BMI/(kg · m^{-2}) (mean±SD)	Diabetes/n (%)	Smoking/n (%)
85+	G1	2	87.65 ± 1.48	127.00 ± 5.19	65.83 ± 6.84	4.85 ± 2.22	1.36 ± 0.58	20.97 ± 0.40	0	0
	G2	3	89.17 ± 3.20	156.67 ± 6.11	89.78 ± 8.39	4.70 ± 1.03	1.55 ± 0.23	23.77 ± 3.63	0	0
t value			–0.604	*U* test**	*U* test	*U* test	*U* test	*U* test	N/A	N/A
P value			0.589	0.400	0.400	0.800	1.000	0.400	N/A	N/A

Notes: Test of difference: For age, blood pressure, TC, and HDL-C independent sample *t* test was performed; for diabetes and smoking rate, Pearson's χ^2 analysis was performed.

*Non-normal distribution, non-parametric test was adopted, range interquartile were listed in the brackets.

**U test means Mann-Whitney *U* test.

Table B2 Characteristics and age-group specific risk factors, comparison of hypertensive population grouping by hypertension control or not, female

Age group	Group	N	Age (mean±SD)	SBP/ mmHg (mean±SD)	DBP/ mmHg (mean±SD)	TC/(mmol · L^{-1}) (mean±SD)	HDL-C/ (mmol · L^{-1}, mean±SD)	BMI/(kg · m^{-2}, mean±SD)	Diabetes/n (%)	Smoking/n (%)
35~44	G1	7	42.49 ± 2.02	131 ± 10	86 ± 4	5.14 ± 1.26	1.31 ± 0.25	24.5 ± 3.36	1 (14.3)	0
	G2	22	40.54 ± 2.82	155 ± 29	102 ± 11	4.65 ± 0.85	1.30 ± 0.23	26.1 ± 4.41	2 (9.1)	〔1 (4.5)〕
t(Chi-squared) value			1.683	2.14	3.51	–1.19	–0.11	0.90	0.155	0.33
P value			0.104	0.05	0.003	0.25	0.91	0.38	0.694	1.00

continued

Age group	Group	N	Age (mean±SD)	SBP/mmHg (mean±SD)	DBP/mmHg (mean±SD)	TC/(mmol · L^{-1}) (mean±SD)	HDL-C/(mmol · L^{-1}, mean±SD)	BMI/(kg · m^{-2}, mean±SD)	Diabetes/n (%)	Smoking/n (%)
45~54	G1	43	50.92 ± 2.82	125 ± 10	82 ± 6	5.30 ± 1.23	1.53 (1.24-1.76)*	24.9 ± 3.37	10 (23.3)	0
	G2	59	51.03 ± 2.87	152 ± 15	97 ± 11	5.22 ± 1.12	1.34 (1.12-1.52)*	26.6 ± 3.74	9 (15.3)	7 (11.9)
t (Chi-squared) value			−0.188	10.29	7.94	−0.35	−2.58*(Z value)	2.45	1.051	5.48
P value			0.852	0.000	0.000	0.73	0.01*(P value)	0.02	0.305	0.02
Age group	Group	N	Age (mean±SD)	SBP/mmHg (mean±SD)	DBP/mmHg (mean±SD)	TC/(mmol · L^{-1}) (mean±SD)	HDL-C/(mmol · L^{-1}, mean±SD)	BMI/(kg · m^{-2}, mean±SD)	Diabetes/n (%)	Smoking/n (%)
55~64	G1	51	60.27 ± 2.86	127 ± 11	81 ± 6	5.24 ± 0.99	1.40 ± 0.51	25.3 ± 3.03	11 (21.6)	1 (2.0)
	G2	128	60.23 ± 2.72	156 ± 15	96 ± 8	5.48 ± 0.97	1.33 ± 0.31	25.7 ± 3.46	32 (25.0)	11 (8.6)
t (Chi-squared) value			0.074	12.36	11.93	1.52	−1.10	0.66	0.235	2.57
P value			0.941	0.000	0.000	0.13	0.27	0.51	0.628	0.18
Age group	Group	N	Age (mean±SD)	SBP/mmHg (mean±SD)	DBP/mmHg (mean±SD)	TC/(mmol · L^{-1}) (mean±SD)	HDL-C/(mmol · L^{-1}, mean±SD)	BMI/(kg · m^{-2}, mean±SD)	Diabetes/n (%)	Smoking/n (%)
65~74	G1	63	70.04 ± 2.94	131 ± 8	79 ± 8	5.24 ± 0.99	1.38 ± 0.37	25.2 ± 3.41	22 (34.9)	〔1 (1.6)〕
	G2	109	70.31 ± 2.89	156 ± 15	90 ± 11	5.27 ± 1.02	1.44 ± 0.30	24.7 ± 4.25	29 (26.6)	〔11 (10.1)〕
t (Chi-squared) value			−0.578	12.05	6.93	0.18	1.10	−0.90	1.323	4.45
P value			0.546	0.000	0.000	0.86	0.27	0.37	0.250	0.06

continued

Age group	Group	N	Age (mean±SD)	SBP/ mmHg (mean±SD)	DBP/ mmHg (mean±SD)	TC/(mmol · L^{-1}) (mean±SD)	HDL-C/ (mmol · L^{-1}, mean±SD)	BMI/(kg · m^{-2}, mean±SD)	Diabetes/n (%)	Smoking/n (%)
75~84	G1	22	78.30 ± 2.26	126 ± 13	79 ± 9	4.87 ± 0.88	1.40 ± 0.35	24.3 ± 4.52	7 (31.8)	0
	G2	60	79.24 ± 2.75	164 ± 24	87 ± 11	5.51 ± 0.88	1.46 ± 0.35	23.5 ± 4.32	15 (25.0)	〔5 (8.3)〕
t (Chi-squared) value			−1.431	7.72	3.30	2.94	0.72	−0.76	0.381	1.95
P value			0.156	0.000	0.003	0.004	0.48	0.45	0.537	0.32

Age group	Group	N	Age (mean±SD)	SBP/ mmHg (mean±SD)	DBP/ mmHg (mean±SD)	TC/(mmol · L^{-1}) (mean±SD)	HDL-C/ (mmol · L^{-1}, mean±SD)	BMI/(kg · m^{-2}, mean±SD)	Diabetes/n (%)	Smoking/n (%)
85+	G1	1	86.50	137.67	75.00	4.04	1.78	19.33	0	0
	G2	4	85.80 ± 0.81	164.08 ± 5.87	87.33 ± 6.37	4.68 ± 1.31	1.38 ± 0.30	23.91 ± 3.39	0	0.25
t (Chi-squared) value			0.771	*U* test**	*U* test	*U* test	*U* test	*U* test	N/A	N/A
P value			0.497	0.200	0.200	1.000	0.800	0.800	N/A	N/A

Notes: Test of difference: For age, blood pressure, TC, and HDL-C independent sample T test was performed; for diabetes and smoking rate, Pearson's χ^2 analysis was performed.

*Non-normal distribution, non-parametric test was adopted, range interquartile were listed in the brackets.

**U test means Mann-Whitney U test.

Table B3 Age-gender urban-rural population mortality rate and structure

Age/gender	Mortality rate/100, 000		Proportion in the whole population/%	
	Urban	Rural	Urban	Rural
Male				
35-	116.12	166.82	2.72	4.08
40-	220.52	268.42	2.61	4.64
45-	274.92	349.22	2.25	3.93
50-	531.18	627.51	1.65	3.05
55-	755.40	830.51	1.49	3.37
60-	1, 227.23	1, 368.67	1.01	2.53
65-	1, 984.41	2, 305.59	0.67	1.79
70-	3, 169.18	3, 725.56	0.57	1.38
75-	5, 167.37	6, 138.59	0.41	0.94
80-	9, 052.67	10, 598.65	0.21	0.49
85-	18, 323.58	19, 594.67	0.11	0.23
Female				
35-	48.04	67.15	2.56	3.92
40-	96.84	109.39	2.43	4.56
45-	118.50	149.91	2.07	3.91
50-	234.83	293.95	1.57	2.92
55-	324.37	393.48	1.50	3.25
60-	606.47	721.00	1.03	2.39
65-	1, 064.47	1, 296.45	0.71	1.71
70-	1, 882.75	2, 290.84	0.61	1.36
75-	3, 509.27	3, 945.77	0.44	1.07
80-	6, 721.27	7, 423.16	0.24	0.66
85-	15, 318.04	15, 928.79	0.15	0.42

Source: China Health and Family Planning Yearbook 2014, China Statistical Bureau 2014.

Table B4 Parameter values for projection in a Markov model of the two groups

Group	Age-gender structure of hypertensive population/ %	CHD					Stroke					Non-CVD mortality/ 100, 000
		Prior CHD/ %*	Incidence of CHD of G1/ 100, 000	Incidence of CHD of G2/ 100, 000	28-days case fatality (proportion)	CHD case fatality (proportion)	Prior stroke/ %*	Incidence of stroke of G1/ 100, 000	Incidence of stroke of G2/ 100, 000	28-days case fatality (proportion)	Stroke case fatality (proportion)	
Male												
35-44	9.36	0.6	130	215	0.12	0.02	1.3	24	49	0.25	0.02	149
45-54	7.13	1.2	135	223	0.21	0.03	3.2	145	298	0.18	0.02	305
55-64	5.23	3.4	220	363	0.29	0.03	8.8	670	1, 378	0.12	0.02	696
65-74	2.71	4.7	500	825	0.33	0.05	14.2	1, 250	2, 571	0.20	0.04	1, 741
75-84	1.28	6.0	2, 010	4, 641	0.48	0.18	15.0	2, 510	8, 314	0.45	0.11	4, 142
85+*	0.21	6.0	2, 010	3, 317	0.48	0.65	15.0	2, 510	5, 163	0.45	0.28	10, 806
Female												
35-44	8.92	0.4	19	26	0.18	0.00	0.9	23	39	0.18	0.01	67
45-54	6.8	1.3	49	69	0.23	0.02	2.4	180	376	0.14	0.01	141
55-64	5.13	3.1	141	198	0.27	0.01	6.0	800	1, 670	0.15	0.02	333
65-74	2.75	4.0	310	432	0.43	0.04	10.0	1, 500	2, 515	0.20	0.04	946
75-84	1.48	6.0	1, 900	3, 276	0.51	0.17	12.0	2, 500	7, 799	0.45	0.11	2, 670
85+*	0.34	6.0	1, 900	3, 248	0.51	0.55	12.0	2, 500	6, 263	0.45	0.30	8, 335

Notes: *The parameters not available for the age group of 85+ were substituted by that of the age group of 75-84, which includes 28-days case fatality of CHD, CHD Mortality, 28-days case fatality of stroke and stroke mortality. CHD mortality and stroke mortality of adults aged 85+ were calculated based on urban-rural age-gender disease-specific mortality from the 2013 Chinese Health Statistic Yearbook and the age-gender structure of the 2010 Chinese Census data.

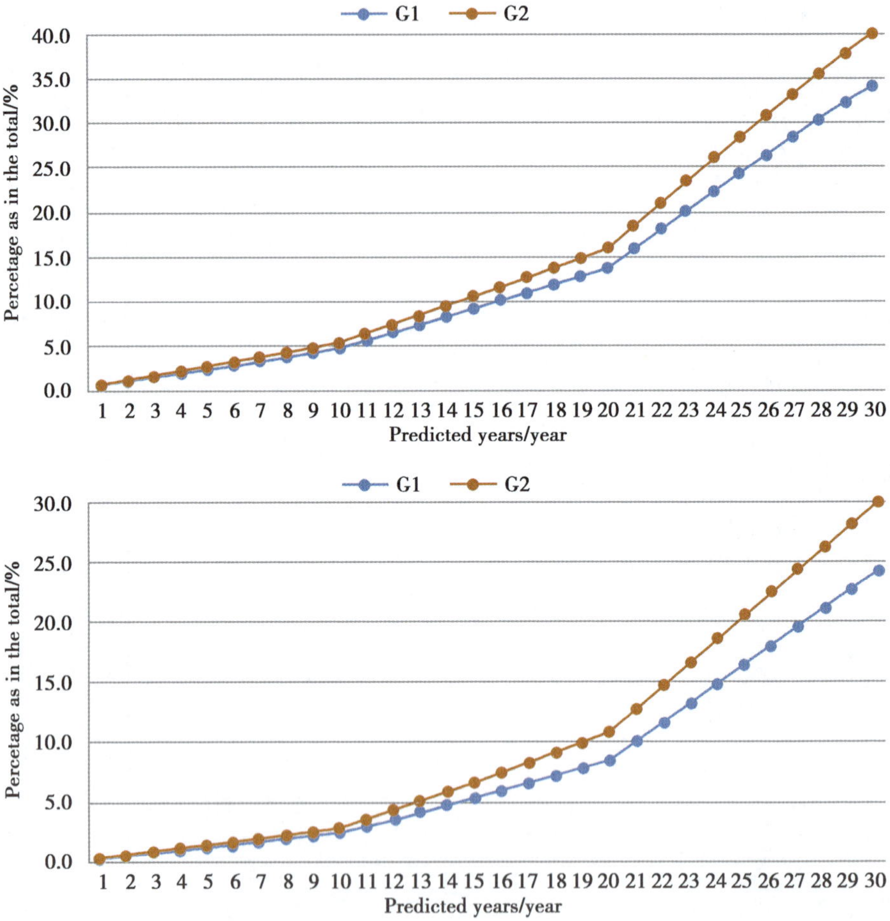

Figure B1 Percentages of deaths in G1 and G2, 45-54-year age group, male (upper side) and female (below side)

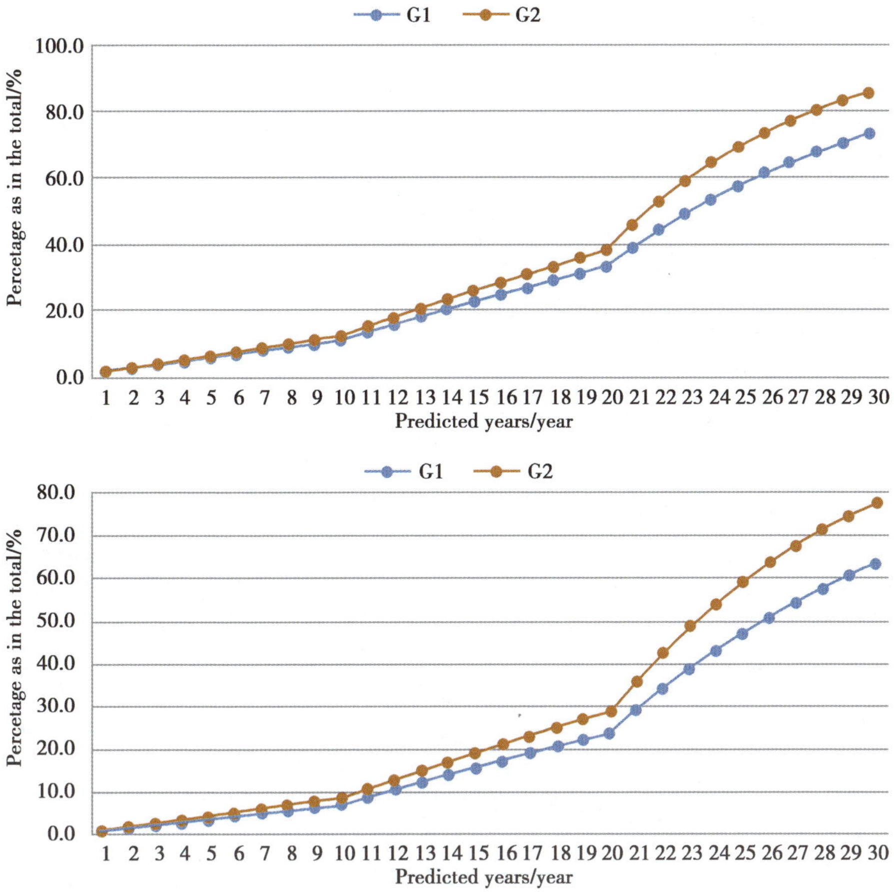

Figure B2 Percentages of deaths in G1 and G2, 55-64-year age group, male (upper side) and female (below side)

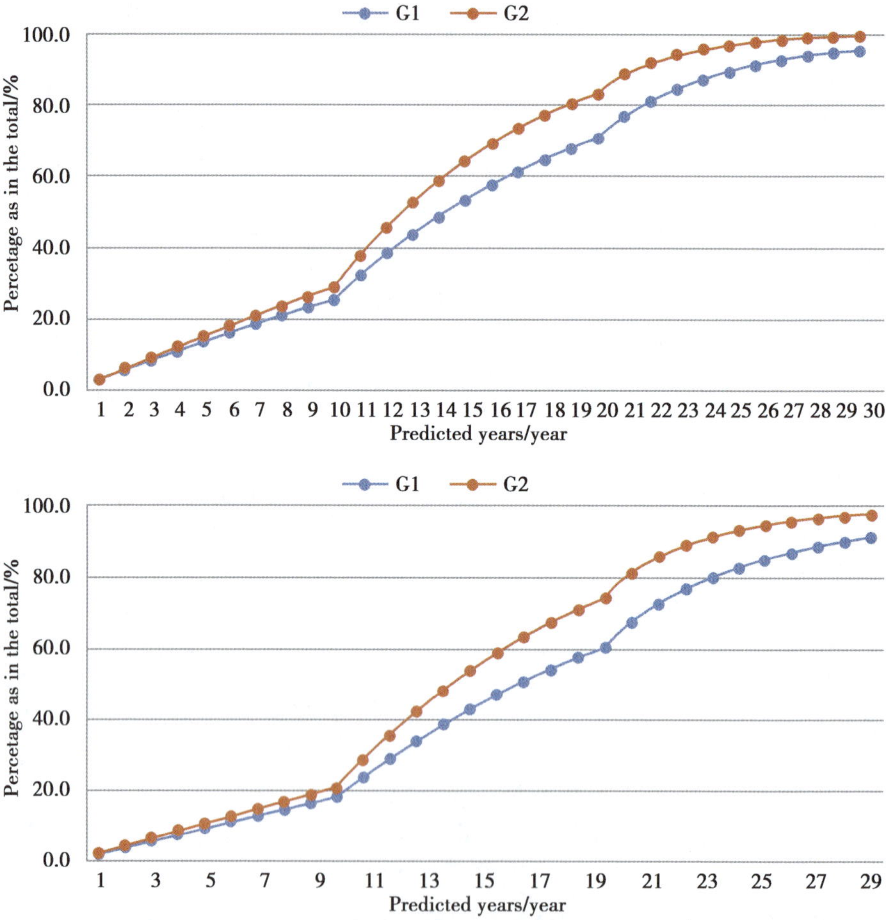

Figure B3　Percentages of deaths in G1 and G2, 65-74-year age group, male (upper side) and female (below side)

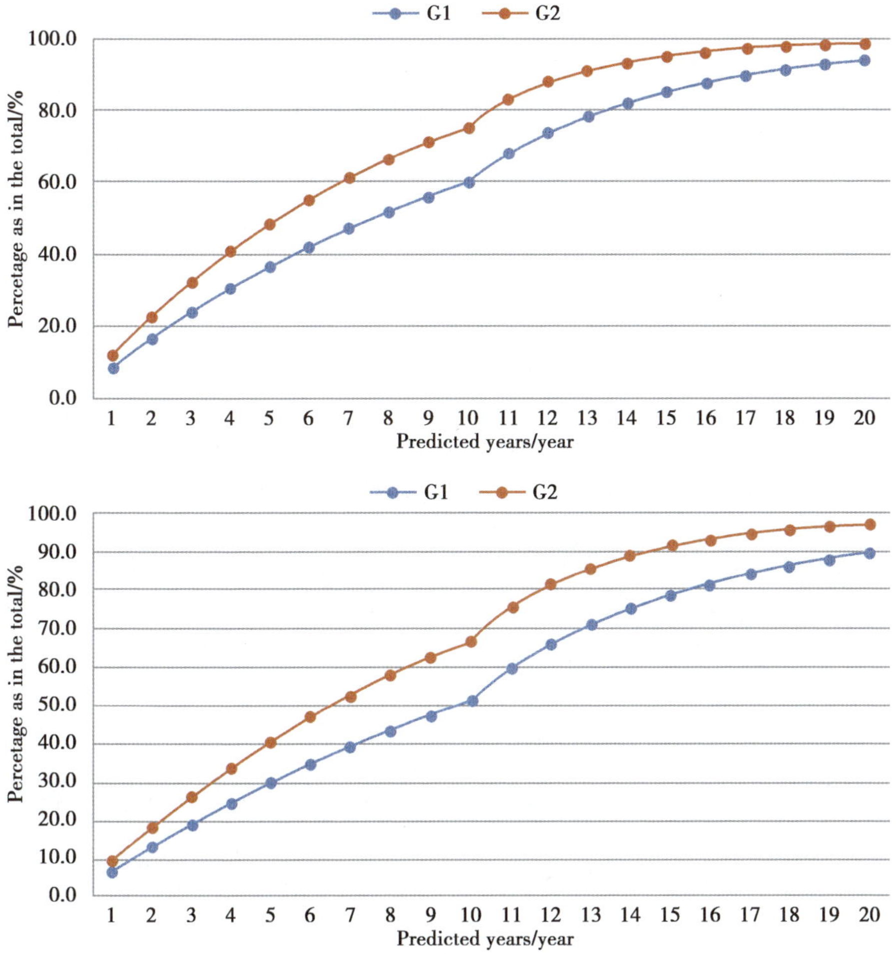

Figure B4 Percentages of deaths in G1 and G2, 75-84-year age group, male (upper side) and female (below side)

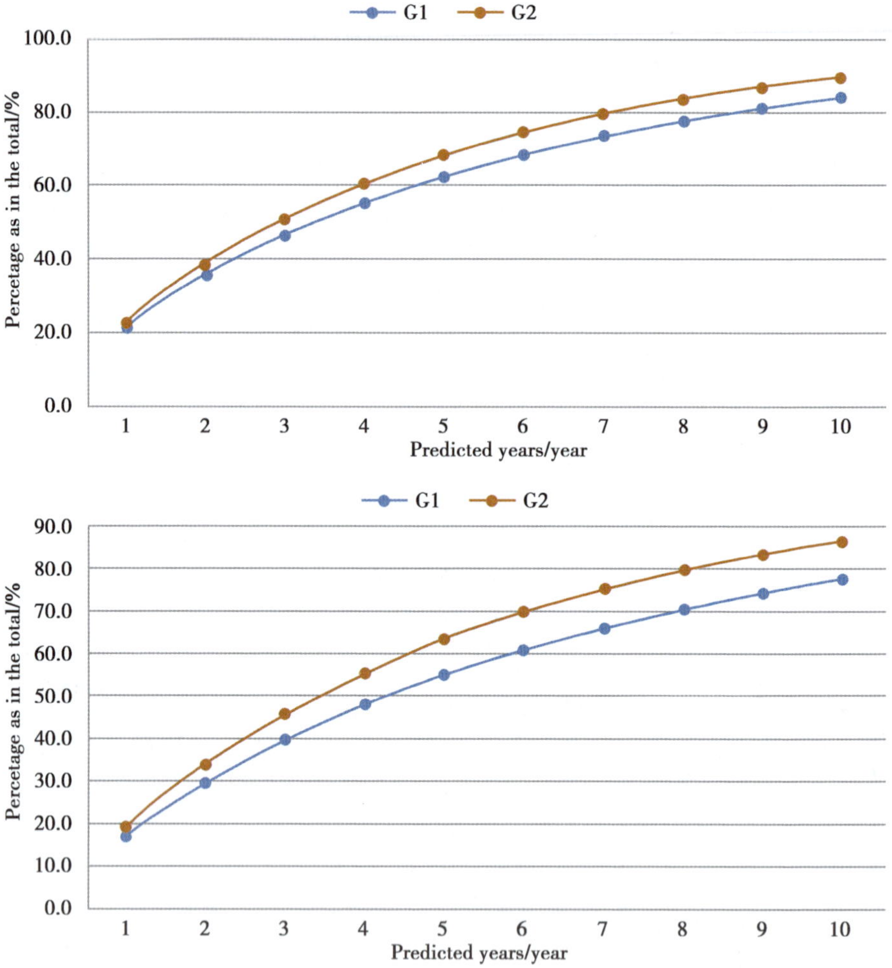

Figure B5 Percentages of deaths in G1 and G2, 84+-year age group, male (upper side) and female (below side)

Appendix C Supplementary material for Chapter 5

In Table C1, HTN means simple hypertension; CHD means hypertension with comorbidity of CHD; stroke means hypertension with stroke.

Table C1 Accumulative probabilities of each illness at the end of predicted 30 years for each group (person-years)

Group	With NBPHS (HTN controlled)			Without NBPHS (HTN uncontrolled)		
	HTN	CHD	Stroke	HTN	CHD	Stroke
Male/yr						
35-44	38, 995, 672	27, 995	1, 383, 296	37, 275, 289	57, 935	2, 354, 312
45-54	78, 488, 850	70, 185	5, 150, 234	73, 006, 122	153, 108	8, 442, 201
55-64	62, 237, 009	74, 190	9, 025, 025	57, 005, 290	152, 649	11, 803, 038
65-74	23, 815, 907	33, 350	4, 940, 132	21, 392, 395	69, 469	6, 020, 998
75-84	2, 854, 003	5, 164	604, 500	2, 568, 392	10, 365	705, 204
85+	19, 126	44	4, 028	18, 115	79	4, 401
Female/yr						
35-44	28, 232, 339	9, 984	605, 057	27, 124, 297	33, 404	1, 297, 875
45-54	69, 464, 945	61, 294	3, 769, 957	62, 434, 246	161, 475	8, 068, 701
55-64	75, 686, 346	122, 564	10, 214, 433	61, 836, 177	283, 756	17, 756, 172
65-74	27, 049, 344	64, 610	6, 100, 186	20, 073, 023	135, 737	9, 370, 996
75-84	4, 193, 453	11, 759	937, 886	2, 942, 426	28, 158	1, 402, 902
85+	29, 168	87	5, 621	23, 291	240	7, 896

Notes: The prediction duration of the age group 75-84 and 85+ is 20 years and 10 years, respectively, because of parameter availability and average life expectancy of the population in China.

Table C2 Mean age of each age group of hypertensives estimated based on CHNS 2015

Group	N	Mean	SD	Group	N	Mean	SD
Male/yr				Female/yr			
35-44	39	41.10	2.761	35-44	36	41.06	2.540
45-54	154	50.06	2.705	45-54	168	50.61	2.606
55-64	296	60.10	2.715	55-64	331	60.34	2.674
65-74	310	69.06	2.824	65-74	337	68.89	2.720
75-84	104	78.23	2.735	75-84	150	78.68	2.781
85+	15	87.33	2.127	85+	17	87.53	21.25

Notes: The prediction duration of the age group 75-84 and 85+ is 20 years and 10 years, respectively, because of parameter availability and average life expectancy of the population in China.

Table C3-1 Deaths of difference in the NBPHS and non-NBPHS groups in projected years, male

Year	35-44 age group		45-54 age group		55-64 age group		65-74 age group		75-84 age group		85+ age group	
	Age	Number	Age	Number	Age	Number	Age	Number	Age	Number	Age	Number
2016	42	94	51	533	61	1, 698	70	2, 956	79	13, 547	88	1, 086
2017	43	102	52	578	62	1, 810	71	3, 085	80	12, 203	89	1, 220
2018	44	110	53	620	63	1, 913	72	3, 176	81	10, 603	90	977
2019	45	118	54	661	64	2, 006	73	3, 233	82	8, 911	91	675
2020	46	125	55	700	65	2, 090	74	3, 260	83	7, 237	92	403
2021	47	132	56	737	66	2, 166	75	3, 260	84	5, 650	93	180
2022	48	139	57	772	67	2, 233	76	3, 237	85	4, 193	94	9
2023	49	146	58	805	68	2, 292	77	3, 194	86	2, 888	95	-116
2024	50	153	59	836	69	2, 344	78	3, 133	87	1, 743	96	-203
2025	51	159	60	866	70	2, 390	79	3, 058	88	758	97	-259
2026	52	379	61	1, 663	71	5, 921	80	22, 089	89	-1, 378		
2027	53	395	62	1, 735	72	5, 865	81	18, 769	90	-5, 064		
2028	54	411	63	1, 800	73	5, 775	82	15, 453	91	-6, 099		
2029	55	425	64	1, 858	74	5, 656	83	12, 289	92	-6, 184		
2030	56	439	65	1, 909	75	5, 512	84	9, 368	93	-5, 880		
2031	57	452	66	1, 954	76	5, 346	85	6, 738	94	-5, 410		
2032	58	464	67	1, 993	77	5, 163	86	4, 420	95	-4, 882		
2033	59	476	68	2, 027	78	4, 966	87	2, 415	96	-4, 349		
2034	60	487	69	2, 055	79	4, 756	88	710	97	-3, 840		
2035	61	497	70	2, 078	80	4, 538	89	-715	98	-3, 368		
2036	62	851	71	4, 963	81	30, 424	90	-5, 625				
2037	63	881	72	4, 874	82	25, 215	91	-10, 257				
2038	64	908	73	4, 762	83	20, 212	92	-11, 421				
2039	65	931	74	4, 630	84	15, 569	93	-11, 260				
2040	66	952	75	4, 482	85	11, 373	94	-10, 541				
2041	67	970	76	4, 320	86	7, 661	95	-9, 594				
2042	68	985	77	4, 146	87	4, 438	96	-8, 583				
2043	69	997	78	3, 963	88	1, 690	97	-7, 590				
2044	70	1, 008	79	3, 774	89	-616	98	-6, 658				
2045	71	1, 016	80	3, 579	90	-2515	99	-5, 807				

Notes: The minus numbers are treated as 0 in calculations, which are the same in Table C3-2, C4-1 and C4-2.

Table C3-2 Deaths of difference in the NBPHS and non-NBPHS groups in projected years, female

Year	35-44 age group		45-54 age group		55-64 age group		65-74 age group		75-84 age group		85+ age group	
	Age	Number	Age	Number	Age	Number	Age	Number	Age	Number	Age	Number
2016	42	14	52	332	61	2, 043	70	2, 307	80	14, 376	89	2, 662
2017	43	14	53	353	62	2, 205	71	2, 451	81	13, 441	90	2, 942
2018	44	15	54	374	63	2, 355	72	2, 569	82	12, 233	91	2, 551
2019	45	15	55	394	64	2, 493	73	2, 663	83	10, 871	92	1, 956
2020	46	16	56	413	65	2, 621	74	2, 736	84	9, 445	93	1, 352
2021	47	16	57	432	66	2, 738	75	2, 788	85	8, 017	94	814
2022	48	17	58	450	67	2, 845	76	2, 823	86	6, 634	95	367
2023	49	17	59	468	68	2, 943	77	2, 841	87	5, 326	96	14
2024	50	18	60	486	69	3, 031	78	2, 844	88	4, 111	97	−254
2025	51	18	61	503	70	3, 111	79	2, 834	89	3, 002	98	−450
2026	52	113	62	1, 744	71	5, 313	80	22, 187	90	2, 262		
2027	53	120	63	1, 843	72	5, 274	81	19, 909	91	−2, 111		
2028	54	126	64	1, 935	73	5, 216	82	17, 477	92	−4, 417		
2029	55	132	65	2, 020	74	5, 141	83	15, 013	93	−5, 572		
2030	56	138	66	2, 097	75	5, 051	84	12, 603	94	−6, 059		
2031	57	144	67	2, 167	76	4, 946	85	10, 306	95	−6, 148		
2032	58	150	68	2, 230	77	4, 831	86	8, 161	96	−6, 002		
2033	59	155	69	2, 288	78	4, 704	87	6, 192	97	−5, 719		
2034	60	161	70	2, 339	79	4, 569	88	4, 409	98	−5, 361		
2035	61	166	71	2, 384	80	4, 427	89	2, 816	99	−4, 966		
2036	62	562	72	4, 017	81	29, 393	90	454				
2037	63	594	73	3, 958	82	25, 698	91	−5, 405				
2038	64	623	74	3, 887	83	21, 988	92	−8, 446				
2039	65	649	75	3, 807	84	18, 383	93	−9, 869				
2040	66	673	76	3, 717	85	14, 964	94	−10, 342				
2041	67	695	77	3, 620	86	11, 784	95	−10, 257				
2042	68	715	78	3, 516	87	8, 874	96	−9, 850				
2043	69	733	79	3, 407	88	6, 246	97	−9, 266				
2044	70	749	80	3, 292	89	3, 904	98	−8, 595				
2045	71	763	81	3, 174	90	1, 842	99	−7, 893				

Table C4-1 The difference in the numbers of hypertensives of CHD in the two groups projected, male

Year	35-44 age group		45-54 age group		55-64 age group		65-74 age group		75-84 age group		85+ age group	
	Age	Number	Age	Number	Age	Number	Age	Number	Age	Number	Age	Number
2016	42	428	51	799	61	1, 370	70	1, 735	79	4, 783	88	405
2017	43	854	52	1, 586	62	2, 677	71	3, 302	80	8, 189	89	648
2018	44	1, 276	53	2, 361	63	3, 925	72	4, 714	81	10, 510	90	777
2019	45	1, 695	54	3, 123	64	5, 114	73	5, 981	82	11, 981	91	825
2020	46	2, 111	55	3, 874	65	6, 247	74	7, 114	83	12, 795	92	820
2021	47	2, 523	56	4, 613	66	7, 326	75	8, 121	84	13, 105	93	781
2022	48	2, 933	57	5, 341	67	8, 353	76	9, 013	85	13, 035	94	721
2023	49	3, 340	58	6, 056	68	9, 328	77	9, 798	86	12, 685	95	650
2024	50	3, 743	59	6, 761	69	10, 255	78	10, 483	87	12, 132	96	575
2025	51	4, 144	60	7, 454	70	11, 134	79	11, 077	88	11, 440	97	501
2026	52	4, 501	61	8, 442	71	12, 882	80	15, 999	89	9, 207		
2027	53	4, 853	62	9, 381	72	14, 430	81	19, 231	90	7, 350		
2028	54	5, 199	63	10, 274	73	15, 794	82	21, 148	91	5, 814		
2029	55	5, 540	64	11, 123	74	16, 988	83	22, 055	92	4, 550		
2030	56	5, 875	65	11, 928	75	18, 024	84	22, 194	93	3, 515		
2031	57	6, 204	66	12, 692	76	18, 914	85	21, 762	94	2, 672		
2032	58	6, 528	67	13, 415	77	19, 669	86	20, 915	95	1, 991		
2033	59	6, 847	68	14, 100	78	20, 301	87	19, 777	96	1, 444		
2034	60	7, 161	69	14, 746	79	20, 818	88	18, 445	97	1, 009		
2035	61	7, 469	70	15, 357	80	21, 230	89	16, 995	98	665		
2036	62	7, 896	71	16, 540	81	26, 675	90	13, 384				
2037	63	8, 301	72	17, 572	82	30, 006	91	10, 425				
2038	64	8, 684	73	18, 464	83	31, 707	92	8, 014				
2039	65	9, 047	74	19, 227	84	32, 170	93	6, 059				
2040	66	9, 390	75	19, 870	85	31, 706	94	4, 485				
2041	67	9, 713	76	20, 404	86	30, 566	95	3, 227				
2042	68	10, 018	77	20, 836	87	28, 946	96	2, 228				
2043	69	10, 305	78	21, 176	88	27, 004	97	1, 443				
2044	70	10, 574	79	21, 430	89	24, 861	98	832				
2045	71	10, 826	80	21, 605	90	22, 612	99	364				

Table C4-2 The difference in the numbers of hypertensives of CHD in the two groups projected, female

Year	35-44 age group		45-54 age group		55-64 age group		65-74 age group		75-84 age group		85+ age group	
	Age	Number	Age	Number	Age	Number	Age	Number	Age	Number	Age	Number
2016	42	17	52	156	61	588	70	623	80	3, 140	89	739
2017	43	33	53	309	62	1, 148	71	1, 197	81	5, 442	90	1, 207
2018	44	50	54	461	63	1, 680	72	1, 724	82	7, 058	91	1, 475
2019	45	67	55	610	64	2, 185	73	2, 208	83	8, 114	92	1, 599
2020	46	83	56	758	65	2, 664	74	2, 649	84	8, 718	93	1, 620
2021	47	100	57	903	66	3, 117	75	3, 052	85	8, 960	94	1, 571
2022	48	116	58	1, 047	67	3, 547	76	3, 417	86	8, 914	95	1, 476
2023	49	132	59	1, 189	68	3, 952	77	3, 747	87	8, 644	96	1, 353
2024	50	149	60	1, 329	69	4, 335	78	4, 045	88	8, 203	97	1, 215
2025	51	165	61	1, 467	70	4, 695	79	4, 311	89	7, 634	98	1, 072
2026	52	214	62	1, 850	71	5, 220	80	7, 539	90	6, 354		
2027	53	262	63	2, 213	72	5, 692	81	9, 757	91	5, 186		
2028	54	310	64	2, 557	73	6, 114	82	11, 156	92	4, 138		
2029	55	357	65	2, 884	74	6, 489	83	11, 894	93	3, 210		
2030	56	403	66	3, 192	75	6, 819	84	12, 107	94	2, 399		
2031	57	449	67	3, 483	76	7, 109	85	11, 905	95	1, 698		
2032	58	494	68	3, 757	77	7, 359	86	11, 383	96	1, 101		
2033	59	539	69	4, 015	78	7, 573	87	10, 618	97	597		
2034	60	583	70	4, 258	79	7, 752	88	9, 674	98	178		
2035	61	626	71	4, 485	80	7, 900	89	8, 605	99	-166		
2036	62	746	72	4, 805	81	11, 029	90	6, 754				
2037	63	861	73	5, 089	82	12, 993	91	5, 114				
2038	64	969	74	5, 339	83	14, 021	92	3, 680				
2039	65	1, 071	75	5, 559	84	14, 304	93	2, 445				
2040	66	1, 168	76	5, 748	85	14, 001	94	1, 393				
2041	67	1, 259	77	5, 910	86	13, 247	95	510				
2042	68	1, 345	78	6, 046	87	12, 152	96	-221				
2043	69	1, 426	79	6, 158	88	10, 808	97	-816				
2044	70	1, 502	80	6, 247	89	9, 290	98	-1, 291				
2045	71	1, 573	81	6, 315	90	7, 660	99	-1, 662				

Table C4-3 The difference in the numbers of hypertensives of stroke in the two groups projected, male

Year	35-44 age group		45-54 age group		55-64 age group		65-74 age group		75-84 age group		85+ age group	
	Age	Number	Age	Number	Age	Number	Age	Number	Age	Number	Age	Number
2016	42	109	51	1, 448	61	8, 365	70	8, 412	79	11, 160	88	870
2017	43	216	52	2, 875	62	16, 389	71	16, 072	80	19, 352	89	1, 408
2018	44	323	53	4, 282	63	24, 080	72	23, 031	81	25, 181	90	1, 709
2019	45	430	54	5, 669	64	31, 451	73	29, 335	82	29, 138	91	1, 842
2020	46	535	55	7, 035	65	38, 510	74	35, 030	83	31, 626	92	1, 860
2021	47	640	56	8, 382	66	45, 268	75	40, 157	84	32, 968	93	1, 802
2022	48	744	57	9, 710	67	51, 733	76	44, 756	85	33, 427	94	1, 695
2023	49	848	58	11, 018	68	57, 916	77	48, 864	86	33, 214	95	1, 561
2024	50	950	59	12, 307	69	63, 824	78	52, 514	87	32, 500	96	1, 413
2025	51	1, 052	60	13, 577	70	69, 467	79	55, 740	88	31, 420	97	1, 262
2026	52	1, 726	61	19, 949	71	78, 047	80	66, 254	89	26, 258		
2027	53	2, 391	62	26, 055	72	85, 725	81	73, 147	90	21, 879		
2028	54	3, 045	63	31, 901	73	92, 565	82	77, 203	91	18, 177		
2029	55	3, 691	64	37, 497	74	98, 626	83	79, 054	92	15, 055		
2030	56	4, 327	65	42, 850	75	103, 964	84	79, 213	93	12, 430		
2031	57	4, 953	66	47, 969	76	108, 630	85	78, 093	94	10, 230		
2032	58	5, 571	67	52, 860	77	112, 675	86	76, 025	95	8, 391		
2033	59	6, 179	68	57, 530	78	116, 144	87	73, 273	96	6, 858		
2034	60	6, 779	69	61, 987	79	119, 080	88	70, 048	97	5, 583		
2035	61	7, 369	70	66, 238	80	121, 524	89	66, 515	98	4, 527		
2036	62	10, 343	71	72, 578	81	131, 652	90	55, 427				
2037	63	13, 191	72	78, 220	82	137, 307	91	46, 092				
2038	64	15, 917	73	83, 215	83	139, 494	92	38, 249				
2039	65	18, 526	74	87, 608	84	139, 027	93	31, 673				
2040	66	21, 020	75	91, 443	85	136, 559	94	26, 170				
2041	67	23, 405	76	94, 761	86	132, 617	95	21, 573				
2042	68	25, 682	77	97, 601	87	127, 620	96	17, 741				
2043	69	27, 856	78	99, 998	88	121, 901	97	14, 554				
2044	70	29, 930	79	101, 987	89	115, 722	98	11, 907				
2045	71	31, 907	80	103, 598	90	109, 290	99	9, 714				

Table C4-4 The difference in the numbers of hypertensives of stroke in the two groups projected, female

Year	35-44 age group		45-54 age group		55-64 age group		65-74 age group		75-84 age group		85+ age group	
	Age	Number	Age	Number	Age	Number	Age	Number	Age	Number	Age	Number
2016	42	43	52	1, 742	61	10, 362	70	7, 335	80	13, 574	89	2, 314
2017	43	87	53	3, 467	62	20, 359	71	14, 163	81	24, 308	90	3, 861
2018	44	130	54	5, 175	63	30, 002	72	20, 513	82	32, 661	91	4, 829
2019	45	173	55	6, 868	64	39, 299	73	26, 407	83	39, 026	92	5, 368
2020	46	216	56	8, 543	65	48, 260	74	31, 870	84	43, 735	93	5, 591
2021	47	259	57	10, 203	66	56, 895	75	36, 924	85	47, 073	94	5, 588
2022	48	302	58	11, 847	67	65, 211	76	41, 592	86	49, 279	95	5, 427
2023	49	344	59	13, 474	68	73, 218	77	45, 893	87	50, 556	96	5, 160
2024	50	387	60	15, 086	69	80, 924	78	49, 846	88	51, 078	97	4, 827
2025	51	430	61	16, 682	70	88, 338	79	53, 472	89	50, 989	98	4, 457
2026	52	982	62	23, 693	71	94, 939	80	67, 971	90	45, 492		
2027	53	1, 528	63	30, 452	72	100, 983	81	78, 969	91	40, 389		
2028	54	2, 070	64	36, 967	73	106, 500	82	87, 054	92	35, 700		
2029	55	2, 606	65	43, 243	74	111, 518	83	92, 723	93	31, 427		
2030	56	3, 137	66	49, 287	75	116, 065	84	96, 399	94	27, 563		
2031	57	3, 663	67	55, 106	76	120, 167	85	98, 441	95	24, 089		
2032	58	4, 184	68	60, 706	77	123, 849	86	99, 152	96	20, 983		
2033	59	4, 699	69	66, 092	78	127, 136	87	98, 787	97	18, 219		
2034	60	5, 210	70	71, 271	79	130, 049	88	97, 563	98	15, 772		
2035	61	5, 716	71	76, 248	80	132, 611	89	95, 661	99	13, 612		
2036	62	7, 938	72	80, 438	81	146, 777	90	84, 513				
2037	63	10, 081	73	84, 250	82	156, 836	91	74, 418				
2038	64	12, 146	74	87, 705	83	163, 499	92	65, 329				
2039	65	14, 135	75	90, 824	84	167, 371	93	57, 187				
2040	66	16, 051	76	93, 625	85	168, 964	94	49, 925				
2041	67	17, 895	77	96, 125	86	168, 709	95	43, 475				
2042	68	19, 669	78	98, 343	87	166, 971	96	37, 766				
2043	69	21, 376	79	100, 295	88	164, 057	97	32, 729				
2044	70	23, 016	80	101, 995	89	160, 225	98	28, 299				
2045	71	24, 593	81	103, 460	90	155, 690	99	24, 415				

Appendix D Age-specific analysis on hypertension control and re-analysis of return on investment and benefit-cost ratio

1. Trend analysis of hypertension control, 1991-2009

Using a Lagrange interpolation polynomial method, age-specific data of hypertension control from 1991 to 2009 were completed, as shown in Table D1.

Table D1 Completed data of hypertension control rates, by age group, 1991-2009

Year	Control rate/%				
	35-44	45-54	55-64	65-74	75+
1991	2.62	2.43	4.55	2.44	2.54
1992	1.86	2.60	5.58	2.41	2.48
1993	1.55	2.67	5.62	2.50	2.52
1994	1.59	2.68	5.00	2.74	2.65
1995	1.87	2.67	4.06	3.14	2.86
1996	2.26	2.70	3.12	3.75	3.14
1997	2.67	2.82	2.51	4.59	3.47
1998	2.71	3.19	3.41	5.96	3.77
1999	2.75	3.66	4.63	7.39	4.15
2000	2.81	4.21	6.00	8.74	4.65
2001	3.22	4.90	6.98	9.29	5.74
2002	3.65	5.61	7.88	9.67	6.87
2003	4.00	6.32	8.68	10.03	7.85
2004	4.17	6.97	9.38	10.52	9.38
2005	3.81	7.50	7.78	11.55	8.30
2006	3.58	7.91	10.50	12.47	8.50
2007	3.68	8.15	10.55	13.13	7.93
2008	4.32	8.21	11.01	13.34	8.16
2009	5.69	8.03	12.02	12.96	8.92

Given that the trend analysis is based on fewer than 20 data points, small sample time series analysis was performed, where pre-treatment was performed on small sample data using the Lagrange Interpolation Polynomial method. With SPSS 22.0, time series predicting analysis was performed using an expert-modeler method in which the difference was used to realize time series stationarity. According to the expert modeler and modelling figures, ARIMA models (2, 0, 1 for ages 35-44 and 65-74; 1, 0, 1 for other age groups) were selected for linear trend prediction, as shown in Table D2.

The residual auto-correlation function (ACF) showed a random distribution with no outliers, which indicates good model fitness (see Appendix B: Supplementary material).

Table D2 Model statistics for the time series prediction of hypertension control rate for people aged, by age group

Control-model_1	Number of predictors	Model fit statistics		Ljung-Box Q (18)			Number of outliers/n
		Stationary R-squared	R-squared	Statistics	DF	Sig.	
35-44	1	0.736	0.955	3.410	3	0.333	0
45-54	1	0.984	0.984	39.293	16	0.001	0
55-64	1	0.882	0.882	11.618	16	0.770	0
65-74	1	0.995	0.995	26.241	15	0.036	0
75+	1	0.949	0.949	18.986	16	0.269	0

Table D3 is the forecasted control rate of hypertension from 2010 to 2015 based on the model established from 1991 to 2009. Both upper control limit and lower control limit are listed. It is predicted that in 2015, the control rate for people aged 35-44 of hypertension would be 11.64%[95%*CI* (8.34%, 14.93%)], 10.39%[95%*CI* (8.99%, 11.79%)]for those aged 45-54, 13.79%[95%*CI*(10.28%, 17.29%)]for those aged 55-64, 17.60% [95%*CI* (15.57%, 19.64%)] for those aged 65-74, and 12.04% [95%*CI*(10.11%, 13.96%)] for those aged 75 and over, based on the trend from 1991 to 2009. Details are shown in Table D3 and Figures D1-D5.

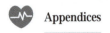

Table D3 Forecasted control rate of hypertension from the prediction model, 2010-2015

Age group	Model	2010	2011	2012	2013	2014	2015
35-44	Forecast	7.34	8.82	9.88	10.54	11.03	11.64
	UCL	6.85	7.58	7.84	7.86	7.94	8.34
	LCL	7.83	10.06	11.91	13.21	14.11	14.93
45-54	Forecast	8.11	8.58	9.04	9.50	9.95	10.39
	UCL	7.71	7.75	7.98	8.29	8.63	8.99
	LCL	8.51	9.41	10.10	10.71	11.27	11.79
55-64	Forecast	12.25	12.47	12.74	13.06	13.41	13.79
	UCL	9.98	9.52	9.50	9.67	9.95	10.28
	LCL	14.52	15.41	15.99	16.45	16.88	17.29
65-74	Forecast	12.74	13.01	13.79	14.96	16.31	17.60
	UCL	12.14	11.77	12.06	12.99	14.28	15.57
	LCL	13.33	14.25	15.52	16.94	18.34	19.64
75+	Forecast	9.56	10.12	10.63	11.11	11.58	12.04
	UCL	8.26	8.41	8.79	9.22	9.66	10.11
	LCL	10.87	11.82	12.47	13.01	13.50	13.96

Notes: UCL = Upper control limit.

LCL = Lower control limit.

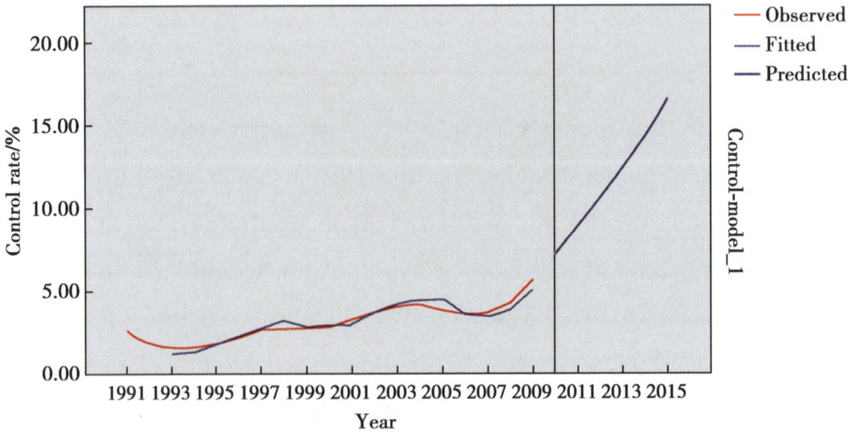

Figure D1 Time series trend of hypertension control rate for people aged 35-44, 1991-2009 and predicted analysis from 2010 to 2015

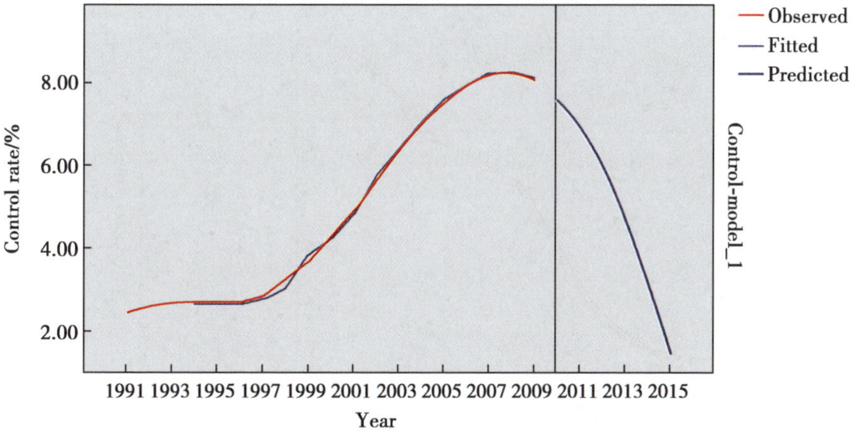

Figure D2 Time series trend of hypertension control rate for people aged 45-54, 1991-2009 and predicted analysis from 2010 to 2015

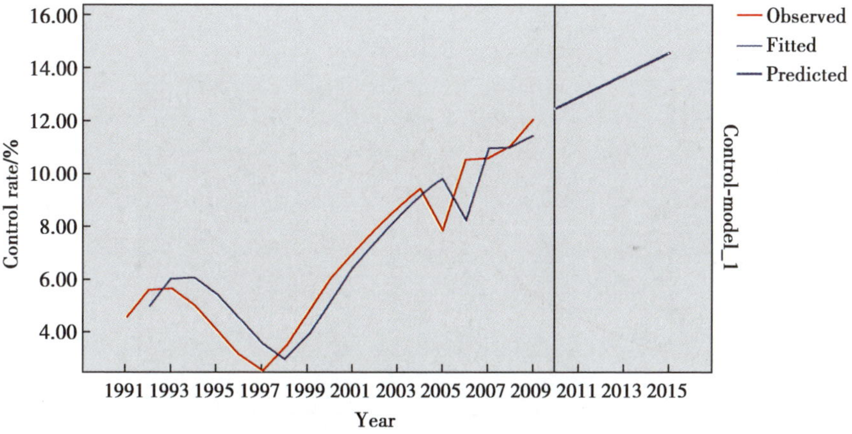

Figure D3 Time series trend of hypertension control rate for people aged 55-64, 1991-2009 and predicted analysis from 2010 to 2015

2. Estimation of hypertension control from the NBPHS

According to the China Hypertension Survey 2012-2015, the prevalence of hypertension among adults aged 35 or above was 32.62% in 2015 (Wang et al., 2018). The predicted control rates and the observed control rate of 2015 for each age group were listed in Table D3. With the same population data and method, it was estimated that from 2009 to 2015, the NBPHS program increased the number hypertensives under control by 0, 1, 635, 397, 1, 564, 164, 170, 388 and 617, 939

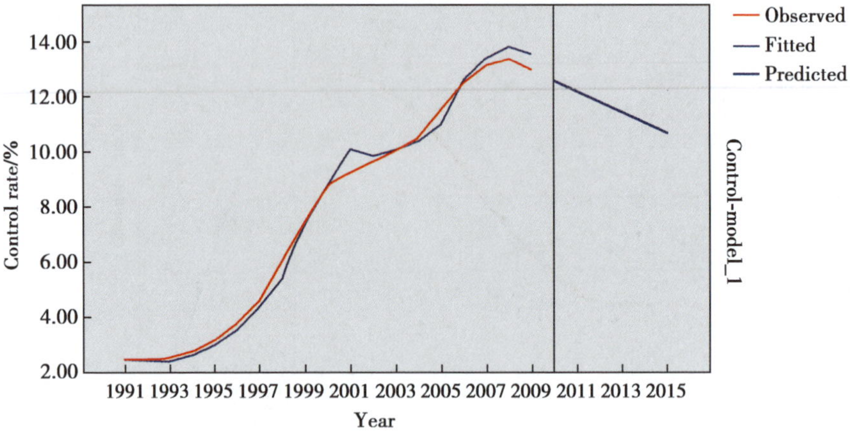

Figure D4 Time series trend of hypertension control rate for people aged 65-74, 1991-2009 and predicted analysis from 2010 to 2015

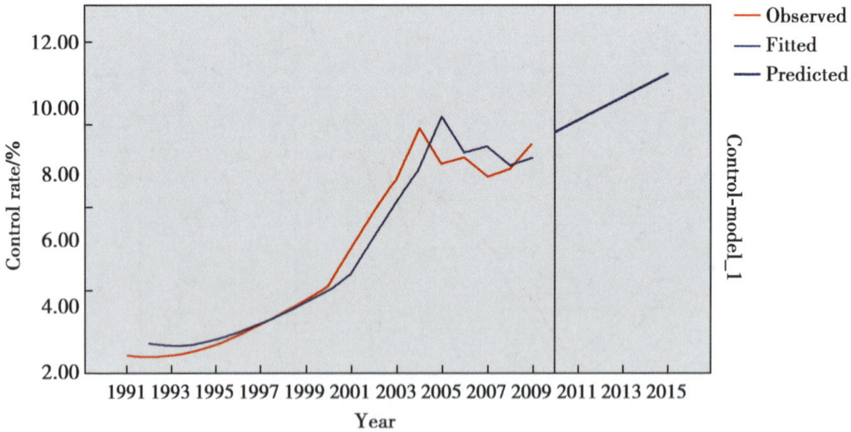

Figure D5 Time series trend of hypertension control rate for people aged 75 and over, 1991-2009 and predicted analysis from 2010 to 2015

for males in age groups 35-44, 45-54, 55-64, 65-74 and 75+, respectively. The numbers would be 0, 1, 568, 221, 1, 523, 002, 169, 167 and 761, 170 for females in each age group, respectively. The total number of hypertensives under blood pressure control increased by the NBPHS would be 8, 009, 449 (1, 581, 856, 13, 065, 018). Details are shown in Table D4.

3. Age-specific analysis of estimates of CVDs and deaths averted

At the end of the 10th projection year in the G1 scenario, compared with G2,

Table D4 Estimation of the number of hypertensives under control through the NBPHS (CHS 2012-2015)

Groups	Number of population	Preva-lence/%	Observed control rate/%	Predicted control rate/%	Number of hypertension controlled through NBPHS/n(95%*CI*)
Males/yr					
35-44	127, 459, 929	15.90	9.90	11.64	0* (−1, 019, 386, 316, 152)
45-54	96, 759, 903	29.60	16.10	10.39	1, 635, 397 (1, 234, 424, 2, 036, 370)
55-64	72, 912, 562	44.60	18.60	13.79	1, 564, 164 (425, 999, 2, 705, 581)
65-74	38, 237, 979	55.70	18.40	17.6	170, 388 (−264, 102, 602, 749)
75+	20, 695, 107	60.20	17.00	12.04	617, 939 (378, 737, 858, 388)
Females/yr					
35-44	122, 114, 836	15.90	9.90	5.1	0** (−976, 638, 302, 894)
45-54	92, 785, 346	29.60	16.10	10.39	1, 568, 221 (1, 183, 718, 1, 953, 723)
55-64	70, 993, 810	44.60	18.60	13.79	1, 523, 002 (414, 788, 2, 634, 382)
65-74	37, 963, 871	55.70	18.40	17.6	169, 167 (−262, 209, 598, 428)
75+	25, 491, 986	60.20	17.00	12.04	761, 170 (466, 524, 1, 057, 351)
Total	705, 415, 330	N/A	N/A	N/A	8, 009, 449 (1, 581, 856, 13, 065, 018)

Notes: N/A is not applicable. *Actual value is −352, 631, to make it fit to reality, negative values were changed to 0. ** Actual value is −337, 843, to make it fit to reality, negative values were changed to 0.

34, 198, 262, 071, and 284, 796 hypertensive patients would have avoided CHD, stroke and death, respectively. At the end of the 20th projection year, 41, 632, 380, 448, and 355, 955 hypertensive patients would have avoided CHD, stroke and death, respectively. At the end of the 30th projection year, 23, 476, 306, 955 and 697, 204 hypertensive patients would have avoided CHD, stroke and death, respectively. Details of these results are provided in Tables D5-D7. In Table D7, there are some

Table D5 Running results for a 10-year horizon

Groups	G1			G2			Number of patients avoiding CVD and death		
	CHD	Stroke	Death	CHD	Stroke	Death	CHD	Stroke	Death
Male/yr									
35-44	0	0	0	0	0	0	0	0	0
45-54	28, 028	58, 081	74, 940	36, 894	74, 975	84, 533	8, 866	16, 895	9, 593
55-64	54, 048	175, 359	164, 325	63, 991	241, 358	185, 745	9, 942	65, 999	21, 420
65-74	6, 787	23, 312	43, 431	8, 284	31, 636	48, 917	1, 498	8, 325	5, 486
75-84	14, 880	38, 654	367, 123	19, 243	62, 137	461, 696	4, 363	23, 482	94, 573
85+	0	0	0	0	0	0	0	0	0
Female/yr									
35-44	0	0	0	0	0	0	0	0	0
45-54	22, 406	54, 314	36, 259	24, 454	77, 383	42, 386	2, 048	23, 069	6, 127
55-64	52, 134	150, 108	102, 949	56, 438	229, 354	129, 034	4, 304	79, 246	26, 085
65-74	5, 883	22, 877	30, 395	6, 460	30, 180	34, 721	578	7, 303	4, 326
75-84	21, 925	52, 314	387, 116	24, 525	90, 065	504, 302	2, 599	37, 751	117, 186
85+	0	0	0	0	0	0	0	0	0
Total	206, 091	575, 018	1, 206, 538	240, 289	837, 089	1, 491, 334	34, 198	262, 071	284, 796

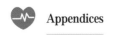

Table D6 Running results for a 20-year horizon

Groups	G1			G2			Number of patients avoiding CVD and death		
	CHD	Stroke	Death	CHD	Stroke	Death	CHD	Stroke	Death
Male									
35-44	0	0	0	0	0	0	0	0	0
45-54	37, 774	117, 997	223, 107	53, 930	198, 647	258, 446	16, 156	80, 650	35, 339
55-64	50, 749	180, 250	512, 768	65, 212	276, 766	588, 904	14, 463	96, 517	76, 136
65-74	2, 908	8, 579	119, 758	3, 377	13, 368	141, 137	469	4, 788	21, 379
75-84	648	2, 350	577, 566	269	1, 608	607, 277	−378	−741	29, 711
85+	0	0	0	0	0	0	0	0	0
Female									
35-44	0	0	0	0	0	0	0	0	0
45-54	31, 915	125, 437	130, 749	37, 784	223, 040	167, 533	5, 869	97, 603	36, 783
55-64	46, 528	196, 755	358, 829	52, 158	292, 013	433, 827	5, 630	95, 258	74, 998
65-74	3, 626	10, 721	101, 975	3, 766	17, 627	125, 479	140	6, 905	23, 504
75-84	1, 418	4, 434	678, 536	701	3, 902	736, 641	−717	−532	58, 105
85+	0	0	0	0	0	0	0	0	0
Total	175, 566	646, 523	2, 703, 289	217, 197	1, 026, 971	3, 059, 245	41, 632	380, 448	355, 955

Table D7 Running results for a 30-year horizon

Groups	G1			G2			Number of patients with avoiding CVD and death		
	CHD	Stroke	Death	CHD	Stroke	Death	CHD	Stroke	Death
Male									
35-44	0	0	0	0	0	0	0	0	0
45-54	44, 586	152, 647	557, 423	61, 918	258, 449	651, 470	1, 7332	105, 801	94, 047
55-64	24, 109	69, 487	1, 139, 026	26, 293	109, 558	1, 331, 195	2, 185	40, 071	192, 168
65-74	128	472	162, 371	45	289	168, 586	−84	−183	6, 215
75-84	648	2, 350	577, 566	269	1, 608	607, 277	−378	−741	29, 711
85+	0	0	0	0	0	0	0	0	0
Female									
35-44	0	0	0	0	0	0	0	0	0
45-54	35, 127	186, 822	378, 264	41, 445	292, 405	468, 063	6, 318	105, 583	89, 798
55-64	30, 054	90, 911	959, 687	29, 015	148, 021	1, 176, 142	−1, 039	57, 110	216, 455
65-74	250	794	154, 590	110	640	165, 295	−140	−154	10, 705
75-84	1, 418	4, 434	678, 536	701	3, 902	736, 641	−717	−532	58, 105
85+	0	0	0	0	0	0	0	0	0
Total	136, 320	507, 917	4, 607, 465	159, 796	814, 872	5, 304, 669	23, 476	306, 955	697, 204

negative figures which are generated mainly from older age groups of both genders in the 30-year horizon analysis (age groups of 65-74 and 75-84 years). This is because in the non-NBPHS group, more patients die from CVD than those in the NBPHS group, which makes less CVD survivors compared with those in the non-NBPHS group, especially for stroke. This section further explains analysis of Chapter 4.

4. Re-analysis of the return on investment and benefit-cost ratio (BCR)

Originally, analysis for all age groups based on the CHS 2012-2015 data was performed. At a discount rate of 3% and given that 14.59% of the NBPHS funding were spent on hypertension management, the BCR would be 6.0. With social benefit included, the BCR would be 15.4. The internal rate of return would be 14.6% and 20.7%.

With age-specific analysis based on the CHS 2012-2015 data, at a discount rate of 3% and given that 14.59% of the NBPHS funding were spent on hypertension management, the BCR would be 5.9. With social benefit included, the BCR would be 15.1. The internal rate of return would be 14.7% and 20.4%. Details are shown in Tables D8 and D9.

Table D8 Cost and return on investment at different discount rates (million CNY)

Discount rate	0(95%*CI*)	2% (95%*CI*)	3% (95%*CI*)	5% (95%*CI*)
GDP-deaths averted, NPV	321, 976 (63, 590, 525, 207)	206, 498 (40, 783, 336, 840)	166, 880 (32, 959, 272, 215)	110, 882 (21, 899, 180, 871)
Social benefit, NPV	597, 498 (118, 005, 974, 639)	343, 187 (67, 779, 559, 807)	263, 261 (51, 994, 429, 432)	158, 597 (31, 323, 258, 704)
Cost				
10% of the NBPHS funding	25, 526	21, 727	19, 499	15, 837
14.59% of the NBPHS funding	37, 243	31, 699	28, 449	23, 107
18% of the NBPHS funding	45, 947	39, 108	35, 099	28, 507

Table D9 Benefit-cost ratios at different discount rates and internal rate of return

Benefit-cost ratios	0 (95%*CI*)	2% (95%*CI*)	3% (95%*CI*)	5% (95%*CI*)	Internal rate of return/%(95%*CI*)
18% of the NBPHS funding as cost					
GDP-deaths averted/cost	7.0 (1.38, 11.42)	5.3 (1.05, 8.65)	4.8 (0.95, 7.83)	3.9 (0.77, 6.36)	12.9 (2.5, 21.0)
GDP-deaths averted plus social benefit/cost	20.0 (3.95, 32.62)	14.1 (2.78, 23.00)	12.3 (2.43, 20.06)	9.5 (1.88, 15.50)	18.6 (3.7, 30.3)
14.59% of the NBPHS funding as cost					
GDP-deaths averted/cost	8.6 (1.70, 14.03)	6.5 (1.28, 10.60)	5.9 (1.17, 9.62)	4.8 (0.95, 7.83)	14.7 (2.9, 24.0)
GDP-deaths averted plus social benefit/cost	24.7 (4.88, 40.29)	17.3 (3.42, 28.22)	15.1 (2.98, 24.63)	11.7 (2.31, 19.09)	20.4 (4.0, 33.3)
10% of the NBPHS funding as cost					
GDP-deaths averted/cost	12.6 (2.49, 20.55)	9.5 (1.88, 15.50)	8.6 (1.70, 14.03)	7.0 (1.38, 11.42)	18.0 (3.6, 29.4)
GDP-deaths averted plus social benefit/cost	36.0 (7.11, 58.72)	25.3 (5.00, 41.27)	22.1 (4.36, 36.05)	17.0 (3.36, 27.73)	24.0 (4.7, 39.1)

Acknowledgements

This book is developed totally based on a PhD thesis. As the editor in chief, I would like to thank my principal supervisor, Professor Peter J. Sheehan, who has always impressed me with his sharp and critical thinking in conceptualizing and addressing problems. I would also like to thank Dr. Kim Sweeny and Professor Qin Jiangmei, my associate supervisors, for the invaluable advice, encouragement and assistance they provided to me in the course of writing this thesis. Kim Sweeny is an excellent supervisor, who is an economist, mathematician, modeler, and writer. I can never forget those weekends we spent together revising and improving my thesis. Professor Qin Jiangmei, who is a multi-discipline expert on health policy making and development in China, especially in primary care, provided critical sources for me to examine while continuing my study in Australia. A special thanks goes to colleagues at the Victoria Institute of Strategic Economic Studies at Victoria University for their advice and support, particularly Bruce Rasmussen and Margarita Kumnick.

Director Fu Wei and Director Zhang Zhenzhong, who were taking a lead in the CNHDRC, provided important administrative support for me to continue my work and studies. Special thanks goes to Director Fu Qiang and Gan Ge, who are Director General and Deputy Director of the CNHDRC, whose encouragement and administrative support is essential to this work.

Many thanks to Mr. Liu Liqun, Mr. Ao Qishun, and Mr. Chen Kai, from the National Health Commission of the People's Republic of China, taking a lead in policy making and the development of primary healthcare in China. They generously provided me with much mentorship support on related policy development.

I want to take this opportunity to thank Prof. Gu Dongfeng, whose work has been cited many times in this thesis. Prof. GuDongfeng, together with Director Zhang Bingli (from the National Health Commission of the People's Republic of China), Prof. Chen Yude and Prof. Wu Yangfeng provided me with valuable suggestions on the methodology and policy recommendations for the thesis.

I want to say thank you to my colleagues, Zhang Lifang and Lin Chunmei, for their spiritual support during my study overseas.

Ms. Sun Fanghong, Mr. Zhong Jianjun and Shan Selina provided great support during my four years of study. My husband, Bai Yongsheng, and my daughter, Bai Yiwen have displayed remarkable forbearance over too many years, and without their support and encouragement, this thesis would not have been possible. I am grateful to my parents, Zhang Qingquan and Xie Guiming. In completing this thesis and book, I have made one of my parents' dreams come true.

I feel deeply fortunate to have met great supervisors, leaders, teachers, colleagues and family members. All your generous help, support and spiritual encouragement were cornerstones, allowing me to complete this book.